UNWELL
WOMEN

UNWELL
WOMEN

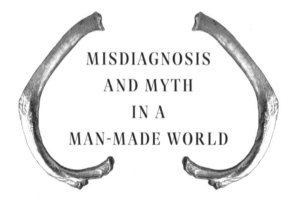

MISDIAGNOSIS
AND MYTH
IN A
MAN-MADE WORLD

ELINOR CLEGHORN

DUTTON

DUTTON

An imprint of Penguin Random House LLC
penguinrandomhouse.com

Copyright © 2021 by Elinor Cleghorn
Penguin supports copyright. Copyright fuels creativity, encourages diverse voices, promotes free speech, and creates a vibrant culture. Thank you for buying an authorized edition of this book and for complying with copyright laws by not reproducing, scanning, or distributing any part of it in any form without permission. You are supporting writers and allowing Penguin to continue to publish books for every reader.

DUTTON and the D colophon are registered trademarks of Penguin Random House LLC.

LIBRARY OF CONGRESS CATALOGING-IN-PUBLICATION DATA

Names: Cleghorn, Elinor, author.
Title: Unwell women: misdiagnosis and myth in a man-made world / Elinor Cleghorn.
Description: New York: Dutton, Penguin Random House LLC, 2021. |
Includes bibliographical references.
Identifiers: LCCN 2020053644 (print) | LCCN 2020053645 (ebook) |
ISBN 9780593182956 (hardcover) | ISBN 9780593182963 (ebook)
Subjects: LCSH: Women—Health and hygiene. | Women—Health and hygiene—History. |
Women patients. | Diagnostic errors.
Classification: LCC RA564.85 .C54 2021 (print) | LCC RA564.85 (ebook) |
DDC 613/.04244—dc23
LC record available at https://lccn.loc.gov/2020053644
LC ebook record available at https://lccn.loc.gov/2020053645

Printed in the United States of America
1ST PRINTING

For Dorothy,
my beloved unwell woman

The history of illness is not the history of medicine—it is the history of the world—and the history of having a body could well be the history of what is done to the many in the interest of the few.　　　　　　　—Anne Boyer, *The Undying* (2019)

You shall have to explore the history of those wonderful functions and destinies which her sexual nature enables her to fulfill, and the strange and secret influences which her organs, by their nervous constitution, and their functions, by their relation to her whole Life-force, whether in sickness or health, are capable of exerting, not on the body alone, but on the heart, the mind, and the very soul of woman.

　　—Charles D. Meigs, MD, "Lecture on Some of the Distinctive Characteristics of the Female" (1847)

You see, he does not believe I am sick! And what can one do?

If a physician of high standing, and one's own husband, assures friends and relatives that there is really nothing the matter with one but temporary nervous depression—a slight hysterical tendency—what is one to do?

　　—Charlotte Perkins Gilman, "The Yellow Wallpaper" (1892)

CONTENTS

PART THREE: 1945—PRESENT

UNWELL
WOMEN

INTRODUCTION

We are taught that medicine is the art of solving our body's mysteries. And we expect medicine, as a science, to uphold the principles of evidence and impartiality. We want our doctors to listen to us and care for us as people. But we also need their assessments of our pain and fevers, aches and exhaustion, to be free of any prejudice about who we are. We expect, and deserve, fair and ethical treatment regardless of our gender or the color of our skin. But here things get complicated. Medicine carries the burden of its own troubling history. The history of medicine, of illness, is every bit as social and cultural as it is scientific. It is a history of people, of their bodies and their lives, not just of physicians, surgeons, clinicians, and researchers. And medical progress has not marched forward just in laboratories and benches, lectures and textbooks; it has always reflected the realities of the changing world and the meanings of being human.

Gender difference is intimately stitched into the fabric of humanness. At every stage in its long history, medicine has absorbed and enforced socially constructed gender divisions. These divisions have traditionally ascribed power and dominance to men. Historically, women have been subordinated in politics, wealth, and education. Modern scientific medicine, as it has evolved over the centuries as a profession, an institution, and a discipline, has flourished in these exact conditions. Male dominance—and with it the superiority of the male body—was cemented into medicine's very foundations, laid down in ancient Greece. In the third century BCE, the philosopher Aristotle described the female body as the inverse of the male body, with its genitalia *"turn'd outside in."* Women were marked by their anatomical difference from men and medically defined as faulty, defective, deficient. But women also possessed an organ of the highest biological—and social—value: the uterus. Possession of this organ defined the purpose of women: to bear and raise children. Knowledge about female biology centered on women's capacity—and duty—to reproduce. Being biologically female defined and constrained what it meant to be a woman. And being a woman was conflated with, and reduced to, the "female sex." Medicine validated these social determinants by constructing the myth that a woman *was* her biology; that she was ruled by it, governed by it, at the mercy of it. Women's illnesses and diseases were consistently related back to the "secrets" and "curiosities" of her reproductive organs. The mystical uterus influenced every conceivable disorder and dysfunction of her body and mind. And ever since, medical knowledge about women's susceptibility to illness and disease has been shaped and distorted by prejudiced beliefs that possessing a uterus defines our inferior position in the man-made world.

Of course, not all women have uteruses, and not all people who have uteruses, or who menstruate, are women. But medicine, historically, has insisted on conflating biological sex with gender identity. Over centuries, medical knowledge about the organs and systems marked "female" have been imbued with patriarchal notions of womanhood and femininity. As medicine's understanding of female biology has expanded and evolved, it has constantly reflected and validated dominant social and cultural expectations about who women are; what they should think, feel, and desire; and—above all else—what they can do with their own bodies. We understand, today, that our biology does not determine our gender identity. For centuries, feminism has fought for the rights of all people to not have their lives limited by their basic biology. But medicine has inherited a gender problem. Medical myths about gender roles and behaviors, constructed as facts before medicine became an evidence-based science, have resonated perniciously. And these myths about female bodies and illnesses have enormous cultural sticking power. Today, gender myths are ingrained as biases that negatively impact the care, treatment, and diagnosis of all people who identify as women.

Health-care providers and the health-care system are failing women in their responses to and treatment of women's pain, especially chronic pain. Biased gender expectations directly affect how real, serious, and deserving of treatment women's pain is perceived to be. Women are more likely to be offered minor tranquilizers and antidepressants than analgesic pain medication. Women are less likely to be referred for further diagnostic investigations than men are. And women's pain is much more likely to be seen as having an emotional or psychological cause, rather than a bodily or biological one. Women are the predominant sufferers of chronic diseases that begin with pain. But before our pain is taken seriously as a symptom of a possible disease, it first has to be validated—and believed—by a medical professional. And this pervasive aura of distrust around women's accounts of their pain has been enfolded into medical attitudes over centuries. The historical—and hysterical—idea that women's excessive emotions have profound influences on their bodies, and vice versa, is impressed like a photographic negative beneath today's image of the attention-seeking, hypochondriac female patient. Prevailing social stereotypes about the way women experience, express, and tolerate pain are not modern phenomena—they have been ingrained across medicine's history. Our contemporary biomedical knowledge is stained with the residue of old stories, fallacies, assumptions, and myths.

Over the past few years, gender bias in medical knowledge, research, and practice has hit the mainstream. Headlines like "Why Won't Doctors Believe Women?," "Doctors Are Failing Women with Chronic Illness," and "Doctors Are More Likely to Misdiagnose Women Than Men" crop up regularly in the UK and US press. Public awareness is growing around the way that women are all too frequently being dismissed and misdiagnosed. We're learning that medical sexism is rife, systemic, and making women sicker. But women are not a monolithic category. The extent to which gender bias affects a woman's health—and life—depends on who she is. I have a chronic disease. But I am acutely aware of my privilege. I am white and cisgender, and I look healthy enough to pass as "well." I also have access to publicly funded, universal medical care through the UK's National Health Service. The discrimination women encounter as medical patients is magnified when they are Black, Asian, Indigenous, Latinx, or ethnically diverse; when their access to health services is restricted; and when they don't identify with the gender norms medicine ascribes to biological womanhood.

In the US, Black, Asian, and other ethnically diverse women face serious barriers to accessing adequate health care, treatment, and services, as well as being approved for medical insurance. Structural racism intertwines insidiously with gender bias: 22 percent of Black women in the United States have experienced discrimination when they visited a doctor or a clinic. As a white woman, I risk having my pain written off as hysterical. But a Black woman will often have to fight to have the very existence of her pain acknowledged. A study in 2016 showed that myths about biological racial differences lead to massive disparities in the medical treatment of Black people's pain. The false but pervasive belief that Black women feel less pain, because they are assumed to have "thicker skin" and "less sensitive nerve endings," originates from dehumanizing falsehoods perpetuated to justify white history's horrific abuses of enslaved Black people. This racist discounting of Black women's physical and psychological pain means they are prescribed fewer pain medications and are more vulnerable to misdiagnosis or to having their diagnoses dangerously delayed. And these disparities are killing them.

In the UK, Black women are five times more likely to die from complications in pregnancy and during childbirth than white women. In the US, Black women have the highest rates of maternal and infant mortality of any country in the industrialized world. And many of the pregnancy and birth complications killing Black women are preventable. Preeclampsia, a hypertensive condition that can occur suddenly during pregnancy, strikes Black women at 50 percent higher rates than white women in the UK and 60 percent higher than white woman in the US. The risk of developing the condition escalates in women with other chronic diseases, including lupus, diabetes, and kidney disease, which

Black women in the UK and US experience at significantly higher rates. If preeclampsia is ignored or untreated, it can lead to eclampsia, which causes potentially fatal seizures, cardiac disease, kidney and liver damage, blood clots (including pulmonary edema, which affects the lungs), fetal growth disorders, and infant and maternal death. The early warning signs of preeclampsia—such as raised blood pressure, headaches, nausea and vomiting, vision disturbances, heartburn, and swelling in the feet, ankles, face, and hands—can easily be mistaken for normal pregnancy symptoms. Black women are not treated with enough respect, attention, and empathy when they report their pain. Their testimonies about what is happening to them—to their own bodies—are invalidated all too often. It's a risk for Black women to tell the truth about their pain. It's not enough for medicine to address the racist biases contributing to this shocking lack of care and empathy. Medicine needs to become actively antiracist, which means facing its complicity in the historic neglect of Black, Asian, and other ethnically diverse women.

The invisibility Black women feel and encounter when they are unwell isn't contained to the emergency room, the clinic, or the doctor's office. Ignorance and mistreatment arise from the implicit—and sometimes explicit—biases held by some medical professionals, but it's never only social. It is deeply historical and systemic, and it pervades knowledge and research as perniciously as it impedes care and treatment. I do not believe the vast majority of doctors are consciously dismissing women out of hand. I truly hope that most medical professionals are not willfully nullifying and obstructing the health concerns of Black women because they are explicitly racist. But the persisting discrimination against unwell women is cast by a centuries-long shadow, which skews perspective and judgment beyond the level of unconscious and individual prejudice. Women's diseases—particularly those that occur differently and more frequently in Black women and other ethnically diverse women—were not historically a priority. As a result, there is a profound gender and race gap in medical and clinical knowledge. From the exemption of women from swathes of clinical and observational trials and studies until as late as the 1990s to the failure to examine how heart disease, certain cancers, and HIV and AIDS manifest differently in female bodies, decades of medical advancements have failed to take women into account. And as rates of diagnostically challenging, incurable diseases rise in women across the world, this culture of neglect urgently needs to be corrected.

Sometimes women's bodies genuinely baffle medicine. Pain and fatigue are the most common "medically unexplained" symptoms. And these symptoms are endured every day by women with mysterious chronic diseases whose very existences are often contested within the medical community. Chronic fatigue syndrome and fibromyalgia both affect more women than men, but not nearly enough research has been dedicated to finding out why. In no small way, the understanding of these complex, diagnostically challenging illnesses has been mired by medical misconceptions and social attitudes toward women's expressions of their physical feelings. Faced with a patient whose illness baffles them, a doctor might consider that the cause is psychological. Since the 1950s, psychosomatic diagnoses have validated the very real ways that the mind can express itself through the body. But those recognized classifications have become entangled with misconceptions about women's tendencies to exaggerate and feign their symptoms. And this dismissal rears its head acutely when it comes to "female complaints" such as gynecological diseases and disorders, which have long been shrouded in shame, secrecy, and mythology.

Endometriosis, a chronic, incurable disease in which endometrial tissue grows and spreads in other places in the body, is an object lesson in male-dominated medicine's historic failures. This disease was named in the 1920s but has existed in medical literature for centuries. Across those centuries, so many punitive fictions and fantasies have been projected onto women's blood and pain. Its symptoms—including excruciating pelvic, back, and stomach pain; pain during sex; and heavy bleeding—have an extremely long history of being pathologized as physical expressions of emotional distress. In the nineteenth century, women's pelvic and abdominal pain, as well as their menstrual "derangements," was met with aggressive and butchering surgeries, accusations of hysteria, and forced admissions to asylums. Today, women are frequently dismissed as neurotic, anxious, depressed, hypochondriac, and even hysterical when they report the early symptoms of endo. Menstrual and gynecological pain, for too long, has been minimized as the "natural" and inevitable consequence of being female.

Today, endometriosis affects an estimated one in ten women across the world. It takes an average of between six and ten years to be correctly diagnosed. Not nearly enough research or time has been spent on figuring out the cause of this debilitating disease, which has led to a woeful lack of care and respect for sufferers. And one of the most prevalent mythologies about who gets endo still has a malign effect. Since the late 1940s, medicine has cultivated an image of the endo sufferer as a white, middle-class, overeducated, and socially and economically privileged young woman who resisted the biological imperative of having children. It was not even recognized as affecting Black women until the 1970s, when it was frequently misdiagnosed as pelvic inflammatory disease—a bacterial infection that can be sexually transmitted. Racist views of Black women's sexuality and pain sensitivity have also obstructed an understanding of other gynecological diseases that affect them more frequently and in different ways, including uterine fibroids, cervical cancer, and polycystic ovarian syndrome. It wasn't until 2012 that a team of research gynecologists studying endometriosis in Detroit, Michigan, revealed that Black women often have more severe growth of endometrial tissue at different places in their bodies than white women do.

Just as the development of medicine and health care sits at the heart of social progress, it has always been deeply political too. The systemic neglect of Black women's gynecological pain is rooted in the exploitation of enslaved and disenfranchised women in the name of medical and surgical research since the nineteenth century. Black women have since been used as medical specimens, as experimental material. Their pain has been constantly disavowed, their humanity continuously denied. Keeping women silent and diminishing their voices are conditions of the man-made world. Medicine, a construct of the man-made world, is androcentric. It assumes male bodies to be the standard and holds male-dominated knowledge in the highest esteem. But it also means that traits of maleness and masculinity are privileged. Throughout its history, medicine has claimed that the defective, deficient, excessive, and unruly nature of female biology means that women are suited only to the subjugated sphere of "femininity." It seems ridiculous now to imagine physicians once believed that women's nerves were too highly strung for them to receive an education and that their ovaries would become inflamed if they read too much. But these outrageous myths are alive and well in a world where menstruation and menopause are still seen by many people as credible reasons why women shouldn't hold positions of political power. When clinical research exempts women from studies and trials on the grounds that female hormones fluctuate too much and upset the consistency of results, medical culture is reinforcing the centuries-old myth that women are too biologically erratic to be useful or valuable.

Androcentrism doesn't only mean that men hold all the power and influence. It also assumes that all people are valued according to "male perspectives [and] standards." The term "androcentric" was first introduced by an American sociologist and women's rights advocate named Lester Frank Ward in 1903. Eight years later, the American feminist writer, lecturer, and activist Charlotte Perkins Gilman published a book dissecting "androcentric culture," *The Man-Made World*. Gilman was a fierce critic of the medical oppression of women's bodies and minds and a vocal detractor of the gender discrimination medicine upheld. She was writing during the fight, unfolding on both sides of the Atlantic, for women's right to vote. Campaigning for suffrage was about so much more than women having a say at the polls. As Gilman put it, it was a movement toward "economic and political equality," toward "freedom and justice," and, most importantly, toward the "humanization of women." To be treated and valued according to only the androcentric view of femininity is to be reduced to a biologically determined gender myth. When androcentric medicine maligns, ignores, belittles, and undermines unwell women today, it is consciously or unconsciously reigniting historical ideas about women's bodies and minds that were invented to maintain the patriarchal status quo. Gilman was writing at a time when many physicians and scientists believed "women were a sex" and, despicably, "a subspecies told off for reproduction only." But the fundamental truth of her argument, that the insistence on women's "femaleness" and "femininity" denies our humanity, is still astonishingly relevant.

Gilman was one of many women who bravely campaigned against androcentric medicine's hold on women's bodies, minds, and lives throughout its history. Real change happened when women spoke on behalf of their own bodies and those of others, when they created knowledge by listening to other women, when they challenged, countered, and resisted oppressive ideas. When women refuse to be silenced, androcentric culture loses some of its power.

Since the 1960s, feminist health campaigners have fought tirelessly against the suppression of drugs' side effects and systemic gender and racial bias in clinical research, from both inside and outside the medical establishment. Women forced changes in law and practice by campaigning from the ground up. Their efforts, ultimately, have made medications, including the contraceptive pill and hormone replacement therapy, safer for all women. And medical feminism has a long, fascinating, and inspiring history of women raising their heads above the parapet to ensure that women are represented, cared for, and listened to. Feminist social reformers denounced medicine's perpetuation of women's "natural" inferiority in the eighteenth century. Grassroots activists in the 1970s empowered women to reclaim the ownership and enjoyment of their bodies from man-made medical mystification, and created knowledge for women, by women. In the decades and centuries in between, feminist physicians, socialists, researchers, and reformers have defended women's body rights and freedoms—from normalizing menstruation and celebrating sexual pleasure to legalizing contraception and defending reproductive autonomy.

In the wake of the #MeToo movement, women have been empowered to share their experiences of sexist and misogynistic abuses of power across all sectors of society. With the rise in authoritarian political ideologies across the world, and the erosion and invalidation of women's body rights and the testimonies that come with them, medicine has recently become a critical frontier for women fighting to have their voices heard and believed. Chronic, incurable, mysterious illnesses and diseases have become touchstones for this growing community of unwell women who are bravely testifying to the discrimination they have encountered on the basis of gender and race. In essays, articles, memoirs, novels, short stories, films, documentaries, blog posts, and chat rooms, women are telling their stories of being pushed to the margins of medicine by their elusive illnesses. Speaking out about your own body is profoundly feminist. It is generous and courageous to revisit and recall the trauma of pain, and a radical gesture in a culture skewed toward doubting and disbelieving women. It's a risk—but at the same time, it's an act of defiance against those power structures in the man-made world that would prefer us not to speak.

Sharing the personal, intimate realities of what it means to be an unwell woman also creates valuable knowledge—knowledge that the objective, evidence-based model of diagnosis can't, or won't, accommodate. For centuries, medicine has claimed that women are defined by their bodies and biology. But we have never been respected as reliable narrators of what happens to our bodies. We are denied agency because the man-made world privileges specialist, sanctioned knowledge over our own thoughts and feelings. There is no space in the professional medical narrative of illness and disease for women's own experiences.

I became an unwell woman more than a decade ago. I had been ill before many times. But in October 2010, the cause of the strange pains that had hounded me for years was finally uncovered. I had been in hospital for ten days before a rheumatologist diagnosed me with systemic lupus erythematosus, a chronic autoimmune disease, but the journey to get to that point had taken seven years of dismissed symptoms and unhelpful misdiagnoses. Like most autoimmune diseases, lupus is incurable, and its cause remains a mystery. A few weeks later, I traveled to St. Thomas' Hospital in London for an appointment at a specialist clinic, the largest unit for lupus and related diseases in Europe. With my three-month-old baby strapped to my chest in a sling, I gave my name to the clinic's receptionist. My breath was still ragged from the inflammation that almost claimed my heart. My pulse raced, nerves agitating already strained muscle. The receptionist showed me into a long corridor that served as the waiting room. A line of chairs faced three closed office doors. To the side of each stood a trolley stacked with patients' files. Intermittently, a consultant would open a door, grab a file, glance through it, and call a name. The waiting room was packed, and almost everyone there that afternoon was a woman.

We had all ended up at the clinic because we had been referred by our general practitioners or hospital doctors. We had all experienced symptoms such as pain, fatigue, fevers, rashes, blood clots, pregnancy disorders, and many others that at first didn't have an obvious cause. Each of those files contained our clinical histories. Mine had begun less than two months earlier, when I struggled into my GP's office and told him I couldn't breathe.

As the years went on and I learned to live with my unpredictable, uncertain disease, I mined medical history for answers. Unwell women emerged from the annals of medicine, like so many Matryoshka dolls. Their clinical histories followed similar patterns: childhood illnesses, years of pain and mysterious symptoms, and consistent misdiagnoses. These women were part of my history. Their bodies contributed to the medical discoveries that meant my body recovered and my disease could be managed. But the observations of their disorders and symptoms in those clinical studies told only a fragment of their stories. Their notes gave clues about their bodies but nothing about what it meant to live inside them. I tried to imagine what it felt like to be an unwell woman struggling with a disease that resisted medical understanding at these different points in history. I felt an intimate kinship with them. We shared the same essential biology. What has changed is not the female body itself, but medicine's understanding of it.

Since living with lupus, I've often wondered if women's chronic diseases wouldn't be so enigmatic if medicine accepted that they can't be understood through biological evidence alone. Our diseases are not elusive to us. But something about our diseases seems to thwart and frustrate medicine at every turn. Maybe all that clinical and biomedical uncertainty about us is just medicine's failure to look for answers in the right places. Maybe our diseases are an example of the way women's bodies communicate, and should be listened to, differently.

So much of this book was written in the spring and early summer of

2020, during the COVID-19 pandemic. A week or so after the UK government initiated a lockdown, in March 2020, I was messaging with a dear friend, who asked, "How do you feel now that your book has come to life?" I mulled over what they were really saying: that the hidden social and cultural realities of illness and gender were now shared realities. The reality of living every day with a disease shrouded in uncertainty and speculation, which impacts one's ability to work, think, move freely, and have easy contact with other people was one that everyone was suddenly having to face. Everyone was now having to juggle the responsibilities of work and caring labor amid the ominous threat of possible illness. In another of the many intense conversations I've had during the past months, another close friend said, "I keep hearing this phrase 'we're living in an unprecedented situation.' But this situation isn't unprecedented. Not when we think about how this pandemic has magnified the question of who deserves health." And she is right. COVID-19 has glaringly exposed existing systemic and structural health inequalities. Those communities who are already socially, economically, and medically disadvantaged have the highest risk of exposure to the virus. Black, Asian, and ethnically diverse people in the UK and Black, Indigenous, Latinx, and other ethnically diverse people in the US have the highest rates of infection and death. For people with unmet, untreated health needs, the impact of the virus is devastating. And for women especially, the tendency to diminish, disregard, and sideline illness symptoms is undeniably alive and well in some medical professionals' responses and attitudes.

Globally, it is estimated that twice as many men as women are dying from COVID-19. Although the reasons aren't clear yet, some researchers speculate that this so-called COVID gender gap has to do with biological variables between male and female immune systems. "Something about being a woman is protective, and something about pregnancy is protective," explained Dr. Sara Ghandehari, an intensive care physician at Los Angeles's Cedars-Sinai hospital, "and that makes us think about hormones." In an article for the *New York Times*, Roni Caryn Rabin revealed how doctors at Cedars-Sinai and the Renaissance School of Medicine, on Long Island, New York, have been conducting trials of the "female" sex hormones, estrogen and progesterone, on male and female COVID-19 patients. Both hormones are thought to have anti-inflammatory and protective immunological properties. Women, it's assumed, have hardier immune systems than men do. The capacity of female biology to mount more robust immune responses is one possible explanation for why more women are diagnosed with autoimmune diseases. It's also fairly intriguing to think that the very aspect of female biology that has exempted women from many clinical trials—our erratic hormones—is now being valued and marshaled to treat a virus more prevalent in males. The gender prevalence of COVID-19 has sparked a flurry of controversy and debate. Many people don't believe that biological maleness is quite as straightforward a precipitating factor. Some have pointed out that men diagnosed with COVID-19 are dying given their social and lifestyle factors, including higher rates of smoking, rather than their essential biology. It seems the unerring focus on biological sex might actually hinder, rather than help, the emerging—and vital—understanding of COVID-19 and gender. "When in doubt, look to social factors first, not biology," declared three women directors of the GenderSci Lab, at Harvard University, in a recent essay for the *New York Times*.

Throughout its history, medicine's unerring focus on female biology as the defining factor of being a woman has clouded understanding of our illnesses and diseases. This book focuses on medical culture in the United States and the United Kingdom, where "Western" medicine dominates our mainstream health-care systems. Its history forms the basis of knowledge taught in medical schools; its discoveries inform the decisions made about our bodies and minds in clinics and offices, laboratories and operating rooms. It can heal us, restore our health, and save our lives. But Western medicine is also a system of power, one that has always privileged male knowledge and professional expertise, and enforced and upheld sex and gender binaries, over its long history.

Sweeping through this fascinating and often infuriating history, this book delves into the ways that androcentric medicine has studied, assessed, and defined the biological and anatomical conditions labeled "female." My focus on the ways that medicine has insisted on pathologizing "femaleness," and by extension womanhood, means that my discussions have not extended to the medical history and experiences of trans, non-binary, and gender-nonconforming people. I do not, by any means, believe that gender identity is defined by the biological sex a person is assigned at birth. But I want to show how medicine, since its very beginnings, has enfolded discriminatory myths of binary gender difference into the formation of its knowledge. From classical medical theories about women's diseases and the earliest whisperings of hysteria to the professionalization of gynecology, the birth of public health, and the development of biomedicine, patriarchal ideologies have clung insidiously to medical culture, practice, and knowledge. The health and lives of *all* unwell women today are profoundly affected by this historical mythologizing. It's there when our pain is minimized, our symptoms dismissed, our illnesses and diseases misdiagnosed, and our own bodies and voices distrusted. This book is a journey through the history of unwell women, which is nothing less than the history of what it has meant to exist as a woman in the man-made world. Medicine has been complicit, for centuries, in the punishment, silencing, and oppression of women. But women have also created knowledge and challenged the status quo, fought back and demanded more, and changed laws and reclaimed rights. In this book, women are not only victims of male-dominated medical orthodoxy; they are also powerful, courageous, and sometimes contentious agents of hope and change.

Medicine is working to revolutionize its practice and protocols, but there is a long legacy to quash when it comes to women's bodies and minds. I know from experience that this legacy continues to stymie effective and timely care, diagnosis, and treatment. In the 1970s, health activists, policy makers, researchers, and community creators called time on medicine's historic blindsiding and pathologizing of unwell women. Their clarion calls are as relevant today as they were then. It is well past time for medicine's checkered past to give way to a future where the fabric of women's experience is recognized and respected in its entirety. I feel so privileged to be telling these stories of women's suffering, resilience, endurance, and activism from the rich, absorbing annals of medicine's history. I believe that the only way to move forward, to change the culture of myth and misdiagnosis that obscures medicine's understanding of unwell women, is to learn from our history. In the man-made world, women's bodies and minds have been the primary battleground of gender oppression. To dismantle this painful legacy in medical knowledge and practice, we must first understand where we are and how we got here. No unwell woman should be reduced to a file of notes, a set of clinical observations, a case study lurking in an archive. Medicine must hear unwell women when they speak—not as females weighed down by the myths of the man-made world, but as human beings. Medicine must listen to and believe our testimonies about our own bodies and ultimately turn its energies, time, and money toward finally solving our medical mysteries. The answers reside in our bodies, and in the histories our bodies have always been writing.

PART ONE

ANCIENT GREECE–NINETEENTH CENTURY

1

WANDERING WOMBS

On the Greek island of Kos many centuries ago, a girl was taken ill. At first, she felt strangely weak, her chest heavy and tight. Soon she began to shiver with fever; pain gripped her heart; terrifying hallucinations swarmed her mind. She was found wandering the streets, so consumed by heat and hurt that she wanted to end her life. Throwing herself down a well or hanging from a tree by a noose would have been pleasant compared with the torment that wracked her body and mind. Her father called for the physician—a man trained in the arts of healing. The physician had seen this illness before in girls who had started to menstruate but hadn't yet married. As they developed into puberty, their plentiful female blood had been used up by growing. Once they had grown into women, all that extra blood accumulated in their wombs, ready to spill out every month. All physicians knew that this was how the female body stayed healthy. This girl was drowning in her own blood. It had no way to flow out, so it had traveled from her womb back through her veins, inflaming her heart and poisoning her senses. The physician urged the girl's father to marry her off without delay. Intercourse would open her body so that her blood would flow out, and pregnancy would make her healthy.

In another home on the island, an older married woman was seized by a violent convulsion. Her eyes rolled back, she ground her teeth, and saliva foamed in her mouth. Her skin was deathly cold; her abdomen wrenched with pain. Her husband called for the physician. This malady often befell women of her age who had stopped having sex and bearing children. He watched the woman writhe and sob and noted that her skin was clammy. The woman's womb, empty and dry because it wasn't being filled, had crept toward her liver in search of moisture. From there it had blocked her diaphragm and robbed her of breath. The woman was being suffocated by her own womb. Soon, the physician hoped, phlegm would flow from her head to moisten her womb and weigh it down. The physician listened to the woman's belly for the gurgling sounds of the womb returning to its rightful place. If it lingered too long near her liver, she would choke to death. If only she had been having sex regularly, she might have been spared this misery.

Women like this haunt *The Hippocratic Corpus*, a collection of medical discourse attributed to Hippocrates of Kos, the Greek physician known as the father of medicine, from the Classical era—the fourth and fifth centuries BCE. As a teacher and physician, Hippocrates revolutionized medicine. He debunked centuries-old superstitions that diseases were punishments doled out by vengeful gods. He taught that ill health arose from imbalances in the body, and he invented the patient case study, writing careful notes about the symptoms and course of a person's illness and prescribing herbal recipes as treatments. He vowed to treat all illness, in all people, to the best of his ability and to never abuse the body of any man or woman. Whether his patient was freeborn or enslaved, he promised to do no harm: Hippocrates's oath became the cornerstone of patient ethics, and it is still sworn by medical graduates today.

Hippocrates emphasized how women's bodies and illnesses needed to be dealt with very differently from those of men. He stressed how important it was for physicians to "learn correctly from a patient the origin of her disease" by questioning her "immediately and in detail about the cause." Many women, he remarked, suffered and died because physicians proceeded to treat their diseases like "diseases in men." But even though he acknowledged that the diseases of women required special and specific approaches to healing, Hippocrates was not exactly championing women's right to body autonomy and informed medical choice. *The Hippocratic Corpus* was written at a time when most women had few, if any, civil or human rights. In the patriarchal social order of ancient Greece, girls were the property of their fathers, and women of their husbands. They had no ownership over land, property, money, or even their own bodies. They were seen as weaker, slower, smaller versions of the male human ideal, deficient and defective precisely because of their *difference* to men. But in their difference, women possessed the most useful and mysterious organ of all: the uterus. Since women's sole purpose was thought to be to bear and raise children, their health was entirely defined by the uterus. Medical ideas reflected and legitimized society's control over the female body and its precious procreative power. Right at the very beginnings of Western medical history, in writings that would become the foundations of scientific medical discourse and practice, unwell women emerged as a mass of pathological wombs.

The Hippocratic Corpus was based on the teachings of Hippocrates, but it was actually written down by different physicians who followed him. In treatises like *Diseases of Women*, *Nature of Women*, and *Diseases of Young Girls*, Hippocratic physicians described many different symptoms that afflicted women, from puberty and the beginnings of menstruation to conception, pregnancy, and menopause. The idea that all women's diseases were related to their reproductive functions seems, today, like the worst kind of misogynistic conspiracy. But in ancient Greece, where women's entire social existence was defined by their uteruses, it made perfect sense that the disorders and dysfunctions of their bodies and minds would be too. And the Hippocratics didn't have much else to go on. Human dissection was prohibited, so they had no knowledge about where organs were precisely located, how blood circulated, or how respiration occurred. They didn't know about cells, hormones, or neurons. Their understanding of female physiology decreed that women's bodies were overly wet because they had too much blood. They came to this conclusion because women menstruate.

Physicians could interpret what was making a woman ill only through what they could see and feel. Limited knowledge and prevailing social attitudes led to a concoction of theories about the influence of the uterus on every aspect of women's health. Sometimes it was diseased; other times it caused diseases in different parts of the body, including the mind. It was both a channel and a vessel, and a woman was kept healthy if it was either releasing moisture or being filled with it. The cure for Hippocratic uterine pathologies, from the madness of suppressed menstruation to the horrors of womb suffocation, was as much social as it was medical: marriage, ideally by the age of fourteen, regular sex with one's husband—who was usually around the age of thirty—and multiple pregnancies. "I assert that a woman who has not borne children becomes ill from her menses more seriously and sooner than one who has borne children," wrote the author of the first tract of *Diseases of Women*. For the uterus would always start causing mischief if it was stifled by virginity, dried up for wont of male "seed," or not weighed down with child.

Women in ancient Greece were no more in control of their uteruses than they were any other aspect of their lives. The womb hungered for intercourse and pregnancy in a way that was always beyond the control of the woman it resided within. To govern women's biological destiny, physicians pushed the message *the womb wants what the womb wants*. From Hippocratic diagnoses such as "suffocation of the womb" came the idea that an unfulfilled, unemployed uterus could move out of place, wreaking havoc on the organs it reached, including the heart and liver, and causing a startling array of symptoms. Convulsions that resembled epileptic fits. Delirious visions. Loss of breath. Pain and paralysis.

Just after *The Hippocratic Corpus* was laid down, around the middle of the third century BCE, Plato, the great philosopher of Athens, described the womb as a living creature that became "vexed and aggrieved" if its desires for childbearing were not met. In his famous dialogue *Timaeus*, about the world, the universe, and everything in it, Plato conflated women's biological purpose with their apparently untamable sexual impulses, creating a mythology of a womb that wandered "throughout the body," blocking "the channels of the breath," bringing the sufferer to "extreme stress," and causing "all manner of disorders."

Around the second century CE, Aretaeus, from the Roman province Cappadocia, took Hippocratic teachings on "womb suffocation" further by proclaiming that the uterus was like "an animal within an animal." Its capacity to move "hither and thither" and its responsiveness to sweet and fetid smells meant Aretaeus decided it had appetites and inclinations all of its own. Herbal fumigations were often used as remedies to entice displaced uteruses back to their rightful place. An animalistic womb was erratic, its movements sudden and violent. It could float up and down and "incline to this side and that, like a log of wood." If a womb wandered enough to compress a woman's intestines or choke her throat, she lost all her strength, her knees collapsed, her head ached and swam with vertigo, and the veins in her nose pulsed with pain. If her womb was actually choking her, her pulse might weaken, and she could lose her speech and breath. In extreme cases, she suffered "a very sudden and incredible death" in which she didn't actually look dead but somehow remarkably brighter than she did when she was alive.

Medical writers of ancient Greece and Rome held many different views on the wandering womb. But the uterus, as the dominant force behind so many illnesses, diseases, and symptoms of women, was woven into them all. Women were under the dominion of male authority, and medical discourse legitimized this by making women's bodies subordinate to the whims of the very organ that defined their social purpose. Whether these physicians believed the womb literally wandered or just imagined it did, the idea that all women with uteruses were susceptible to becoming unwell because their bodies were hell-bent on making babies persisted for centuries.

As human civilization lumbered into the Middle Ages, the womb wandered with it. The decline of the Roman Empire plunged Europe into the Dark Ages. With the rise of Christian theology and mythology across the Western world from the first century CE, interpreted and spread through the gospel of Saint Paul, new punitive beliefs about women and their bodies ushered forth. The ancient Greeks had blamed all the sickness of the world on Pandora, the mythological first woman, who was too weak to resist opening the forbidden jar of evils that her husband, Epimetheus, was taking care of. Christianity spun a different story about women and their bodies being responsible for all the sin in the world. The book of Genesis decreed that Eve, the original woman, imperfect and incomplete from the get-go—and an afterthought spawned from Adam's rib—ruined everything because of her desirous

and disobedient ways. Medical writings that survived the fall of
Rome were closely sanctioned by the Church, so those very men who
proselytized that women were universally deviant were also the ones in
charge of teaching texts that claimed the female body was inferior, defective, and always governed by the whims of the womb.

Latin translations of ancient books on the diseases of women, housed
in monastery libraries, taught male physicians—*medici*—about the influence of the uterus on women's illnesses. For most women of the common classes in the early Middle Ages, medical care was provided by
female healers or midwives within their communities, who tended ailments and provided remedies along with delivering babies. But when a
woman did see a *medici*, her symptoms were generally blamed on the
"manifold and diverse" forces of the womb. Thankfully, some of the
sources on women's diseases at least tried to offer a less dramatic view.
One of the most popular volumes at the time was *Gynecology*, an ex-
haustive text attributed to Soranus of Ephesus, a Greek physician practicing in Rome around the first or second century, and first translated
into Latin in the sixth century. Part practical guidebook for midwives,
part treatise on the many and various disorders of the uterus, *Gynecology*
derived from Soranus's more balanced, holistic view of human health.
He didn't subscribe to the notion that women's biological differences
meant they were naturally inferior and defective creatures, and he de-
parted from the Hippocratic idea that women needed an entirely separate branch of medicine. This meant he didn't promote menstruation,
sex, and pregnancy as catchall cures for women's diseases, although he
did believe that a proper understanding of gynecological complaints was
crucial when caring for women.

Illness, for Soranus, was a universal human condition caused by different states of relaxation and constriction within the organs and systems
of the human body. He found the notion of the wandering womb fairly
implausible: "For the uterus does not issue forth like an animal from a
lair." Attributing such impulses to the womb was, in his teaching, an
impediment to women's healing. He found the ancients' belief that the
uterus would return to its rightful place if a woman inhaled "bad
odors"—including cedar resin, burned hair and wool, extinguished lamp

wicks, charred deer horns, and squashed bedbugs—faintly ridiculous. And he held a dim view of the ancient Greek philosopher Xenophon, who, around the time of Hippocrates, suggested banging metal plates together and making a huge racket so the uterus would flee back in fright. Diseases like "womb suffocation" were caused by the uterus being constricted with inflammation from menstrual problems, difficulties in childbirth, miscarriages, and menopause. This could cause intense sympathetic pain in the abdomen, fevers, weakness in the limbs, and "convulsive contractions" that "seized the senses." But it didn't drive a woman into a fit of apoplectic mania resembling epilepsy, as the Hippocratics claimed. In fact, Soranus thought that the whole fumigation business actually caused many of the symptoms associated with womb suffocation, like torpor, and that remedies including "forcing air by means of the smith's bellows into the vagina" damaged rather than healed "the inflamed parts." His suggested treatments were altogether more sensible. He recommended laying the woman down in a bright, warm room "without hurting her," placing warm compresses on her belly, and gently straightening out her cramped limbs. If the "paroxysm" continued, he didn't send her off for a roll around the marital bed. He encouraged restoring her health through exercise and "promenades," light gymnastics, baths, anointments with oils, various "pungent" foods, vocal exercises, and reading aloud.

Medieval Christian moral laws forbade *medici* from physically examining any woman. The female body was shrouded in secrecy and shame, and not only to the eyes and hands of male physicians. Women themselves wouldn't have dared reveal intimate details to men about what was going on in their own bodies. Some medical writers of the time echoed these sentiments, including one who referred to women's gynecological complaints as "her disgrace." In the foundational Hippocratic writings in *Diseases of Women*, the shame felt by women patients, especially those who were young and lacking in experience, was identified as a barrier to their receiving accurate care and treatment. Although the Hippocratic authors advised physicians to ask women about the cause of their illnesses, they also believed that their sense of shame—coupled with their ignorance about medical matters—meant they should not necessarily be trusted as reliable narrators of what was happening in their own bodies. The "diseases of women . . . are dangerous . . . and difficult to understand because of the fact that women are the ones who share these sicknesses . . . For women are ashamed to tell even if they know, and they suppose it is a disgrace, because of their inexperience and lack of knowledge." Without the kind of intense questions that only the authoritative male physician could ask, a young woman's disease might well become incurable. But if she was older and had a decent amount of experience with "diseases that come from the menses," then her own testimony might be taken more seriously. But ultimately, even when medical men were forbidden to touch women's bodies, it was male-authored knowledge that determined how they might be healed.

Soranus's *Gynecology* provided extensive instructions to midwives, who had more access to women's bodies. And it's clear that he wanted to relieve women's pain and suffering and not punish them with weird "cures" based on even weirder religious and cultural superstitions. But his works were translated and taught at a time when women were subservient to men, and their primary role was marriage and motherhood. Illness was a punishment for sin, and women's bodies, and their reproductive organs, were the original source of that sin. The transmission of ancient Greek medical ideas about women's defective bodies and delirious temperaments meant the Middle Ages continued to be dominated by the dimmest views of female biology. In the coming centuries, as new learning was layered upon old, the oppressive mythologies of the wandering womb would continue to shape attitudes toward women's susceptibility to illness, their bodies, and their lives.

From the eleventh century, the town of Salerno in southern Italy became the most important institution of medical teaching and learning since the time of Hippocrates. It was also the first to train women as physicians. The masters of Salerno based their teaching of women's medicine on many different sources, including the works of Hippocrates, Soranus, and Galen of Pergamon—the most influential physician to come out of the Roman Empire—and translations of Arabic medical handbooks and encyclopedias. The most famous woman at Salerno was Trota, a physician who lived around the middle of the twelfth century. She is thought to be the author of *The Trotula*, a compendium of three books on the symptoms and treatments of women's illnesses, which became a popular and widely used source throughout the Middle Ages. The first book, called *Conditions of Women*, begins with the author explaining that women, "from the condition of their fragility, out of shame and embarrassment, do not dare to reveal the anguish of their diseases (which happen in such a private place) to a physician."

Based on readings and interpretations of the works of Hippocrates and Galen, *The Trotula* doesn't deviate from prevailing wisdom that women are physiologically weak, biologically inferior, and always prone to ill health, thanks to their childbearing apparatus. Following Galen's theory of humorism, where illness is caused by imbalances in the four essential substances of the body—black bile, yellow bile, phlegm, and blood—the author maintains that women menstruate because they can't make enough heat to get rid of bad and excessive humors. Symptoms of excessive, suppressed, and retained menstruation, along with that old favorite "suffocation of the womb," are all described in the book, although the author doesn't imply that the suffering makes women throw themselves down wells, hallucinate horrors, or lose their minds. As for the wandering womb, the uterus does ascend enough to cause abdominal pain, and descend if it prolapses, but as the author impresses, it can't actually float about causing mayhem here, there, and everywhere.

The figure of Trota herself appears in the second book, *Treatments of Women*, in which the author talks about a young woman suffering from what seemed to be a rupture in either her uterus or intestines. Trota, "called in as the master of this operation," came to the house "so that in secret she might determine the cause of the disease." The young woman was saved from the surgeon's knife because Trota discovered that she actually had "windiness" in her womb. Trota instructed her to spend a long time in herbal baths, have her limbs massaged, and apply a warm "plaster" made of wild radish juice and barley flour to her vagina "to consume the windiness." The young woman was cured.

Trota's practical, humane treatments ultimately sought to help and heal women, not punish and condemn them. The books of *The Trotula* shed light on the mysteries of women's illnesses in an era when women were dying because of society's—and their own—profound sense of shame around the female body. Sadly, Trota's efforts, in the coming centuries at least, would be in vain. By the fourteenth century, women physicians were prohibited from practicing professionally across Europe. Medicine was once again dominated by religious men who propagated the belief that the female body was the vessel of sin. Religious superstition about disease as divine punishment entangled with medical attitudes about the destructive potential of women's bodies. Now that medicine was armed with religious justification that women were contaminating and depraved, fascination and fear around the secrets of female biology took a sinister turn. And the consequences for far too many women would be harrowing.

2

POSSESSED AND POLLUTING

I n Paris in 1405, Christine de Pizan, the only professional woman of
letters in France, decided she'd had enough of the "awful and damning things" being written by men about women and their bodies. De
Pizan was respected and successful. She was a writer in the court of
King Charles VI and had composed ballads and poems for members of
the French royal family. She was also an esteemed historian, a whip-
smart political thinker, and a feminist visionary. Having spent her life
studying women's contributions to every field of human endeavor, she
felt truly miserable about the ways that "female nature" was represented
by male philosophers, poets, and orators as defective and deranged. So
she wrote *The Book of the City of Ladies*, with its imaginary forum where
female saints and prophets, scribes, poets, inventors, artists, and warriors are rescued from the wastes of history and celebrated and championed on their own terms.

Early in *City of Ladies*, de Pizan explains that the female sex has
been left defenseless for too long, "like an orchard without a wall," and
that it is high time women's nature is protected and defended, especially
from certain male writers who denounce women's bodies as depraved
and corrupt. One offender was Francesco degli Stabili, known as Cecco
d'Ascoli, a notoriously misogynistic thirteenth-century Italian physician,
poet, and astrologer. Cecco d'Ascoli wrote encyclopedic poems about
heaven and earth containing memorable verses like "Women's bodies
are inferior to men's / they menstruate every month because / they are

by nature imperfect beings" and "A woman has less faith than a wild beast / proud, greedy, stupid, crazy and aloof / a poison that infects the body's heart." By the time Christine de Pizan wrote her book, Cecco d'Ascoli had been burned at the stake as a heretic for reading Jesus Christ's horoscope. De Pizan ventured that "he got what he deserved."

Cecco d'Ascoli's beliefs about women's bodies were neither unusual nor novel. Medieval physicians and natural philosophers upheld the "wisdom" that female biology was universally weak and inferior because of its difference to the male ideal. But when de Pizan was writing in the late Middle Ages, medical men were shining a new theological light on the ancient teachings. All human women were daughters of Eve who had to endure God's punishment by submitting to their husbands and suffering the pain of childbirth. De Pizan was a devout Christian. At the beginning of *City of Ladies*, she asks how her trusted God could have made such a horrendous mistake when he allowed the creation of women. But the problem, she knew, wasn't God; it was mortal men who manipulated Christianity's foundational myths to justify society's subjugation of women.

For de Pizan, one of the most offensive examples of pseudomedical misogyny was "a little book in Latin" called *De secretis mulierum* (*On the Secrets of Women*), which "states that the female body is inherently flawed and defective in many of its functions." *Secrets of Women* was a popular treatise written by an unknown follower of Albertus Magnus, the German Catholic bishop and friar—a.k.a. Saint Albert the Great—sometime in the late thirteenth or early fourteenth century. This author, referred to as "pseudo-Albertus," wrote his treatise in the style and tradition of a "book of secrets," a kind of practical guidebook popular throughout the Middle Ages that explained the mysteries of life to many different audiences, from householders to scholars, priests to physicians. And in the thirteenth century, life's most perplexing but essential mystery—how babies were made—lay hidden inside a place shrouded by shame and superstition: the female body. Ostensibly, *Secrets of Women* was meant to instruct churchmen in matters of fertility, conception, and pregnancy without the fear of their getting their hands dirty. But it was also a way of enshrining derogatory beliefs about women and their bodies, laid down nearly two thousand years earlier, into a new regime of professional—and religious—medical knowledge.

The author of *Secrets of Women* delighted in the idea that menstruation meant all women were fragile, faithless, and faulty. He believed he was doing a great service by revealing the sordid and sensational truth about what went on in the darkest recesses of the female body. And he had a very specific audience in mind: celibate monks and priests. "To my dear companion and friend in Christ," he begins. "Since you asked me to bring to light certain hidden, secret things about the nature of women, I have set myself to the task of composing this short and compendious treatise. I have done this despite the youthful frailty of my mind, which tends to be attracted to frivolous things."

After this introductory humblebrag, the author wastes no time getting to the crux of the matter. Women are monstrous. Their "infirmities" lead them to do sinful things. For menstruation is the root of all women's evils. When a woman is menstruating, she can poison animals with a glance, infect children in the cradle, dirty the cleanest mirror with her vile reflection, and transmit leprosy and cancers to men. It's very important that priests understand such things, for "evil cannot be avoided unless it is known." If an "infirm" woman should confess some fleshly sin, her priest needed to understand exactly what physical process led her to commit it in order to give suitable penance. *Secrets of Women* wasn't intended to help women understand their bodies; it was a guide to how to punish them.

Secrets of Women covered all the basics: how embryos are generated, aids and impediments to conception, how sperm is made, how to really tell whether she's a virgin, wandering wombs, womb suffocation, the formation of the fetus by celestial influences including the position of the planets, divine conception, and why monsters get born. Safe to say, this is no midwifery manual. But beneath the absurdity of the author's revelations, countless sinister accusations are made about the depraved female organs and their devilish influence on women's character and temperament. Women are to blame for all infertility, miscarriages, and birth defects. And the abhorrence of their bodies also drives them to commit immoral acts of the most grievous kind. When menstruating, women become so vindictive toward men that they seek out the most inventive ways to harm them. Consumed by lust and cunning, a bleeding woman will lure a man into having sex; but unbeknownst to him, she will have inserted pieces of iron inside her vagina to mortally wound his penis. And women's impressionable imaginations mean they are not strong enough to resist evil images coming into their minds during sex. If a woman imagines a monster, she will cause hideous, monstrous deformities in her unborn child. When pregnant, some women may have an appetite so peculiar that they demand certain foods, and if refused will go on a hunger strike and abort the baby. In this particular story, the food in question happens to be an apple—Eve's snack of choice.

Nothing in *Secrets of Women*, aside from the odd rumor or secondhand yarn, comes from the author's experience of women or their bodies. Nor does it bear any relation to the testimony of women themselves. All his "secrets" were drawn from the writings of the classical fathers of medicine, principally Aristotle and Hippocrates, and extrapolated through Catholic theology and astronomical ideas. *Secrets of Women* was written by a man for an audience of men—men who had vowed never to have intimate contact with a woman's body, much less learn about what it was actually like to live inside one.

Christine de Pizan called out one particular passage in which the author claims that "one of the popes excommunicated any man found either reading the book out loud to a woman or giving it to her to read for herself." This was the reason de Pizan despised *Secrets of Women* so much. It was a text that not only mystified women and their bodies but spread vicious fictions and titillating lies, which women had no ways or means of disputing. "You shouldn't need any other evidence than your own body to realize this book is a complete fabrication," de Pizan wrote. "Any woman who reads it can see that, since certain things it says are the complete opposite of her own experience." If a woman did read it, "she would pour scorn on it and recognize it for the utter rubbish it is."

No matter how fervently de Pizan defended her sex, she could do little to disrupt medicine's promotion of this kind of pseudomedical religious dogma. *Secrets of Women* was, indeed, utter rubbish. But the bases of its ideas were by no means unusual. Medical knowledge in the Middle Ages, as it had been for centuries, was a way of confining women to marriage and endless child-rearing. And the male writers espousing this nonsense understood only too well that women had to be exempted from the hallowed halls of medicine if men were to maintain their stranglehold. By the early fourteenth century, many medical universities in Europe that had previously admitted women, like the Schola Medica Salernitana, were banning them from studying and practicing as physicians. As medicine became more professionalized, and women were barred from obtaining professional status as medics, any woman practicing medicine could potentially be tried in a court.

One such physician was Jacqueline Félicie de Almania, known as Jacoba Felice, who had studied at the University of Paris. In 1322, Jacoba was put on trial for practicing medicine without a license. She was a respected healer who had successfully cured many men and women. In her defense, she argued that the era's virtues of chastity and modesty meant that women were not receiving the care and treatment they so desperately needed. "It is better and proper and more suitable that a woman wise and experienced in the art should visit sick women," she wrote, "and that she should examine them and inquire into the secrets of nature and its hidden things . . . It used to be that a woman would die, rather than reveal her secret illness to a man." Jacoba's defense fell on deaf ears. She was found guilty, fined, excommunicated, and barred from practicing medicine again.

By silencing women and persecuting the women who would care for them, religious purveyors of medical ideas could spout and spread their ideas unhindered by inconvenient facts. Monks, priests, and clerics taught and transmitted material such as that in *Secrets of Women* across Europe in universities instructing scholars in science and philosophy. Men like the author of *Secrets of Women* weren't reinventing the wheel; they were simply putting a new spin on it. But if women were so full of poisonous substances that could cause illness and injury, destruction, and death, how come they weren't poisoning themselves? After all, they weren't suited to learning anything because their internal toxicity sent up vapors that addled their brains. And women cried so much because they must leak all those damnable humors out somehow. But according to *Secrets of Women*, women are immune to their own poisons, like snakes to their own venom; and "venom doesn't act on itself, but on the object." Ancient medical writers had already determined that women's humors were more polluting to the world around them than to themselves. Hippocrates, and later Pliny the Elder, thought menstrual blood could make men ill, ruin crops, kill bees, and drive dogs mad. But in light of Christian gospel teachings that women's bodies had violated the world, the medical wheel was starting to spin dangerously out of control. Attitudes about the ruinous nature of female biology were escalating into beliefs that women were not only harmful but demonic.

In 1346, the bubonic plague swept through Europe, devastating the population. Over four years the Black Death killed an estimated twenty million people. The symptoms and course of the disease were terrifying. Swollen glands caused hemorrhaging under the skin, and high fevers and delirium ensued before sufferers died, more often than not, from septic shock. There was very little understanding in the Middle Ages about how diseases were transmitted, and no knowledge about bacteria and the process of infection. The scale and force of the epidemic were unprecedented. Many believed it was a punishment from God, a pestilence of biblical proportions. Others who followed Galen thought it was caused by foul humors amassing in the air or a violent collision of the planets. Some blamed members of the Jewish faith, believing they were purposely trying to poison Christians. The plague heightened the fear of disease across Europe, enflaming religious and medical superstitions about the ungodly nature of corrupt human biology.

Over seven years, the plague wiped out between 30 and 50 percent of the entire population of Europe. In the wake of the plague, poverty was rife, infertility was high, and birth rates were at an all-time low. Against this backdrop of intense fear and superstition around the causes of this catastrophic decimation, the Church, and society at large, searched for scapegoats. If the population was to be replenished, then women—the very vessels of conception, birth, and new life—had to be scrutinized, regulated, surveilled, and controlled. By the fifteenth century, the attitudes toward women's bodies espoused in material like *Secrets of Women* were embedded in the minds of authoritative men across Europe, men who had the power to determine how women should live and behave. As authors like pseudo-Albertus had made quite clear, women, as reproductive and sexual beings, were corrupting and corruptible. Accepted beliefs about women's dependence on men, their innate physical and mental weaknesses, and their unruly, uncontrollable organs and biological processes made it all too easy to frame women as architects of sin, as instruments of destruction. Suspicion around women's deviant and demonic potential rose stealthily across Europe, especially through the teachings of Catholic churchmen who upheld the religious and social sanctity of marriage.

One such man was Heinrich Kramer. From a young age, Kramer had been educated in Alsace in the Dominican Order of Catholic preachers. The Dominicans were renowned for their intellectual tradition and their teaching of philosophy and theology. They were also dedicated to spreading the Gospel and to identifying, denouncing, and punishing any acts and behaviors that contravened it. In 1474, when he was thirty-four, Kramer was granted permission by Pope Innocent VIII to act as an inquisitor and bring to justice any person committing an act of heresy. His jurisdiction covered Tyrol and Salzburg, as well as Bohemia and Moravia (now part of the Czech Republic). Since the twelfth century, heretics had mostly been Catholic dissenters, Protestants, and Christian spiritualists. But in 1484, the pope included another group of heretics in his decree, known as the papal bull: witches. It was now permissible to try and punish people in a court of law for acts of witchcraft. The Catholic Church had confirmed it: witches roamed the earth, consorting with the devil to bring about disease, death, and destruction. Kramer had found his calling. For years he had enthralled crowds with his fire-and-brimstone sermons, damning to hell all the wicked souls who dared to sin against his faith. Kramer was no longer confined to his pulpit; now he was free to hunt down heretics and rid Europe of demonic influences. And what people in particular were weak, depraved, and deceitful enough to abandon their faith and do the devil's bidding? Of course, it was women.

Kramer began his hunt in 1485. Leading a band of inquisitors, he traveled to Innsbruck to investigate anyone who might be practicing the dark arts. Among the many he brought to trial was Helena Scheuberin, a woman with a smart mouth and loose morals. There were rumors that she had made a woman ill so that she could steal her husband and that she had inflicted disease and death upon a knight who'd rejected her advances. Kramer decided she must have used sorcery—"love magic," to be precise. There was no evidence for this other than the fact that Scheuberin was an adulteress. But adultery, in his opinion, *was* witchcraft. Scheuberin was also friends with a group of women Kramer believed to be witches. Still, his only "facts" were that a woman got ill, a man died, and Scheuberin was somehow connected to both of them. In court, Kramer fixated on Scheuberin's sexual behavior, asking questions to "prove" she possessed animalistic urges. "It is a general rule," he declared, "that all witches have been slaves from a young age to carnal lust and to various adulteries, just as experience teaches." He believed she'd had sex with the devil. The local bishop was so offended by the nature of Kramer's accusations—and his graphic line of questioning—that he feared the reputation of the town would be tainted. So he brought in a lawyer, who also happened to be a physician, to act in Scheuberin's defense. On the basis of Kramer's obvious sexual obsession with Scheuberin, which the lawyer took umbrage with, the trial was thrown out, and she walked free.

Kramer returned to his home in Cologne. His reputation as an inquisitor was tarnished, but his fervor to eradicate witchcraft was undeterred. He decided to write a book explaining how to identify, try, and punish suspected witches. Published in Germany in 1486, the *Malleus maleficarum* (*The Hammer of Witches*) declared that women practicing witchcraft should suffer the same fate as all heretics: execution, by being burned at the stake. For pages upon pages, Kramer set out his case for the existence of witches and the reality of witchcraft. He left no stone unturned when explaining exactly why the Catholic Church should take action. The devil, he claimed, needed agents on earth, instruments to afflict evils on his behalf. And the pact the devil must make was with the human body. In order for the devil to "infect," as Kramer put it, a woman with witchcraft, she must have any one of three specific vices: infidelity, ambition, or lust. The more insatiable the woman, the more likely the devil is to take the form of an incubus and lay with her. According to Kramer, the papal bull named the principal acts of women's witchcraft as inciting passion in men, obstructing the "generative act," removing men's penises, changing men into beasts, preventing other women from conceiving, procuring abortions, and killing babies as offerings to devils. Anyone taking Kramer's thesis seriously would have been hard-pressed not to point the finger at female healers and midwives, unmarried women, women married to infertile men, women who cheated on their husbands, women who wanted to learn or read or speak for themselves—in fact, any woman whose lifestyle, behavior, or personality didn't conform to the highest virtues of chastity and faith.

The *Malleus* was crammed full of the most outrageous and extreme stories Kramer could concoct from his time as an inquisitor. He reserved a special hatred for those witches who, as he wrote with remarkable solemnity, "do marvelous things with regard to male organs." In one story, a young man from Ratisbon dumped a woman he was having an affair with, only to discover, to his horror, that she had "cast some glamour" over his penis so that he could neither see nor touch it. Kramer also claimed that some witches collected penises, put them in bird boxes, and fed them oats and corn. But far more serious, and chilling, was Kramer's assault against midwives.

Female healers were already pushed to the margins of medicine. And since most women couldn't afford to see professional physicians, midwives and wisewomen provided essential support to those who were pregnant and in labor. Since these women were already going against the law and had to operate clandestinely, Kramer crafted a narrative of secrecy and deviance around their practices. Childbirth, at the time, was perilous and fraught with danger. Women and their babies frequently died during labor. Kramer attested that infant death and miscarriage weren't a natural occurrence but the devil working through possessed midwives to slaughter innocents. Among his more egregious tales—of witches stealing newborns, drinking their blood, devouring them, and offering them to the devil as a sacrifice—he strongly implied that any instance of failed pregnancy in a woman attended by a midwife should be suspected as witchcraft. Procuring an abortion, after all, was one of the seven methods of witchcraft Kramer defined. "No one does more harm to the Catholic faith than midwives," he wrote. Toward the end of the *Malleus*, he declared that witch-midwives "surpass all other witches in their crimes" and that such evil was so rife that "there is scarcely a tiny hamlet in which one has not been found."

The Dominican leaders of the Catholic inquisition considered Kramer an ethically dubious crank who was deliberately manipulating Catholic theology to his own ends. But Kramer was tenacious about ensuring that his work was read and used. The availability of the newly invented Gutenberg printing press from 1500 meant that the *Malleus* was circulated widely across Europe. As the fear of witchcraft was beginning to grip the continent, the *Malleus* proved to be an essential guidebook. For Kramer laid down, in scrupulous detail, exactly how suspected witches should be interrogated, tried, and sentenced in both religious and secular courts. While acts of heresy must be dealt with by appointed inquisitors, any person suspected of witchcraft who didn't constitute a crime against the Church could still be brought to justice by any means necessary.

Kramer broadened the scope of what witchcraft actually entailed and who was likely to practice it. Any ordinary person, but especially women who transgressed strict social and moral boundaries, could be accused of practicing witchcraft by members of her community if she was in any way connected to an inexplicable event. Ordinary folks living cheek by jowl in rural villages and farming towns were already inherently superstitious about how dark forces might be behind all sorts of occurrences, natural and social, that threatened their precarious livelihoods. Damage to property, mysterious weather, disputes and arguments, one's cows having more milk than one's neighbors, and buckets moving about on their own were all mentioned in Kramer's judicial proceedings, alongside more acts of bewitching, like illness, injury, and fornication. Fears around everyday unknowns meant that fingers were quickly pointed at anyone perceived to be up to no good—particularly if they were already vilified for being obstreperous, angry, deviant, solitary, or strange. Once any suspected person, usually an older woman, was brought to trial, the court would listen to the witnesses' accusations, search her home for any implement even vaguely related to witchcraft, and then interrogate her with questions like "And why did you touch the child before it got sick?"

While the court was considering the evidence, the accused would be imprisoned, stripped of her clothes, and shaved. Kramer believed that witches often sewed articles of their craft into their garments and even onto their skin. "Articles" included a pock or scar thought to be inflicted by the tongue or claw of the devil. Any mole, birthmark, wart, or blemish could be diagnosed as the "witches mark." If none was found, inquisitors sometimes ordered male physicians or respected midwives to search for other unusual traits, like protruding nipples or enlarged clitorises. Once the offending feature had been identified (as it inevitably was), the court could extract a confession. If an accused woman pleaded innocent or kept silent—both signs of the devil's influence—Kramer recommended torture. Women would be bound, pierced with needles, dunked in water, deprived of food and drink, denied sleep, made to carry red-hot iron, or have hot fat smeared on their vaginas. These sadistic procedures were meant to force women to confess, but they often induced hallucinations and dissociation, which were interpreted as proof of possession. If found guilty on a "light suspicion," the accused may have been made to do penance. If guilty of a more serious offense, she may have been held in prison and tortured daily until a confession was extracted. But if her crime was grievous, or heretical, Kramer said, the judge should "sentence her to flames."

Kramer and his *Malleus* were by no means solely responsible for inciting the mounting fear of witchcraft, which took its most devastating hold across Europe during the sixteenth century. But the *Malleus*, and the many other witchcraft tracts that appeared in the late fifteenth century, certainly inflamed the culture of horrifying persecution that was rigged against women from the very beginning. During the sixteenth and seventeenth centuries, an estimated forty-five thousand people were executed for the crime of witchcraft, of which 80 percent were women, many over the age of forty. The motivations behind this unmitigated war against womankind were a complicated collusion of religious, social, political, and economic forces. Anxieties around the influence of dark magic, sorcery, and demonology were rife across a continent that had been so horribly decimated by disease, upheaval, and unrest. In the witch-hunts and trials that took place, mostly in Germany, France, England, and Scotland, women—especially those who were unmarried, old, poor, involved in healing, or practicing midwifery—were maliciously scapegoated as the vectors of death and destruction. And the ideologies behind this unimaginable campaign of extermination didn't come out of nowhere.

Over centuries, religious doctrine and medical discourse had claimed that women's bodies and minds were defective and dangerous. Ancient physicians had decreed that women were at the mercy of their uncontrollable, unruly reproductive organs. Christian theology had woven these foundational ideas into a new dogma of female inferiority, in which women's physical and mental weakness were proof of their susceptibility to channeling demonic forces and committing evil deeds. Where writings like *The Hippocratic Corpus* maintained that women should marry early and procreate frequently to stave off diseases of the body and mind, the Church insisted on marriage and reproductive sex as a kind of state protection against women unleashing their original sin. Accusing women of witchcraft was a powerful way for social and religious authorities to maintain male dominance and supremacy in their villages and towns. And trying and executing women was a measure to cleanse communities of those who were not performing the marital and reproductive duties assigned to them under patriarchy. Independent women, solitary women, women past childbearing age—in fact, all women who were not subordinated by marriage and motherhood—were a threat, a hazard, a scourge.

In 1542, under the rule of King Henry VIII, the Witchcraft Act was passed in England, which meant accused women could now be punished by death. Implemented after the English Reformation, which wrested control of the Church of England from the authority of the pope and the Catholic Church and instituted the monarch as its supreme religious leader, the Witchcraft Act empowered ecclesiastical courts to exercise responsibility for such ungodly crimes. The year after James I—who ruled Scotland as James VI since 1567—ascended the throne as king of England and Scotland in 1603, he passed the "Act Against Conjuration, Witchcraft and dealing with evil and wicked spirits." James I's act meant that any person accused of "Witchcraft, Inchantment, Charme, or Sorcery" could be tried in the common, rather than religious, courts.

James I's obsession with and acute anxiety around the influence of witchcraft led to between four thousand and six thousand people being prosecuted for witchcraft in Scotland from the late sixteenth to mid-seventeenth centuries, 75 percent of whom were women. In England, around five hundred people were executed—again, almost all women—for witchcraft between 1560 and 1700. Although witchcraft abilities were still believed to originate in supernatural copulation with the devil, the kinds of crimes witch-women could apparently commit soon became terrifyingly ordinary. Now communities had the power to try any suspicious woman in a local court.

In 1682, in a close-knit farming town named Beckenton, Somerset, a forty-four-year-old woman was accused of bewitching a young man and a young woman, both about eighteen years of age. Passing by an almshouse, a residence for the poorest and most "indignant" people, the young man spotted the woman and called her a witch. Understandably, given the climate of superstition, she was enraged. She called immediately for the justice of the peace to admonish the man, and he promised never to insult her again. But that night, according to his statement, he suffered an attack of the fits and remained ill for two weeks. Wracked with fever, he hallucinated that the woman was in his room, laughing at him, waving her fists, and grinning with all her teeth. Meanwhile, the woman reportedly asked a young woman named Mary to help her collect her spinning work from a nearby town, but Mary refused, for this "old woman" frightened her. Mary then came down with the fits, stronger and more violent than those suffered by the young man. Delirious with fever, she also claimed the old woman appeared in her room to jeer at her. Mary was an acquaintance of the afflicted young man, but no one cried conspiracy.

As her fits subsided, Mary said she felt a pricking in her stomach. She told the court she vomited up a crooked pin. Over the course of eight days, she reported throwing up an alarming collection of objects: more pins, some in clusters tied with yarn; nails; several spoon handles; lumps of iron, tin, brass, and pewter; the lead from a window; and inordinate amounts of blood. The alarmed townspeople forced the old woman to visit Mary. At the sight of her, Mary apparently fell into her strongest fit yet. At the trial, the old woman was stripped by a jury of women and scrutinized for the witch's mark. They found her body scored with purple bruises. She was bound with ropes, led to the river, and dunked under. The jury attested that she floated like a cork. Only good Christian women would sink, for water was so sacred that it immediately repelled a witch. The old woman was tortured this way three more times, and each time, the court maintained, she floated. Her guilt was unassailable. She was hanged. Mary continued to vomit up pins for ten more weeks.

There's no way of knowing if Mary's inexplicable illness was real or not; no physician actually witnessed her throw up all that metal. Maybe Mary hallucinated it; maybe she made it up to exact some petty vengeance. Whatever the truth, the old woman of Beckenton was incriminated because of her age, appearance, low social status, and temperament. There's very little information about what she was like, outside of her erratic and supposedly vengeful behavior. Like so many women accused of witchcraft, she was probably going through menopause. The end of fertility didn't only signal the end of the female body's primary social use; early modern medicine interpreted menopause as a depletion of humors, which made the body impure and riddled with poison. Menopause was both a physical and a psychological pathology; women going through the change were seen as unstable, querulous, ill-tempered, and intent on doing harm. Menopausal symptoms, so poorly understood, were often interpreted as diagnoses of witchcraft.

In England, at the beginning of the seventeenth century, a physician and chemist named Edward Jorden was called as a medical witness in the trial of Elizabeth Jackson, an older woman accused of bewitching a shopkeeper's fourteen-year-old daughter, named Mary Glover. Jorden was a respected and successful doctor. He had attended Queen Elizabeth I and was a fellow of the Royal College of Physicians. He was called to act in defense of Jackson, a woman reportedly known for her unpleasant temper and acid tongue. While doing an errand for her mother, Glover ran into Jackson, who accused the girl of making nasty remarks about her daughter's clothes. The court heard that Jackson then "rayled at her, with many threats and cursings, wishing an evill death to light upon her."

That evening, Glover's throat and neck began to swell, and she fell into a "dead senseless fit." A physician was called. He suspected Glover had tonsillitis but couldn't find any physical evidence. Her fits were so strange that he decided she must have been possessed. During one of her fits, Glover was heard to whisper, "Hang her." At the trial, Jorden suggested at first that Glover might have been feigning possession. He later argued that Jackson was not possessed of supernatural powers at all, because Glover was suffering from a natural disease called *passio hysterica*, a condition very similar to "suffocation of the womb." Sadly, he couldn't convince the courts of his diagnosis. Jackson was sentenced to one year in prison, but the controversy surrounding her conviction meant she gained the support of the public, and soon she was pardoned and released. Meanwhile, Glover still suffered her mysterious fits, until she was finally exorcized by a group of Puritan clerics who still believed— as Glover herself did—that she had been possessed by the devil.

Jorden's efforts to denounce demonic intervention as an explanation for Glover's illness were not in vain. The following year, inspired by his findings during Jackson's trial, he wrote *A Briefe Discourse of a Disease Called the Suffocation of the Mother*, a treatise on the "natural" disease "womb suffocation" and the ways it could affect the bodies and minds of women, young and old. "Mother" was an early modern term for the uterus, and according to Jorden, it was capable of causing such extreme symptoms that "simple and unlearned people" would assume an afflicted woman was possessed by the devil.

Briefe Discourse is also considered the first work in English on symptoms associated with disorders of the uterus, which in the coming centuries would be diagnosed according to the all-encompassing medical model of hysteria. As a way of pathologizing the relationship between women's bodies and minds, the idea of hysteria had existed for centuries. The name came from *hystera*, the ancient Greek for "uterus." Hippocrates, Plato, and Aretaeus set the hysterical scene long ago by dramatizing the effects of different illnesses of *hystera* on women's physical and mental health. In an era when religious superstition dominated perceptions of "hysterical" symptoms, like the convulsions and contortions suffered by Mary Glover, gynecological theories were important milestones in medicine's more rational and humane approach to women's bodies, minds, and illnesses. But these new ideas about the uterus and its myriad "natural" disorders were written in the context of reigning social and cultural assumptions that women were inferior, weak, and impressionable because of their "naturally" defective bodies. "The passive condition of womankind," Jorden wrote, "is subject unto more diseases and of other sorts than men are; and especially in regard of that part from whence this disease that we speak of doth arise." By the seventeenth century, women might not have been demonic, but their "diseased" uteruses certainly behaved as if they were.

3

UNDER HER SKIN

In early modern Europe, intense suspicion still hovered around the deviant potential of the female body and mind. Even when women weren't accused of witchcraft, their impressionable imaginations and corruptible wombs were often regarded as instruments of deviance and depravity. But many physicians believed that women's apparent involvement in inexplicable events was more a matter of medicine than magic. As the witch trials raged, a culture of medical fascination was emerging around the inner workings of women's organs and systems. Racing to stake their claims as purveyors of new knowledge about female physiology, physicians conjured novel theories about the material realities of the uterus. For centuries, the uterus had embodied the knotty paradox of womanhood and femininity. On the one hand, it defined women's divine purpose as hosts to the organ of creation. But on the other, it was an unruly cauldron, constantly brewing up disorders that disturbed ideal feminine states of body and mind.

By explaining what might be happening beneath a woman's skin, physicians of "women's diseases" were at least trying to shine a light of reason into the darkness of superstition. But the motives of doctors like Edward Jorden were hardly feminist. They all agreed that an unwell womb could affect women's health in "monstrous and terrible" ways. The more they argued that uterine troubles were medical problems to be cured—not possessions to be exorcized—the more bizarre their symptoms became. Jorden piled every conceivable "strange

accident"—including breathlessness, convulsions, paralysis, and frenzies of laughing, singing, and weeping—onto his descriptions of "womb
suffocation." His suffocation sufferers were all young maids or older,
often widowed women who lacked the blood-purging benefits of regular intercourse and frequent menstruation. When idle or underused,
their uteruses would send up poisonous vapors that "perturbed their
minds." Once she'd taken leave of her senses, a woman might start
barking, hissing, or perhaps croaking. Jorden's ideal cure was marital
sex and pregnancy—just as Hippocrates prescribed more than two
thousand years earlier. If she was in the grip of a fit, Jorden recommended holding her down by her throat and belly and tying up her
legs. To "allure" her mind away from "perturbations," he prescribed fasting, sleeping, not drinking wine, and praying all day. If her thoughts,
desires, emotions, and life choices were strictly policed, then a disease
like "womb suffocation" was "easily overcome."

For Jorden and his contemporaries, the uterus reigned supreme over
almost all women's body functions, from breathing and digesting to
dreaming and thinking. They thought it was in close communication—
or consent—with other organs, especially the heart and liver. So, they
endowed it with the power to radiate its dysfunctions to almost any part
of the body—causing truly terrible symptoms along the way. No matter
how intently these physicians insisted that its diseases were not caused
by the hand of God or mouth of the devil, they still upsold the uterus's
wild pathological potential. And just because they emphasized natural
rather than supernatural causes, it didn't mean they denounced superstitious attitudes toward women and their behaviors. Jorden, after all,
admitted that the more manic uterine symptoms could easily be mistaken for some "metaphysical" or "demonical" intervention. Only the
most scientifically minded physician, like him, could appreciate the
manifold ways that the "rareness and strangeness" of the uterus was
expressed.

The uterus, for so long, had remained inaccessible and out-of-bounds,
resisting scrutiny and evading understanding. During the antiquity and
throughout the Middle Ages, dissection of human cadavers was forbidden on religious and cultural grounds. Prevailing ideas about the

anatomy of the female reproductive organs, until the sixteenth century, were based on the schema laid down by Galen. Galen had studied women's organs during surgeries, but his vision of female anatomy was based mostly on dissections of macaque monkeys and pigs, as well as sheep, goats, and dogs. Although he made many errors, his comparative observations did enlighten him as to the structure of the human uterus. He described the "thin, fibrous appendages" connecting it to the bladder and rectum, and its "sinewy muscular bonds" to the sacrum. A woven network of nerves furnished it with sensation; veins and arteries nourished the organ itself, and the fetus during pregnancy. These bindings allowed the uterus to "change its natural position very gently," but they weren't loose enough to enable it to roam around. Galen essentially disproved the idea of the "wandering womb," but he was resolute that female genitalia were weaker, smaller, and colder facsimiles of the mighty penis and testes. According to his humoral theories, sex difference was determined by heat. As a fetus developed, it needed to generate enough heat to descend the testes out of the body, or they would stay inside as meager little ovaries. Galen's "turned outside in" vision was replicated in anatomical illustrations in the fourteenth and fifteenth centuries. Guides such as the *Disease Woman* represented the female body not as it really was, but as it was imagined by men transmitting and translating knowledge across the centuries. And the uterus's structures remained frustratingly obscured; unsurprisingly, it was usually drawn occupied with a fetus.

The uterus defined women's physiological difference from men; understanding of that difference prompted a raft of theories about its influence on women's health and illness. The uterus also held all the secrets of how human life began and developed. While men's sex and generative organs were distinctly visible, women's were shielded by flesh and propriety. And unlike the stalwart testes, the uterus changed through menstruation, conception, and pregnancy. Searching for the truth about this mysterious and mutable organ was like discovering a foreign land. And beyond the uterus, the entire female anatomy—for a coming generation of medical men—was like a new frontier to colonize with knowledge.

It was one thing to imagine the anatomy of the uterus in writing, and quite another to get one's hands and eyes on it. In Europe, human dissection for medical research was being performed from around the fifteenth century. But a map of the newly chartered territory of the female body wasn't created until the sixteenth century, in Renaissance Italy. In 1543, the Flemish anatomist Andreas Vesalius published a series of seven books, *De humani corporis fabrica* (*On the Fabric of the Human Body*), which illustrated for the first time the organs and systems of dissected corpses. Female bodies were highly prized for dissection, but because cadavers were often the bodies of criminals, and women were convicted less often, they were in scarce supply. Vesalius was tenacious when it came to finding subjects. While studying in Paris in 1536, he dissected the body of a young sex worker, who had been hanged, to try to figure out the processes of menstruation. If the corpses of executed people were not readily available, Vesalius was not averse to a bit of grave-robbing and other dubious tactics.

One of the women Vesalius studied had been the lover of a monk who "died suddenly, as if from suffocation of the uterus or some other fulminating illness." The woman's relatives hadn't given permission for her to be dissected, so Vesalius's students "pulled" her "from her tomb" and "removed all her skin from her body with amazing industry" so that she wouldn't be recognized by her family, who had reported her missing corpse to city authorities. Little is known about who she was. Vesalius described her only as an "attractive whore." Her illicit relationship with the monk reduced her to the disreputable status of a sex worker, and Vesalius clearly believed this meant her body was an object to be used—in death as in life.

Several female bodies that Vesalius dissected during lectures and represented in the *Fabrica* had been sex workers or women condemned for unknown crimes. One had claimed to be pregnant to try to stay her execution because hanging, at the time, was postponed until after an accused woman had given birth. Again, virtually nothing is known about who she was, how she lived, or what circumstances led to her conviction. Vesalius stated that she was very tall, middle-aged, and "had often given birth." Midwives who questioned and examined her decreed that she was not, in fact, pregnant. She was hanged, and her dissection was luridly dramatized on the title page of the *Fabrica*. Rendered in a woodcut, she is splayed open on the anatomist's table before hordes of onlookers. Vesalius's hand points toward her uterus. Her body is diminished to a spectacle of knowledge, theatrically unveiled and meticulously scrutinized by men, for men.

The representations of female anatomy in the *Fabrica* show how the uterus was positioned and its relationship to other organs, including the bladder. But when it came to how the organ actually worked, Vesalius's rich visuals came up short. He wasn't able to properly explain the physiology of menstruation, and he had to rely on animal dissections to figure out the changes the uterus went through during pregnancy. But unlike Galen, Vesalius had created knowledge by venturing inside real human women. His insights went beyond comparative animal observations—so he claimed authority and posterity. But this didn't mean his understanding of female genitalia was in any way objective. His interpretations were still influenced by the dominant medical ideas that the vagina and ovaries were paltry excuses for the penis and testes. The vagina illustrated in the *Fabrica*, based on that of the grave-robbed lover of the monk, looks just like male genitals turned inside out: it resembles an erect penis with a spout for a urethra; the uterus, sliced and opened out, is perched on top like two inverted pears. Vesalius also neglected to acknowledge the existence and purpose of an extremely important organ: the clitoris.

The clitoris has been contested, debated, ignored, demonized, and mythologized in medical discourse since antiquity. But in 1559, the surgeon and anatomist Realdo Colombo—Vesalius's successor at the University of Padua—claimed he was the first man to discover this "principal seat" of women's sexual pleasure. That year he published his own anatomy tract, *De re anatomica* (*On Things Anatomical*), in which he described a "process" inside female genitalia that emerged in a "certain small part" just above the urethra. He named this "part" "the love" or "sweetness" of Venus, because, as he informed his "dearest reader," it enabled women to actually enjoy intercourse. When it was rubbed with a penis or touched with a finger, women experienced such intense physical pleasure that "their seed" flowed "forth in all directions, swifter than the wind, even if they don't want it to." Colombo's insinuation that women's physical manifestations of sexual arousal were so strong that it didn't matter whether they had consented is chilling. He was basically implying that the clitoris had a mind of its own—and women had no control over its impulses. His detached fascination is reinforced by the fact that he didn't mention anything about who he was deriving this knowledge from. Only when he encountered a clitoris that deviated from what he deemed normal did he reveal even the slightest information about the woman herself.

Writing "on those things rarely found in anatomy," Colombo described a female patient, an "Ethiopian gypsy," who possessed a "penis" almost the length and width of a little finger. The opening of her vulva was too narrow to admit even the tip of said finger. Her "penis," of course, was her clitoris. In Colombo's opinion, its size meant she was a "hermaphrodite"—a now obsolete and offensive term for people born with reproductive and sexual biology or anatomy that doesn't conform to normative "male" or "female" standards. Colombo considered his patient "wretched" because her "disadvantage" prevented her from enjoying sex as either the "active" male "giver" or the "passive" female "receiver." Sixteenth-century medicine wasn't exactly appreciative of the sexual identity and body experiences of people who might today identify as intersex. Colombo's idea of sex was limited to cisgender heterosexual penetrative intercourse. As an anatomist keen on defining sex differences, he pathologized his patient's clitoris because he thought it prohibited her from being truly feminine. A diminutive, submissive clitoris, to Colombo, was a "beautiful thing"; but a larger one that might threaten to emasculate a man—or render him sexually redundant—was a dangerous deformity.

Colombo was full of pride at being the self-appointed discoverer of the "processes and working" of the clitoris. He was frankly astonished that no anatomist had detected it before. But the claim to the discovery of a hitherto overlooked female pleasure organ, analogous to the penis, had already been made in 1550 by Gabriele Fallopio, a student of Vesalius's who succeeded Colombo at Padua in 1551. But Fallopio didn't get around to publishing his magnum opus, *Observationes anatomicae*, until 1561, and by then Colombo had beaten him to the punch. Fallopio performed many dissections of men, women, and children, which afforded him more insights than Vesalius had gleaned. As well as describing the clitoris, which Vesalius turned a blind eye to, he was the first to correctly identify the ducts connecting the uterus to the ovaries, which he called "*tuba uteri*" because they looked like little trumpets. Later these would be named the fallopian tubes. One of Fallopio's students tried to charge Colombo with plagiarism for his clitoris claims, but Colombo was dead by the time *Observationes anatomicae* was published, so there wasn't much point. Vesalius, angered by Fallopio's accusation of omission and error, snapped, "It is unreasonable to blame others for incompetence on the basis of some sport of nature you have observed in some women." He acquiesced to the idea that "hermaphrodites who otherwise have well-formed female genitals" might possess a "tiny phallus." Otherwise, he fumed, "you can hardly describe this new and useless part, as if it were an organ, to healthy women."

Whether it was celebrated, denied, or vilified, the clitoris, for these sixteenth-century anatomists, was seen as a device for sexual pleasure only. And whether it was being rhapsodized by Colombo or pathologized out of existence by Vesalius, the clitoris was always assumed equivalent to the penis. These anatomists fixated on the part they could actually see, the glans, which to them was a defective and inferior version of its proud male counterpart. They didn't have the faintest idea that this was an organ extending deep inside the body. It wasn't until the seventeenth century that the term "clitoris"—from the ancient Greek for "little hill" and imbued with meanings like key, sheathe, ladder, and even nail—was used. Until then, its nomenclature was as undefined and contested as medicine's understanding of its size, purpose, and function. Anatomical ignorance about the clitoris wasn't consigned to Renaissance history. Shockingly, the clitoris has been misrepresented, suppressed, and even completely omitted from anatomical and gynecological literature until very recently. It was only in 2005 that Professor Helen O'Connell, Australia's first female urologist, revealed that the glans makes up only about a fifth of this wishbone-shaped organ that extends its legs, or crura, into the tissue of the vulva. Beyond the skin on either side of the walls of the vagina nestle two triangular bulbs containing masses of erectile tissue, all full of nerves. The entire clitoris extends to seven centimeters or more in length—making it quite the match for the average penis.

O'Connell's research shows how important the clitoris is for women's health, which has been summarily ignored by medicine across its history. If its many nerves and blood vessels are properly mapped, then they might not end up being severed during pelvic surgeries. The understanding that the clitoris is more than the sum of its visible part has also led to groundbreaking advances in sensation-restoring surgeries for victims of female genital mutilation, injury, and sexual violence. And for trans people undergoing gender affirmation, accurate knowledge about the clitoris's anatomy and "neurovascular" structure helps preserve and heighten sexual sensation and satisfaction after surgery. Busting the myths behind clitoral secrecy and shame means understanding that we're still grappling with a centuries-old legacy of women's sexuality being marginalized, trivialized, and demonized. As O'Connell writes, "The tale of the clitoris is a parable of culture, of how the body is forged into a shape valuable to civilization despite and not because of itself."

For the Renaissance anatomists, the clitoris confused the physiological differences between men and women that they were so eager to define—men were supposed to be sexual agents, and women the reproductive vessels. The clitoris also proved women could enjoy physical sexuality without having a man involved. Imagine how threatened, not to mention envious, men must have been to realize women had a capacity for pleasure they just couldn't come to grips with. This was reason enough not only to ignore the clitoris but to malign and mythologize it as a pathology, a deformity, an aberration.

While surgeons, anatomists, and physicians in Europe were busy debating the innermost recesses of women's bodies, England's medical community was struggling with the moral implications of unveiling those most secret and shameful parts. Dissection had been prohibited under the Catholic Church until the Protestant Reformation, so

England lagged behind in the race to map the body's mysteries. In 1540, King Henry VIII passed an edict allowing the newly formed Royal Company of Barber-Surgeons to obtain four cadavers a year. Thanks to Queen Elizabeth I's charter of anatomies in 1565, the Royal College of Physicians was permitted to obtain six a year. These strict limits were also imposed on *who* the bodies had belonged to. Anatomists were allowed to obtain the corpses of only hanged criminals. Queen Elizabeth stipulated that these had to come from Tyburn, a village in the parish of Marylebone where horrific public executions had taken place for centuries. Female cadavers, as in Renaissance Italy, were highly prized by anatomists since fewer women were sent to the gallows. Even though dissection was now legal, scientific understanding of women's organs and systems was still hampered by hand-wringing.

The first comprehensive volume on human anatomy in English, *The History of Man*, composed by John Banister in 1578, avoided mentioning female genitalia completely because it was far too indecent to lift "up the vayle of Nature's secrets, in womens shapes." In 1615, Helkiah Crooke, a physician in the court of King James I, and the first appointed keeper of London's psychiatric asylum Bethlem Royal Hospital, caused a stir when he published *Mikrokosmographia, a Description of the Body of Man*. Crooke believed that diseases of women's reproductive organs were the most "fearful and fullest of anxiety," and because of medicine's "modesty," they remained the most difficult to cure. His detailed descriptions and illustrations of dissected female genital organs greatly upset John King, the bishop of London, who thought Crooke was acting indecently by revealing such shameful content to medical and lay readers. *Mikrokosmographia* was published despite protestations from the College of Physicians—which Crooke was a member of—that the offending sections of the book should be burned.

As the century progressed, anatomical understanding of women's bodies progressed beyond its prudish and censured beginnings. In 1626, King Charles I allowed the lead physician of Oxford University's school of anatomy to obtain the body of any person executed within twenty-one miles of the city. But as physicians and surgeons expanded knowledge about the mysteries that lurked under women's skin, interpretations of women's illnesses and diseases were still skewed by punitive social attitudes about who they were and how they should live. As the enlightened eighteenth century beckoned, medicine would finally begin to shed some of the oppressive superstitions of its darker past, and with it the biological tie between unwell women and wild wombs. But while the mystifying insides of the female body emerged into the scientific light through continued dissections and experimentations, women would become even more vulnerable to pathological ideas about their feeble minds and inferior constitutions.

4

ON HER NERVES

In the 1640s, Anne Greene went to work as a scullery maid in a grand house in the Oxfordshire village of Duns Tew. Greene was born in 1628 in the nearby parish of Steeple Barton. Her master was Sir Thomas Reade, a lord of the manor and former county high sheriff. Reade's grandson Jeffrey, strong and tall for a sixteen-year-old, started making "amorous enticements" to Anne. One fateful day in 1650, when she was twenty-two, Anne "consented to satisfy his unlawful pleasure." She was raped and became pregnant. Four months later she went into labor in an outhouse. Her woefully premature son was stillborn. Terrified, she buried his body near the cesspit. But soon it was discovered by another member of the household. She was sent to Oxford jail, "a place as comfortless as her condition," for three weeks to await her trial.

Anne was prosecuted under the Act to Prevent the Destroying and Murdering of Bastard Children, passed in 1624 by King James I, which made any attempt to conceal the death of an illegitimate infant a crime punishable by death. This offense applied only to unmarried or, as the act stipulated, "lewd" women, who drowned or buried their newborns "to avoid their shame and to escape punishment." Regardless of the circumstances of a woman's pregnancy, or the reasons she was desperate to keep her secrets, she would be treated as a murderer. Only if a reliable witness confirmed that the infant was born dead would she have a chance of escaping her fate.

Anne was tried, found guilty, and sentenced to hang. She was taken to the gallows at first light on the freezing morning of December 14, 1650. She sang a psalm before justifying her actions and protesting the "lewdness" of the Reade family. Then she was pushed from the hangman's ladder. After half an hour she was pronounced dead by the prison physician. Laid in a humble wooden coffin, Anne's body was taken to the house of William Petty, an anatomist from Brasenose College, who had been granted permission to dissect her body with fellow experimental anatomists Ralph Bathurst, Henry Clerke, and Thomas Willis. Oxford University was then the country's most important site of anatomical research. Petty and his peers relished this rare opportunity to enhance their knowledge—and reputations—by inspecting the organs of a young childbearing woman. But when Anne's coffin was opened, she appeared, very faintly, to be breathing. Believing she was in the final throes of death, a male servant stamped on her to put her out of her misery. The next morning, Petty and Willis were ready to begin the dissection. Scalpels poised, they noticed a crackle, barely a whisper, from Anne's throat. She had been hanged, stamped on, and laid in a cold house for hours. But she wasn't dead.

Petty and Willis, now joined by Bathurst and Clerke, sat Anne up and forced her mouth full of a hot cordial. Her pulse was faint. They tickled her throat with feathers, applied warming ointments to her skin, administered an enema, and let nine ounces of her blood. Hot poultices were placed on her breasts, and her limbs were massaged to get her blood flowing. A servant woman lay with her throughout the night, rubbing her body and keeping her warm. The next morning, Anne could speak, drink, and even laugh a little. Visitors flocked to see this woman miraculously returned from the dead. Anne's father raised enough from donations to pay for her medical treatment and lodgings. After a month of recovering in the very room she would have been dissected in, Anne was walking, eating, and sleeping normally. The bruises around her neck from the noose were fading. She retired to Steeple Barton to recover and took her coffin with her as a souvenir.

While Anne was being revived, the justice of the peace was petitioned to grant a reprieve until she might be pardoned. The midwife who examined the infant's corpse had confirmed that it was indeed stillborn, and too small and unformed to have lived anyway. Other servant women from Reade's household told the court that Anne had "certain Issues for about a month before she miscarried." They also explained that Anne's periods stopped for only ten weeks, leading her to believe her bleeding was "nothing else but a flux of those humors." Doubt was cast over whether Anne actually knew she was pregnant. Only when the anatomists corroborated their testimonies were Anne's witnesses taken seriously. The fact that Anne was raped—sadly, but not surprisingly—went unmentioned in her defense. Her prosecutor, Thomas Reade, had in any case died three days after she was hanged. Anne was pardoned. Her incredible escape from the hangman's noose and the anatomists' scalpels was declared an intervention from God, and from medicine.

Between the anatomists, the midwife, and Reade's domestic staff, different forms of knowledge about the female body tussled for legitimacy during Anne's trial. And this tension between personal, domestic, and professional understandings of what was happening beneath a woman's skin was writ large in mid-seventeenth-century medical culture. The anatomical explorations of the past century, and the explosion of new gynecological writings about "diseases of women," meant that the female body was now the subject of serious medical inquiry. Dissection and scholarship were, inevitably, the domains of men, since women were barred from receiving formal medical education. But this didn't mean there was a moratorium on women knowing about and caring for other women.

Some midwives, like the one who testified during Anne's trial, were highly respected for their hands-on understanding of maternity and childbirth, which was traditionally the domain of women. It was the midwife, after all, who aided Anne's acquittal by confirming that her baby was not "vital." And while many ordinary women didn't have the level of literacy needed to read medical treatises, that didn't mean they were illiterate about their own bodies. Much of women's everyday care, in health and sickness, happened in the home. Practical experience of herbal recipes and wound dressing and fever relief was shared between mothers and grandmothers, sisters and daughters. The women servants of the Reade household were familiar with the rhythms and flows of menstruation, because they revealed that Anne missed only two periods and probably didn't know she was pregnant. But even though privileged knowledge from women, about a woman, was listened to and taken seriously during Anne's trial, her freedom was secured by the objective hand of "scientific" prowess. And this prowess was almost exclusively wielded at the time by learned men. Although women's intimate, familial healing expertise was so essential for unwell women during the seventeenth century, the rising professionalism of medicine meant that women practitioners were often relegated to the unsanctioned margins. In both the Oxford courtroom and the wider medical community, it was men—with all their access to historical learning, lectures, and anatomy tables—who in the end claimed authority over the female body.

Anne, the woman who actually suffered the terrible ordeal, was granted no authority at all. When recounting what had happened to her, to her body, she was an unreliable witness. And when she became a patient, her body was still regarded as untrustworthy—only those four physicians were able to decipher life in it. Since antiquity, discourse about "women's diseases" had been full of tales about physicians discerning life in women who appeared to be very dead indeed, especially when they were afflicted with "womb suffocation." By the seventeenth century, these anecdotes had become quite the tradition in gynecological literature. Petty and Willis weren't suggesting Anne was playing dead because she'd been strangled by her faulty uterus. But at the time, medicine definitely believed there was something inherent in women that was powerful enough to suspend vital faculties and remove signs of life. Like those ancient and early modern women's physicians, the Oxford anatomists held the prized and privileged ability to revive a woman who was seemingly dead.

From the year after the trial, and throughout the century, Anne Greene's "cure" was immortalized in woodcuts, weird doggerel verses, and popular pamphlets. Women were expected to uphold the virtues of modesty and innocence when it came to the grubby business of bodies. But Anne wasn't afforded such moral protection. In the eyes of the law and the public, she was "lewd." And when she became a medical sensation, it was the anatomists who were afforded reverence and respect, not Anne. Each technique and remedy used to resurrect her was celebrated as a wonder of professional—male—medicine. Anne was reduced to a medical specimen, an object of scientific fascination. The anatomists might have missed an opportunity to improve their knowledge by dissecting a dead body, but they were publicly exalted for "restoring to the world a living one."

Poets penned verses about raising pyramids in the anatomists' honor, while Anne was merely a lucky wench or a cunning cat. Others made bawdy quips about adultery and virginity; some fixated luridly on her execution and "abortive fruit." One proclaimed that no one should be shocked by Anne cheating death because all women are mysterious and devious: "Well, for this trick I'll never so be led / as to believe a Woman, though she's dead." Anne was the victim of an unjust law rigged against women of her class and circumstances. But she was also condemned by cultural and social attitudes about the dangerous and deceptive nature of female biology and sexuality. No one accused Anne of consorting with the devil. But those old ideas about how women's bodies and minds were untrustworthy, pathological, and beyond their own control were nevertheless alive and well—in society and in medicine.

The professionalization of medicine throughout the seventeenth century was established through books and the men who wrote them. The increase in book publishing and the rise of the commercial book trade in England and Europe meant that texts and treatises on health and illness were becoming more widely available—not just to medical practitioners but to the public. By the time of Anne's trial, medical books for lay readers, written in vernacular English rather than in Latin, had become especially popular. A number of self-help books addressed specifically to women patients appeared from the earlier decades of the 1600s. It's hard to know how many women would have been able to read these books, or how they might have used and applied the knowledge contained within. But it's clear that male authors of this material, including Norwich physician John Sadler, whose *The Sicke Woman's Private Looking-Glasse* was published in 1636, regarded women as completely naive about medical matters. Sadler, a self-described "wellwisher" of health, wanted to reveal the truth about the "manifest distempers . . . which yee women are subject unto through your ignorance and modestie." Lacking "instruction" in the "state of her own body," Sadler's imagined female patient suffered silently through every terrible malady her body manifested. And her modesty meant she couldn't bear to "divulge" her troubles to a physician; by concealing her "griefe," she "encreaseth her sorrow." And why did Sadler think women were so hampered by humiliation? Because all their disorders and diseases arose from their shame-filled uteruses: "Among all diseases incident to the body, I found none more frequent, none more perilous than those which arise from the ill affected wombe."

As a practicing physician, Sadler professed to having treated and cured all the "evil qualities" of this mystifying organ. But most of his information about the "nature, cause, signs, prognostics and cure of uterine diseases" was cribbed from classical Greek and Latin texts. Situating oneself as a professional medic wasn't just a matter of concocting new theories. Men like Sadler were consciously inserting themselves into a historical tradition of male medical authorship that began with *The Hippocratic Corpus*. The great fathers of medicine had decreed that the uterus was the unruly site of so many of women's afflictions. Sadler was building on this tradition by spotlighting his own expertise as a "conservator" of women's health. The extent of female readership for a work like *The Sicke Woman's Private Looking-Glasse* is uncertain. But any woman who did read it, or maybe had excerpts read to her, would have come away believing her uterus was constantly stewing up "convulsions, epilepsies, apoplexies, palsies, hectic fevers, dropsies, malignant ulcers," and countless other "woeful experiences."

Whether his motivation was profit or professional esteem, Sadler's message was crystal clear: all women were unwell by virtue of having a uterus. And women who failed to put their uteruses to good use also risked losing their minds. The theory that out-of-work wombs made women mad and sad was as old as medicine itself. But by the middle of the seventeenth century, new ideas had arisen about how the uterus, through its close sympathy with the brain, was responsible for a range of feminine mental illnesses like "passion of the heart, anxiety of the mind," and "dissolution of the spirit." William Harvey, the renowned English physician and anatomist, proposed in 1651 that "unnatural states of the uterus" could cause mental symptoms of the most "grievous" kind. By "unnatural" he meant empty and inactive—not menstruating, not having marital sex, not receiving male seed, and not carrying a child.

Harvey had served as physician to King James I and in 1628 made the first detailed descriptions of blood circulation. It was because of Harvey's discoveries that Petty and Willis knew how to revive Anne Greene. He was also skeptical of the existence of witchcraft. In 1634, he was asked by King Charles I to oversee the examination of a group of accused women from Pendle, Lancashire—the site of England's most famous witch trials—for evidence of the witch's mark. Seventeen women, including Mary Spencer, age twenty, and Margaret Johnson, age sixty, had been found guilty by a jury in Lancashire on the strength of a wild story told by a young boy named Edmund Robinson. One evening, on his way home, Robinson came across two greyhounds. One of the dogs, he claimed, transformed into a witch who spirited him away on a black horse with a magic bridle to a witches' feast, where he met the devil. Robinson was believed, and suspicion was soon aroused in the village about the occult powers of the local women. Mary Spencer was accused of enchanting a pail of water up from a well. Although the jury had returned a guilty verdict, sufficient doubt was cast over Robinson's story, and the judge referred the matter to the king. Spencer, Johnson, and two others were transported to London by the high sheriffs of the neighboring counties to await the physicians' inspection and try to prove their innocence. Harvey—accompanied by surgeons, physicians, and ten midwives—found nothing more suspect, on any of the women, than a leech bite. Robinson subsequently confessed that he had made up the whole story to avoid getting a beating from his father for getting home late.

Thanks in no small part to Harvey's expertise, all four women were pardoned. But despite his more humane attitudes, he still believed that women could be so overcome by "mental aberrations"—such as melancholy, delirium, and "paroxysms of frenzy"—that they often appeared "as if under the dominion of spells." And the source of these derangements was, invariably, the uterus, particularly when it rose, fell, or spasmed in the body because it was "in want of action." Edward Jorden had already argued against witchcraft by claiming that an afflicted uterus could affect seemingly occult alterations to a woman's temperament. But the "perturbations" Jorden saw as primarily physiological were, in Harvey's opinion, more distinctly mental. As he was England's most acclaimed research physician, Harvey's ideas held credence. The stage was set for renewed "scientific" theories about how disorders of the uterus manifested in the mind.

Whether physical or mental, most symptoms thought to be caused by an unwell or unemployed womb were, throughout the century, termed "hysteric." The word literally means "of or from the uterus." But in the age of anatomical inquiry, some physicians had already questioned whether the uterus was to blame for the fits, furies, and frenzies that men thought so common in women.

Thomas Willis, who earned his fame bringing Anne Greene back from the dead, had worked as a physician in an Oxfordshire parish during the English Civil War. He encountered several girls and women with bizarre symptoms that appeared to be hysteric—convulsions, intense melancholy, unexplained pains, violent manias, and even inexplicable fits of leaping. As a follower of Galen, he assumed such symptoms were caused by foul humors emanating from their uteruses. But his interest in the causes of extreme behavioral and emotional states shifted as he became fascinated by the way the mind and body communicated. At the time, philosophical questions about human nature, behavior, and emotions intertwined with new medical ideas about animal spirits. Animal spirits had been pondered since antiquity, and by the seventeenth century these invisible, weightless substances, believed to be made in the blood, were imagined as tiny messengers trafficking soul and consciousness—think neurotransmitters loaded with feelings. Willis, who had been a chemist, believed the brain purified spirits into particles, which were then distributed through the body via the nervous system. After he was appointed professor of natural philosophy at Oxford in 1660, Willis revolutionized the anatomical study of the brain by removing it intact from the skull. This meant he could study its component parts—the vessels and arteries that supplied it with blood and the intricate network of nerves that connected it to the body's organs and muscles. He began to consider how spirits triggered the body's nerve functions and also transferred impressions from outside the body that were processed as thoughts, memories, feelings, and sensations. In 1664, Willis coined the term "neurology" in his magnum opus *Cerebri anatome*, then the most detailed and accurate study of the brain and nervous system. His findings formed the basis of many theories about illnesses and diseases that affected the mind, including "the passions commonly called hysterical." For Willis, women's hysteric symptoms weren't caused by "the evil influence of the womb" but by disorders of the nerves and spirits.

In 1667, Willis performed an autopsy on a woman who had been tormented by "convulsive passions" for years. This married noble lady of an Oxfordshire parish, virtuous in "mind and manners," had conceived many times, but most of her pregnancies had ended in miscarriage. When Willis met her, she was nine weeks pregnant and suffering horrible pains in her pelvis and belly. After enduring fevers, contractions in her face and limbs, more intense pains, vomiting, and a miscarriage, she died after a "very horrid convulsive fit" left her "insensible and speechless." Other physicians assumed the convulsion must have been hysterical, because the loss of her baby strongly suggested some "distemper of the womb." Willis found her uterus in its rightful place and all its parts healthy. But the membranes covering her brain—the meninges—were distended with blood. The rest of her brain's "enfoldings and crevices" were overflowing with a watery, serous substance. And the "choroides"—the choroid plexus, where cerebrospinal fluid is made—were "discolored and half-rotten." From Willis's descriptions, it seems as if his patient might have died from complications of encephalitis, an inflammation of the brain that can cause the kinds of symptoms she had, including fevers, vomiting, and convulsions. Today encephalitis is known to be triggered by viruses, bacterial infections, or an immune system reaction. It would be centuries before these forms of encephalitis were documented and their causes understood. For Willis, the inflammation that had swelled the lady's brain was "morbific matter"—a term meaning a disease-causing substance. This "matter," he concluded, had flowed from her brain, infiltrated her nerves, and caused her pains, convulsions, fevers, pregnancy loss, and eventually death.

"Hysteric passions" had by now become a panacea for almost all diseases befalling women. Everything from heart and breathing troubles, liver complaints, muscle weakness, and pregnancy complications to dizziness, weeping, laughing, absurd speech, and even eye rolling had been lumped together with the customary chokings, fainting, convulsions, and contortions in the diagnostic behemoth that was hysteria. Before Willis severed the connection between hysteria and the reproductive organs, it seemed that by simply having a uterus, a woman was claimed to be hysterical. But even though the uterus was no longer the breeding ground for this maddeningly broad and vague medical category, hysteria remained a distinctly female disease. Hysteric "passions" and "affections" were caused not only by nerve deficiencies and dysfunctions but also by the impact of the spirits on emotions like sadness, fear, grief, and anger. Women, universally believed to be utterly at the mercy of feelings, were always predisposed to illnesses and diseases incited by emotional lability. Seen as weak, sensitive, and impressionable, women were thought to simply not possess the male qualities of reason, rationality, and strength needed to protect their bodies and minds from life's more nerve-trembling experiences.

This certainty about the fragility of female spirits was shared even by physicians who weren't on board with Willis's "doctrine of the nerves." Thomas Sydenham, his contemporary at Oxford, also believed the cause of hysteric illnesses wasn't to be found in the womb. But unlike Willis, Sydenham didn't go searching for its alternative location in the body itself. He denounced dissection because of his puritanical belief that God intended the etiology—the cause—of diseases to be diagnosed and treated only according to what man could naturally perceive. Sydenham, who became Willis's rival, preferred a patient-centered approach, which earned him the moniker "the English Hippocrates." Despite refusing to look inside a female body, he certainly had plenty to say about how and why hysteria manifested in it. In 1681, Sydenham declared that "hysteric disorders," second to fevers, were the most common chronic conditions of the time: "For few women (which sex makes half of the grown persons) . . . are quite free from every species of this disorder."

Sydenham crammed almost every conceivable symptom into his "hysterical" grab-bag. He claimed the disease was so multifaceted that only physicians of utmost "judgment and penetration" could distinguish it from any other disease of "this or that particular part." Considering himself highly qualified in the judgment and penetration department, Sydenham decided hysteria could affect any part of a woman's body, depending on how the nerves and spirits were impaired or obstructed. Unless they were hardy and working-class, women were always vulnerable because "kind nature has given them a finer and more delicate constitution of body, being designed for an easier life" and "the pleasure of men."

By rejecting the association between the uterus and hysteria, Sydenham had to admit that men could suffer from it too. But only "such male subjects as lead a sedentary or studious life, and grow pale over their books and papers" were vulnerable to hysteria—and when men were afflicted, Sydenham preferred to diagnose them with "hypochondriasis." He neglected to mention whether medical study induced "hypochondriasis" in men of his noble profession. In the seventeenth century, being a "hypochondriac" didn't mean one was enduring an imagined illness. Hypochondriasis described a deep melancholy caused by disordered spirits that manifested in physical as well as mental symptoms—and it was reserved for men. Female hysteria and male hypochondria had affections in common, namely "lowness," "disordered mind," and "incurable despair." In men, these were thought to be far rarer, because their constitution was seen as robust enough to withstand such nervous and emotional deterioration—unless, of course, they chose to pursue a decidedly more "feminine" life of the mind. But in women, such symptoms were practically epidemic because female spirits were *always* defective. Sydenham insinuated that women could even induce hysteric symptoms with their inconvenient feelings: "Whenever I am consulted by women concerning any particular disorder, which cannot be accounted for . . . I always inquire, whether they are not chiefly attacked with it after fretting, or any disturbance of mind." Hysteric women, he believed, always exaggerated and catastrophized—no matter what their physicians told them. "They cannot bear with patience to be told there are any hopes at all of recovery," he wrote; they "easily imagine they are liable to all miseries that can befall mankind . . . presaging the worst evils to themselves."

By the beginning of the eighteenth century, humankind's philosophical and cultural fascination with sensibility and emotion was embedded in new medical theories about women's nervous temperaments. Sydenham expanded the definition of "hysteria" to such an extent that it became a diagnostic dumping ground for any illness in any woman that was even slightly tricky to explain. New medical theories about women's nervous delicacy came thick and fast. In England and Europe, women emerged into the age of emotion enslaved by their nervous deficiencies. Women's illnesses were easily interpreted—and dismissed— according to blanket assumptions about the weakness and inferiority of the female body and mind. Hysteria then became whatever male physicians and medical writers wanted it to be. The only definitive diagnostic sign was being a woman.

Ignited by the social and political movements sparked by the French Revolution, from 1789, dissent was stirring against the way that medicine validated the subjugation of women's bodies, sexualities, and social roles through these new definitions of nervous illnesses. One woman leading the charge for women's rights outside hearth and home was the English philosopher and women's rights activist Mary Wollstonecraft. Inspired by the campaigns in France led by activists like Olympe de Gouges for women's rights to intellectual activity and political participation, Wollstonecraft wrote *A Vindication of the Rights of Women: With Strictures on Political and Moral Subjects* in 1792, one of the earliest, and now most influential, feminist texts in history. Wollstonecraft knew women's bodies and minds were by no means naturally feeble and weak. Rather, the subordination of women in the age of sensibility was cultivating the "weak and wretched" conditions of womanhood. Having worked as a governess and teacher, Wollstonecraft saw how the private, domestic education of middle-class girls stunted their intelligence and encouraged the infantile, frivolous qualities valued as marriageable.

"Exquisite sensibility" was prized in women because it made them dependent on men. By being told they had to fashion themselves into inferior helpmates, women were no longer seen as rational human beings. Equal education, to enliven the mind and strengthen the body, was, in Wollstonecraft's opinion, the cornerstone of the highest moral virtues a woman could possess.

Medicine at the time viewed the education of girls as either a pathological tax on their fragile nerves or a treacherous path to deviance and immorality. Wollstonecraft passionately disagreed. "Taught from infancy that beauty is woman's scepter," she wrote, "the mind shapes itself to the body, and roaming around its gilt cage, only seeks to adorn its prison." Such superficial traits were the most insignificant part of a woman's worth. By liberating and enlarging their minds, women could become so much more than the delicate, flimsy accessories society—and medicine—molded them into.

Wollstonecraft understood from bitter experience just how damaging these new diagnoses of nervous disorders, and medicine's supposed "cures," could be. Ten years before she wrote *Vindication*, her younger sister Eliza suffered from an illness that today would be diagnosed as postpartum depression. Eliza's husband, Meredith Bishop, was wealthy, respected, and emotionally abusive. Eliza endured "raving fits," disturbing thoughts, hallucinations, and deafness over her prolonged illness, which was deemed incurable. Bishop hadn't been so cruel to Eliza—by the standards of English law at the time—for her to be granted a divorce. Wollstonecraft knew her sister would recover only if she escaped her marriage. So the sisters fled, leaving Eliza's infant daughter, legally Bishop's property, behind. Once they were on the road, Eliza bit her wedding ring clean off her finger.

Eliza's recovery inspired Wollstonecraft to write *Thoughts on the Education of Daughters* in 1786, in which she argued that an active, curious mind was fundamental to the mental and physical health of girls and women. Wollstonecraft's views vehemently opposed medicine's, which supported society's view that not only were women unsuited to intellectual and professional activities, but also that such pursuits were completely detrimental to their health. She understood only too well that no relief was to be found in the social cure of unequal marriage. "Weak minds fall a prey to imaginary distress," she wrote, "to banish which they are obliged to take as a remedy what produced the disease."

In 1797, less than two weeks after giving birth to her second daughter—who became Mary Shelley, the legendary author of *Frankenstein; or the Modern Prometheus*—Wollstonecraft died. In the hours after Mary's birth she lost too much blood, and within days the shivering set in. She had developed puerperal, or "childbed," fever, a disease that, for centuries, killed thousands of women and children. Named in the eighteenth century, puerperal fever reached epidemic levels in London and other parts of England between the 1760s and 1780s. Once the fever took hold, death was almost inevitable. Mystery and misconception surrounded the possible causes until the mid-nineteenth century. Some believed the fever was aroused by inflammation and poisoned humors; others thought it was exacerbated by the impact on women's delicate nerves of being tended by a male physician.

In 1847, Ignaz Semmelweis, a Hungarian physician who came to be called "the savior of mothers," discovered that rates of puerperal fever on the maternity wards of Vienna General Hospital, where he served as obstetrician, were drastically reduced when physicians attending births washed their hands in solutions of chlorinated lime, which had disinfectant properties. Although he was unable to explain why, handwashing prevented physicians—who had been performing autopsies—from transferring group A streptococcus bacteria to women during labor. Semmelweis's wisdom was mocked and derided until after his death in 1865. Around that time, Louis Pasteur was introducing his world-changing research into disease-causing microorganisms, and medical pioneers including Joseph Lister began applying the emerging science of germ theory to surgical practice and revolutionizing antiseptic techniques. Wollstonecraft likely contracted puerperal fever when Dr. Poignand, physician and "man-midwife," reached his hand inside her to extract her placenta. Throughout her life she defended women against notions of biological and intellectual inferiority that medicine validated and upheld. Her death, caused by medical ignorance, was a tragedy. "I firmly believe that there does not exist her equal in the world," wrote her husband, William Godwin, the evening she died. As the nineteenth century drew in, the medical attitudes Wollstonecraft tried to dismantle—the doctrine of nervousness that limited women's lives and rights—prevailed in medicine's advancing understanding of women's diseases, bodies, minds, and pain.

5

FEELING PAIN

In 1807, a seventy-seven-year-old woman from Liverpool died after enduring mysterious pain for nearly fifty years. J.S. was middle class, very close to her sister, and liked to take rides in carriages. For most of her early life she was healthy and well, apart from the occasional "hysterical affection" common in young women of her social class who enjoyed "sedentary habits." She married when she was twenty-seven and became pregnant the following year. The labor was "difficult, lingering and laborious." Her first and only baby was stillborn. She contracted puerperal fever, which left her extremely weak, and a year later she discovered a lump deep in the left side of her pelvis. Within a year this lump—an infected abscess that swelled to the size of a "child's head"—burst inside her. For the next twenty years, she had fevers, palpitations, nausea, breathing problems, and unrelenting pain in her pelvis that radiated to her back, head, and sides. After going through menopause at fifty, J.S. felt a new ache, hot and sore, in her uterus near where the abscess had been. This ache became a pain that tormented her every day. As she approached the end of her life, J.S. could barely speak, move, or breathe. She asked her close friend, a Liverpool physician named John Rutter, to promise she would be autopsied so the "nature and cause of her severe and uncommon sufferings" could finally be explained.

Rutter asked two Liverpool surgeons to perform her autopsy and to pay close attention to her pelvis and abdomen. The surgeons found damage in her colon, an egg-sized tumor in her abdomen, a tubercle in her gut, and a cyst between her rectum and uterus. All these disorders would have caused J.S. severe pain. But Rutter was certain that none were destructive enough to have triggered the "degree of sensibility" she had confessed to. Rutter didn't think J.S. was exaggerating her pain. Nor did he presume she was "mistaken in her belief" that she felt it every day for more than twenty-five years in her uterus. Her uterus was small and slightly blistered, but Rutter could see no sufficient evidence of damage or disease. Her ovaries and fallopian tubes appeared to be healthy. Rutter was baffled. "If this pain was not occasioned by an organic affection of the uterus," he asked during a presentation to the Medical Society of Liverpool in 1808, "to what cause is it to be ascribed?"

J.S. had made Rutter the executor of her papers. Searching through the extensive collection, he discovered numerous letters from physicians she had consulted about her "complaints." One London doctor had attributed all her pain to abnormal leukorrhea, or vaginal discharge. Despite the fact that she also suffered muscle weakness, stomach problems, tinnitus, and paralysis on top of her other symptoms, he had refused to consider any other cause. And this "continual . . . discharge," apparently, was as much a drain on her mind as her body. J.S. had also been subject to fainting spells, restlessness, "agitations," and "fluttering and surprise from little things." Rutter noticed that she became unbearably anxious before her pain began to flare. She had terrible "depression of spirits" and would "forebode the worst termination of her complaints." It was J.S.'s intense emotions, Rutter believed, that were really to blame for her "horrid pain."

Rutter decided J.S.'s pain was hysterical. After all, she was "disposed to hysterical affections well before her troubles began. It didn't matter that she had suffered untreated and misdiagnosed gynecological illnesses for most of her life. Her nervous "constitution" was clearly pathological, because the physician who attended her labor placed the blame for her baby's death on her "excessive terror." Rutter gave her the posthumous diagnosis of "hysteralgia," a medical term for uterus pain first introduced in the eighteenth century by French physiologist François Boissier de Sauvages de Lacroix. Although the word is very close to "hysteria," Sauvages wasn't implying that uterus pain was always caused by uncontrollable feelings. "Hysteric affections" were only one of Sauvages's sixteen "species" of hysteralgia, along with disordered menstruation, ulcers, cancer, prolapse, abscesses, contractions after birth, and suppressed lactation when breastfeeding. Though J.S. had an abscess, a cyst, and a tumor, to Rutter her "hysterical" instability was a far more credible cause of her pain than any of her awful "organic" disorders.

If J.S. were alive today, she might have been diagnosed with chronic pelvic pain, hysteralgia's modern successor. This syndrome, thought to affect as many as one in six women of childbearing age in the UK and US, and around 30 percent worldwide, describes any persistent pain in the ovaries, uterus, and lower abdomen that lasts for six months or longer. Although medicine acknowledges that it can be caused by many diseases, including endometriosis, irritable bowel syndrome, ovarian cysts, pelvic inflammatory disease, fibroids, abscesses, and uterine prolapse, the actual cause can be difficult to identify, and many sufferers are misdiagnosed. Frustratingly, the long association between women's pelvic pain and their emotions continues to stymie understanding. Although medicine now recognizes how the trauma of sexual abuse, sexual violence, and difficult childbirth can lead to chronic pelvic pain, the ingrained connection between women's mental health and their reproductive organs means the syndrome is often interpreted as a symptom of depression or anxiety.

The burden of living with "hysteralgia" must have had a profound effect on J.S.'s mental health. She had also been through the unimaginable trauma of losing her baby after an incredibly difficult labor. But physicians like Rutter didn't have a clue about the complex ways that chronic pain can lead to mental ill health. Symptoms like "depressed spirits" and "agitations" were commonly seen as pain's causes, not its consequences. And medicine's ongoing fascination with the pathological power of women's impressionable nerves and delirious emotions meant that their pain was considered almost always more a matter of psychical feeling than physical fact. At a time when even women's autopsied bodies were not reliable proof of their pain, imagine how dimly their own expressions of pain were viewed.

"Horrid pain" were the only words of J.S.'s that Rutter quoted in his study. Rutter was so close to J.S. that he considered them "nearly related," and he felt genuine compassion for her. But while playing medical detective, he focused only on his and other physicians' assessments. He would be the judge of the severity, manifestations, and causes of her pain.

Five years after J.S. died, the author and playwright Frances "Fanny" Burney revealed, in intimate detail, what it felt like to endure pain. In a letter to her sister Esther, written in 1812, Burney recalled the torturous experience of undergoing a mastectomy for suspected breast cancer. While in Paris in 1810, aged fifty-eight, Burney "began to be annoyed by a small pain" in her right breast. Soon she felt a hard spot, and her pains became "quicker and more violent." In 1811, after consulting three doctors and hoping in vain for a cure, Burney was "formally condemned to an operation." She consulted with the revered French surgeon Antoine Dubois, who insisted the cancer was already "internally declared" and surgery would only "accelerate" her frightful death. But after other doctors recommended that she have the operation, Dubois agreed to perform it. He told her she should expect to suffer.

Three weeks after Dubois relented, he arrived at Burney's home with six doctors all dressed in black. She was given a wine cordial to soothe her nerves. Having been assured the operation would take place in an armchair, Burney was terrified when Dubois demanded she be placed on a mattress. A cambric handkerchief was laid over her face, but through it she could see the "glitter of polished steel." When the surgeon "plunged into the breast, cutting through veins—arteries—flesh—nerves," Burney "began a scream that lasted unremittingly . . . so excruciating was the agony." After the knife was withdrawn, "the air that suddenly rushed in to those delicate parts felt like a mass of minute but sharp and forked poniards . . . tearing the edges of the wound." When she felt the knife "rackling against the breastbone," she remained "in utterly speechless torture." For twenty minutes she "never moved . . . nor resisted, nor remonstrated, nor spoke."

Her memories of what happened afterward were lost to fainting. When her wounds were dressed, she was carried to bed, pale and weak.

The physicians' report stated that the roots of a scirrhous tumor showing signs of cancerous degeneration had been successfully removed during an operation that "was very painful and . . . tolerated with great courage." Burney recovered and lived to the age of eighty-seven. But she was haunted by her experience. She wrote her letter nine months after the operation, and it took three more to complete; "the recollection is still so painful." Reading her account is harrowing. But it is also a privilege. She had the courage to revisit and record the memory of her ordeal, and in doing so she gave a rare insight into a woman's medical experience at a time when women's voices were so undervalued and discredited.

When Burney was diagnosed, theories about what caused breast cancer included injuries, heredity, diet, climate, air quality, and, of course, women's thoughts, feelings, and fears. In 1815, the Scottish surgeon John Rodman argued that the "feeble structure of the female constitution" greatly "encouraged" the development of breast cancer. Women, he surmised, were so easily aroused to states "of unsafe sensibility" that their moods could exacerbate lymph-gland swelling and other morbid changes that led to malignant tumors. He thought the very idea of breast cancer was so "afflicting" that women could induce it by feeling sympathy for others who had it. "They reflect upon the calamities of this distemper with feelings of horror . . . while they anxiously compassionate the state of the patient." Compassion turned to fearful brooding, which "unhinged the mind" and disturbed the body to such an extent that "disorder commences in their own breast." Women, Rodman believed, were so "sharpened by sympathy" that the symptoms of a growing tumor could arise in a matter of hours.

One patient, described only as an "unmarried lady," felt darting pains, heat, and swelling in her left breast after a friend told her about her mastectomy. All the details were "fitted to produce feelings of horror in the female mind." Apparently she had manifested a phantom tumor with her overblown feelings. While she was definitely cancer-free, she was left with a "great . . . irritability of mind . . . [and] afflicting thoughts, which distempered her frame for a long time after." Rodman treated another "lady" who had recovered after developing a tumor the size of an "ordinary plum" in 1797 from the "accidental stroke of a man's elbow." In 1809, the lady's "intimate friend" had a mastectomy. "Instantly alarmed" by their similar experiences, the lady felt pain in her previously diseased breast. Once Rodman "gained ascendancy over her perturbed imagination," her pain abated and "in a few weeks all was well."

For Rodman, the "dispositions of mind" that incited breast cancer were endemic among the middle and upper classes. Like many physicians, Rodman viewed characteristics such as sensitivity, sympathy, and delicacy as biological and social symptoms of modern womanhood. Nervous deficiencies and emotional fragilities were being nurtured at every turn by the excitements and anxieties of leisurely lifestyles. More concern was being placed on the social conditions exacerbating diseases like breast cancer than on figuring out their physical causes. Women were effectively being blamed for inflicting such diseases on themselves, or at least for cultivating the mental states thought to kindle them.

Women have always risked having their pain written off as an exaggerated mental "passion" that male physicians could cajole them out of. But in the early nineteenth century, exquisite sensitivity to pain was a highly prized marker of civility. The more civilized a woman was, the more pain she was capable of feeling. And by "civilized," Rodman and his ilk meant women who enjoyed the spoils of England's colonial wealth. The association between class and sensibility was already embedded in medical discourse about women's nervous diseases. Thomas Trotter, a physician in the Royal Navy, delighted in explaining how "nut brown country girls" living in straw-clad cottages were invulnerable to the "airs and duplicities" that affected "the sisterhood in every great town." Innocent rustics were rarely subject to "mental disquietudes" and the "bodily ailments" that came with them. But people of the "savage state," as Trotter grimly put it, were immune not only to nervous afflictions because of their "health and vigor of body" but also to the sensibility that engendered feeling—particularly physical pain.

The distorted and dehumanized perception of hierarchies of sensation across different races had been perpetuated since the seventeenth century. But by the early nineteenth century, these beliefs had expanded into racist assessments about how the color of a person's skin determined their capacity to feel and tolerate pain. White, wealthy, Western European women were highest on the pain pecking order. Even if such women's pain was thought to be a symptom of civility, physicians still viewed it as a matter of *who* rather than *what* they were. Medical writing of the time emphasized how diagnoses should be made according to women's individual thoughts, feelings, and mental perturbations. But *all* "savage" women's pain was characterized according to their "sameness."

Racist assumptions that Black women feel less pain than white women echo insidiously through medical practice today. In the nineteenth century, with its focus on social status and sensibility, these assumptions became firmly entrenched. In 1827, Henry James Johnson, a British surgeon and the editor of the *Medico-Chirurgical Review*, reported on five surgeries by American surgeon Ephraim McDowell in Kentucky, "a black settlement of America," on women with diseased ovaries. These surgeries were deemed a success because only one of the five women died. But Johnson didn't believe McDowell's methods would have quite the same success when performed on the sensitive white women of Britain, because McDowell was operating on "negresses" who "will bear cutting with nearly, if not quite, as much impunity as dogs or rabbits."

The mid-nineteenth century ushered in a new focus on male professionalism in obstetric and gynecological medicine. In the American South in the 1840s, international progress in obstetrics and gynecology forged forth; but this progress was enabled and fueled by the most dehumanizing attitudes and motives. James Marion Sims, a US physician, treated men and women working on the plantations in Montgomery, Alabama, where two-thirds of the population was enslaved. One afternoon, in 1845, a plantation owner named Westcott asked Sims to attend to his servant who had become ill five days after giving birth. Her name was Anarcha, and she was seventeen. Back in 1808, President Thomas Jefferson had passed an act prohibiting the importation of slaves. But this didn't mean slave owners couldn't multiply those they already had. Anarcha's agonizing days-long labor, which Sims had attended, left her seriously injured and incontinent. Her "soft parts" were sloughed away by the pressure of the baby's skull, and it seemed she was "hopelessly incurable." Sims told Westcott "Anarcha has an affection that unfits her for the duties of a servant."

Sims understood that Anarcha had a vesicovaginal fistula, which damages the bladder and causes urine to leak through the vagina. At the time there was no cure. It was often caused by obstructed childbirth and was common in enslaved women whose poor diets and grueling work regimens deformed their pelvic bones. But it could also be caused by inept medical interventions and, chillingly, rape. Sims professed to have no interest in the diseases of women—in fact, he was repulsed by their "soft parts." But then he was persuaded to examine one Mrs. Merrill, whose pelvis was damaged when she was thrown from her pony. Sims discovered that Mrs. Merrill had a retroverted uterus. The pressure of air rushing into her vagina when he distended it with his fingers enabled him to return her uterus to its rightful place. It occurred to Sims that with this method he might be able to treat Anarcha after all. Sims had been asked by another plantation doctor to examine a young servant named Betsey, who also had a fistula. He had intended to send her away from his hospital, situated in his backyard, because her condition was incurable. But after his success with Mrs. Merrill, he asked Betsey to stay for another examination. After improvising a speculum with a bent pewter spoon, Sims dilated Betsey's vagina and "saw everything, as no man has seen before."

Sims requested that Betsey stay, along with another enslaved girl named Lucy who was suffering the same injury. He called Westcott to request that Anarcha be returned. He then made a bargain with all the girls' owners: they would hand them over for Sims to experiment on, and in exchange he would "not charge a cent for keeping them." His first operation was on Lucy. She was naked, on her knees, and given no anesthesia. The pain she was subjected to during the operation was horrific, and she was left with blood poisoning and a high fever. The sponge placed in her bladder to encourage her catheter to stay put had hardened and needed to be wrenched out. After enduring so many experiments,

Lucy needed to recover. Meanwhile he operated on Betsey. When her operation also failed, he started on Anarcha. Sims's descriptions of Anarcha's state are graphic and humiliating. "Her life was one of suffering and disgust," he wrote. She had no control over her bladder, and her fistula was so large that it had forced an opening in her rectum. "Death would have been preferable," Sims stated. "But patients of this kind never die; they must live and suffer." By the time he finally perfected his operation, by using a silver wire to suture the catheter, Anarcha had been experimented on thirty times, always without anesthetics.

There are no records of what Anarcha, Betsey, or Lucy felt and experienced—no accounts in their own words of what they endured. To Sims, they were not human beings but medical specimens, objects used to innovate his procedure and further his professional reputation. The reproductive and physical abuse Anarcha, Betsey, Lucy, and other women suffered in the fields and homes of plantation owners under chattel slavery was continued by Sims in his backyard surgical hospital, where he colonized their bodies for personal profit and professional gain. And he felt justified in his actions by the dehumanized perceptions of Black women's diminished sensitivity to pain. He valued only *his* efforts and exhaustion, having made "one of the most important discoveries of the age for the relief of human suffering." In his 1853 clinical paper he doesn't mention that his subjects were enslaved women. It would be a few years before anesthetics were widely used during surgery, but nonetheless Sims's practice, even by the standards of the time, was brutal. He used enslaved women to "perfect" his procedure for the benefit of white women, whose pain he thought deserved newly available anesthetics. The barbaric realities behind Sims's methods made him one of medical history's most controversial and derided figures. In 2018, after years of protests, a memorial statue of Sims that had stood in New York's Central Park since the 1920s was removed from public view to his burial site.

While Sims was performing his torturous experiments, another American obstetrician, Charles Meigs, was engaged in a war of words with Scottish obstetrician James Young Simpson about the pain of childbirth. Since 1841, Meigs had been professor of obstetrics and "diseases of women" at Jefferson Medical College in Philadelphia, from which Sims graduated in 1835. Meigs saw women as domestic martyrs ordained only for mothering. He thought the "pain of parturition" was a God-given agony that helped mothers love their babies, a myth that still exists today. Simpson didn't believe there was anything virtuous about women enduring pain. In 1847, he administered ether—a gas inhaled to relieve pain—to a woman enduring an excruciating labor. She wasn't able to deliver without the aid of forceps, so Simpson allowed her to inhale ether so that she could bear the procedure. That same year, Simpson became personally acquainted with the benefits of chloroform, a sweet-smelling liquid narcotic that was being tentatively used as an anesthetic.

While larking about with friends one evening (purely for research purposes, of course), Simpson discovered that chloroform delivered a euphoric high before a blissful peace-out. A few days later, Simpson was called by a retired physician friend to attend his wife, Jane Carstairs, who was due to have their second baby. Jane's first labor had lasted three grueling days. Dreading going through it again, Jane, anxious and sleep deprived, started having contractions. After three and a half hours, she was fully dilated. Simpson wetted a handkerchief with half a teaspoon of chloroform, rolled it into a funnel, and placed it over her nose and mouth. She fell peacefully to sleep. Within half an hour Simpson delivered Jane's baby girl. She slumbered on through her daughter's squalls. When she awoke, she exclaimed, "I've enjoyed such a comfortable sleep! Now I'm ready for the work before me." She couldn't believe her eyes when the nurse appeared with her baby. "Is it really over?" she exclaimed. "Is this my living baby?" The story goes that Jane christened her daughter Anesthesia.

Meigs objected to Simpson's attempts to popularize obstetric chloroform. In a letter to Simpson in 1848, Meigs declared labor pain the "most desirable, salutary, and conservative manifestation of life-force." He believed women needed only the "cheering counsel" of male obstetricians to relieve them. This, by the way, came from a man who decided that women suffered pain only during contractions, and that during an (entirely unrealistic) average labor of four hours, women had no more than fifty contractions lasting thirty seconds apiece. So according to Meigs's calculations, laboring women endured only twenty-five minutes of pain—and that was hardly worth expending morality-ruining chloroform for, was it? As well as believing labor pain was perfectly tolerable, Meigs also saw women's expressions of pain as a helpful guide for obstetricians during complicated births. Simpson argued that any obstetrician who needed the guidance of women's cries and grunts ought not to be wielding forceps. Simpson was more progressive and compassionate, but he still shored up his arguments for obstetric-pain relief against Black women's perceived invulnerability. Chloroform, he claimed, allowed the "civilized female" to enjoy as fast and easy a labor as women of the "savage state."

Many obstetric physicians objected passionately to chloroform. Some, like Meigs, argued that labor pain was natural and necessary; others thought chloroform was highly dangerous and resisted its use on religious grounds. Some feared its intoxicating properties would rid women of inhibition and reduce them to sexually depraved beasts. English gynecologist Tyler Smith disagreed; he thought pain neutralized the "sexual emotion" of childbirth. No decent woman would *dream* of abandoning her chastity and self-control during such an intimate occasion.

On April 7, 1853, Queen Victoria gave birth to her eighth child. For all her previous births, Victoria had endured childbirth like all the other mothers of her kingdom, from workhouse to palace. But she did not agree that labor pain was a moral or physical necessity. She loathed pregnancy, which she called the "shadow-side" of marriage, and thought giving birth was "a complete violence to all one's feelings of propriety." Having endured the ordeal seven times already, Queen Victoria was now able to slumber through it, all thanks to chloroform. Her physician, the anesthetist and public health advocate John Snow, poured a carefully measured dose into the canister of a brass vaporizer and attached it to a velvet-lined face mask. The queen inhaled steadily for fifty-three minutes, her pains evaporating with the liquid. In her journals, Queen Victoria reflected: "I was taken ill early on the morning . . . and a boy was born to great happiness to me. Dr. Snow administered 'that blessed

Chloroform' & the effect was soothing, quieting & delightful beyond measure."

Queen Victoria's use of chloroform popularized pain-free labor as not just a possibility but a right. After all, it was hard to argue that it was immoral if the queen was an advocate. But chloroform was available only to middle- and upper-class women who could afford to be attended by those physicians who agreed and were trained to administer the magic potion. Childbirth remained agonizing and dangerous for poor women in the lying-in hospitals, and even more so for those forced into the squalid, cramped wards of workhouse infirmaries. But for those who could get it, obstetric pain relief was a revolutionary liberation from the suffering women had been obliged to endure. There were very few freedoms afforded to women in Victorian society, and this freedom, from pain solely known by the female body, was incredibly significant.

Chloroform also enabled medicine—and society—to frame childbirth as a pleasant, peaceful, and even effortless experience. But this experience was reserved for women whose sexuality existed within the bonds and bounds of marriage. Sexual feeling for the purposes of anything but bearing children and pleasing one's husband remained a scourge. The Victorians felt strongly that if patriarchal order was to be upheld, women's most private impulses and desires had to be rubbed out like a stain. Female sexuality was a disease, they claimed, and feared it was becoming epidemic. And to stop a disease from spreading, medicine must find a cure.

6

CONTAGIOUS PLEASURES

In 1850, the physiologist and neurologist Marshall Hall attended a woman who had come to London seeking help for her mysterious uterine illness. This wife of a humble village curate had been urged by an aristocratic lady friend to visit her personal physician, who was particularly keen on using an instrument Hall found repellent: the vaginal speculum. Writing in *The Lancet*, Hall couldn't bear to describe exactly what went on during this offensive procedure. But the physician would have inserted the metal blades, opened them up, screwed them in place, and closely scrutinized her vulva, vagina, and cervix for ulcers, lesions, and inflammation. When her cervix was dilated, remedies could be applied. Caustics to burn away diseased tissue. Injections of water or bicarbonate of soda to purge infection. Leeches to draw out excess blood.

This money-hungry "speculumiser" had, according to Hall, induced "a new and lamentable form of hysteria" by intruding upon the curate's wife with his monstrous tool. After her course of examinations and treatments, she became obsessed that something terrible was happening *down there*. Her temperament was "moody and perverse," her sentences "unintelligible." As far as Hall could tell, her "uterine organs" were perfectly healthy. But her mind was horribly poisoned. The speculum made her conscious of the secret recesses of her body, and now she could think of little else. And for the decent wives of Victorian England, even a little body awareness was a dangerous thing. Hall diagnosed "uterine hypochondriasis" bordering on *furor uterinus*. The unwitting victim was the poor woman's husband, for whom Hall couldn't conceive of "a case of more complicated misery." To save other beleaguered men, the cause had to be wiped out. Abettors of the speculum must put down their tools and never again disturb the modesty of female patients.

The speculum had become increasingly popular in gynecological and obstetric practice in England since the 1830s. By enabling physicians to look inside women's bodies, it was an invaluable aid in diagnoses and treatments. In the past they had relied on palpating a woman's abdomen or, if necessary, examining her internally with their fingers. This method, "the touch," was performed—by upstanding physicians—without so much as a glimpse in the direction of her genitals so as not to risk blurring polite doctor-patient boundaries. But the speculum replaced the fumbling assumptions of touch with the objective power of vision. Now physicians could actually cast their eyes over those organs that were the mystifying source of so much female suffering.

Despite its benefits for saving women's lives, the speculum was hotly contested. Using it meant literally penetrating and exposing the most forbidden parts of a woman's body. And for vehement detractors like Hall, this violated the decency and propriety gynecologists should scrupulously uphold when treating "women's diseases." Hall's belief that being "speculumised" would turn women erotically hysteric seems like quite a reach. But his attitudes reflected those of many members of the Victorian gynecological community. A woman's modesty was aligned with her moral character and her health, so the speculum represented a transgression of fiercely guarded social and bodily boundaries. The need to preserve modesty was all too often prized over objective knowledge about women's bodies, diseases, and pain. After being opened up and scrutinized, Hall gravely declared, a woman "was not the same person in delicacy and purity as she was before."

Thankfully, not all physicians prioritized moral codes over medical care. William Jones, a midwifery specialist, recognized how essential the speculum was for understanding women's bodies beyond the ignorance and superstitions of the past. Others appreciated its benefits for treating the "Proteus-like" diseases of the uterus and cervix, and thought it far more effective than touch for making diagnoses. Without seeing with his own eyes, how could a physician figure out exactly what was causing the pelvic pain or menstrual problems a patient confessed to? Even though supporters of the speculum were slightly more forward-thinking, they still discredited patients' own descriptions of their symptoms. How Jones lamented the "futile" efforts of gullible physicians who trusted the "vague information" women imparted. The attitudes of Jones and other advocates were firmly of the time; but on the whole, they were more concerned about relieving women's suffering than silencing them. Still, the speculum was an instrument of power and control. It enabled physicians to gain knowledge that was inaccessible and out of bounds to women themselves. And a major advantage of the speculum, beyond preserving women's health, was that it helped diagnose many causes of infertility. For a healthy fecund womb was a happy fertile woman.

Speculum-gate reached its peak in 1850, when Robert Lee, the speculum-denouncing professor of midwifery at St. George's Hospital in London, gave a lecture at the Royal Medical and Chirurgical Society. On the evening of May 28, more than three hundred members—all men, naturally—crammed into the library to hear the esteemed physician's opinion on this hot topic. Lee acknowledged that the speculum was by no means a modern invention. He mentioned some wince-inducing contraptions, like the bronze three-bladed horror found by archaeologists excavating the ruins of Pompeii in 1818 and the equally disturbing sixteenth-century version used to treat cervical ulcers and lacerations. He failed to credit the innovations of Marie Gillain Boivin, the French obstetrician who beat James Marion Sims to the invention of the bivalve speculum by at least two decades. In 1825, only twenty-five years before Lee gave his potted history, Boivin developed the precursor to the "duck bill" speculum commonly used by gynecologists today, to enable her to treat disorders of the cervix. But speculum history wasn't Lee's primary concern. He was mostly alarmed by the threat its improper use posed to professional gynecology. Jones recoiled when Lee claimed disorders of the cervix were an overdiagnosed fad among women willing to line the pockets of quacks. He knew that speculum examinations meant physicians could identify and treat early "altera-tions" that might lead to serious diseases. But Lee was insistent that genuine cases of cervical ulceration and erosion were extremely rare. Besides, there was no tumor, cyst, polyp, or fibroid that *he* ever failed to find using his fingers.

When treating "nervous affections" in young and unmarried women, like painful, heavy, irregular periods and unusual discharge, Lee thought the speculum was useless, and even dangerous. For it risked "destroying the structures"—breaking the hymen. Hall agreed that us-ing the speculum on unwed women was tantamount to stealing their virginity. For married women who were infertile or childless, Lee justi-fied its use as a last resort for treating life-threatening diseases. But even then, he reserved judgment; in uterine cancer he thought the speculum was injurious and should never be used. But Lee protested too much that speculum examination was unnecessary and harmful. What really lay behind detractors' objections was the fear that the speculum would unravel the tightly laced sexual morality of Victorian women.

For some gynecologists, the speculum threatened to unlock Pando-ra's box. Many believed that if a woman's vulva, vagina, or cervix were stimulated by the speculum, her body would unleash a torrent of sexual urges that she couldn't control. Hall went so far as to claim that most women contrived a "revolting attachment . . . to the practice and to the practitioner." The fact that men like Hall denounced the speculum be-cause they feared it would turn women on is hard to stomach. We know today how internalized shame can make pelvic and gynecological exams especially difficult for many people. In the UK, since 2018, rates of cervical-screening Pap smears have been the lowest in twenty years. The National Health Service and charity campaigns have worked to allay fears that smear tests are embarrassing and painful, and to normalize gynecological exams as a straightforward part of routine health care. But for anyone who endures chronic pain in their vulvas and vaginas, including sufferers of endometriosis or vulvodynia, a poorly understood condition that causes burning, stinging, and intense discomfort, smears can be unbearable. Many people with vaginismus, where the muscles of the vagina tighten and spasm, find smears anxiety-inducing, if not physically impossible. And for survivors of sexual violence and abuse, being subjected to the speculum can be overwhelmingly traumatizing.

Even though most physicians in the mid-nineteenth century were oblivious to women's feelings about medical procedures, some at least acknowledged how distressing the prospect of the speculum could be. After Lee's lecture, Dr. Thomas Litchfield recalled how a married patient suffering "some obscure uterine mischief" told him she would rather die than submit to such intrusion. Nonetheless, he interpreted her terror as more to do with the preservation of modesty than the violation of her body. Some tried to minimize women's shame by allowing a husband or family member to be present during examinations. Others, including Queen Victoria's personal obstetrician Charles Locock, insisted that the speculum posed "no immorality or danger to purity" if it was appropriately used. And if the patient was lying on her side with her skirts strategically gathered, the procedure was no more exposing than a glance down the throat. Still, he was concerned mostly about maintaining his respectability rather than putting his patients at ease.

To Lee and Hall, it didn't matter how discreetly examinations were conducted. English modesty was defenseless against an instrument tainted with degeneracy and vice. Many speculum advocates studied in Paris during the 1830s, where they watched and performed examinations on women sex workers. Since 1810, when the French government passed laws regulating prostitution across Paris, women sex workers had to attend special dispensaries, often once a week, for vaginal and rectal examinations to check for venereal diseases like syphilis and gonorrhea. If any suspicious ulceration was found on the vulva or inside the vagina or cervix, they were detained in a venereal ward of a women's lock hospital like Saint-Lazare, basically a medical prison, until they were "cured." Philippe Ricord, then chief surgeon of Paris's Venereal Hospital, chillingly called the speculum "a measure of medical police." Among the women, the violating blades were "the government's penis."

The fear that female sexuality could destroy middle-class social values simmered beneath medical ideas about the influence of the reproductive organs on women's emotions and behaviors. Hall was one of many physicians who believed that hysteria, along with its unruly sister nymphomania (sexual obsession), was a spurious collection of emotional and behavioral symptoms caused by the nervous system becoming over-excited in response to some vague disorder of the reproductive organs. In other words, a rehash of the old equation *defective womb* x *delicate nerves* = *deranged woman*. Hall's major medical contribution was his theory, developed from 1833, of reflex action, which explained how the nervous system induces involuntary responses to stimuli in the glands or muscles. According to reflex logic, if a woman's genitalia or uterine organs were stimulated, her nervous system would trigger a plethora of uncontrollable symptoms.

For the physician and ophthalmologist Robert Brudenell Carter, hysteria was a disorder of the nervous system caused by women's excessive emotions. Men were immune because they were gifted with reasoning and intellect. But women were "under the dominion" of feelings, so they were incapable of mustering the rational control needed to stave off diseases of the body and mind. And if you added "sexual desire" to the "forces bearing upon the female," then she would succumb to hysteria, because social mores dictated that women conceal such feelings. Men had the option of seeking "gratification" to take the lid off the proverbial pressure cooker. One might hope Carter would have recommended that women were allowed similar indulgences for the good of *their* health. But he was a zipped-up conservative who believed women's ardor must be dampened by any means necessary. His treatments for taming a woman's nervous system included making her wind a heavy wheel for hours, confess her secrets, play chess, go to bed early with a short candle, pretend others believe she is pregnant, practice a bit of light astronomy, and avoid reading.

Any attention a woman paid to her own reproductive and genital organs, Carter insisted, had dire consequences for her physical and moral health. The speculum incited exactly this kind of attention, especially in young girls seeking to indulge their "prurient desires." And the symptoms these girls often complained of, like abdominal swelling and pain, menstrual disorders, and "womb heaviness," were hypochondriac delusions "arising from the habit of contemplating and discussing the sexual organs." Such afflictions were usually caused by sexual frustration and "cured" with marriage. But now girls were so fixated on the speculum that their moral characters were completely destroyed. "I have, more than once," Carter confessed, "seen young, unmarried women of the middle-classes . . . reduced, by the constant use of the speculum, to the mental and moral condition of prostitutes; seeking to give themselves the same indulgence by the practice of solitary vice."

By "solitary vice" Carter meant masturbation. Physicians who believed that undue sexual feelings were causing women's diseases thought that masturbation was the most damaging habit imaginable. "Healthy" sexual fulfillment was confined to the marital bed. And wives were expected to bear it obediently for the purposes of procreation, and not strictly for their own pleasure. By passively enduring their husbands' advances, married women wouldn't ignite their destructive propensity for sexual excess. But if they dared pleasure themselves, they wouldn't only be eroding their moral decency but inflicting terrible symptoms. Reflex theory supported the rationale that bothering at one's clitoris led to nervous derangements. And because the clitoris, since at least as early as the sixteenth century, was deemed useless for anything except female pleasure, it was still pathologized as an instrument of depravity.

According to Samuel Ashwell, gynecologist at Guy's Hospital, "sexual passion" provoked by an unusually sensitive clitoris "subdues every feeling of modesty and delicacy" in young and unmarried women. He had treated many "tormented" girls, "aggravated by digitation," who caused their "part" to become inflamed and ulcerated. The symptoms Ashwell observed included headaches, menstrual problems, memory loss, sentimental thoughts, attention seeking, and hysteric attacks. If left unchecked, masturbation would lead to full-blown nymphomania, which, according to Ashwell, originated "exclusively from an excited, enlarged, and sensitive clitoris."

The glans of the clitoris contains around eight thousand nerve endings. Its sensitivity, when engorged, is a biological fact. But at a time when women's sexual feelings were so pathologized, the size of the glans and its sensitivity were diagnostic proof that an illness was self-inflicted. If the glans was slightly swollen, Ashwell recommended rest, cold baths, bland foods, chemical douches, and vegetable tonics, presumably to bore the patient out of her erotic fever. For more serious cases, he advised trying a caustic or a couple of leeches. But if it was too large, or so "unduly sensible" that she continued to seek "mechanical annoyance," then she was beyond medical help. The only option was to cut it off.

Clitoridectomy, the surgical removal of the clitoris glans, is one of the most shocking "cures" enforced on women in the history of medicine. Its association with the control and limitation of women's sexuality dates back to the Roman era. But for some Victorian gynecologists, this despicable practice was not only medically necessary but morally justified. In 1858, Isaac Baker Brown, a London gynecologist and obstetrician, took on the practice as a moral crusade. Brown was a fellow of the Royal College of Surgeons and one of the founders of London's St. Mary's Hospital, where he served as chief obstetrician in 1845. Despite his glowing reputation, Brown was a fame-hungry puritan who forged his career by mutilating women. In the early 1850s, he was a pioneer of ovariotomy, an operation to amputate ovaries diseased with cysts and tumors. Among the more cautious gynecological community, ovariotomy was highly controversial. Women often died on the table, and in many cases an ovariotomy was needlessly performed when no evidence of ovarian disease, cysts, or tumors could be found.

Brown wasn't the only gynecologist who performed ovariotomies, but he was certainly the most vociferous. In his opinion, the operation wasn't only legitimate but merciful. Several women died under his hands at St. Mary's between 1852 and 1854. Twenty-three-year-old M.A.B., married with no children and suffering an ovarian tumor, bled to death. Mrs. D., thirty-seven, her abdomen swollen with a cyst, died four days after the operation from "shock and exhaustion." Elizabeth D., a twenty-nine-year-old married mother of one young child, "labouring under ovarian dropsy," died just four weeks after surgery, her wound infected, her body emaciated. Of the few patients he claimed to have cured, one was his own sister.

In 1858, Parliament passed the Medical Act. The General Medical Council was formed to ensure that medicine was practiced only by qualified and licensed physicians. This meant men, since women were

forbidden from receiving medical education. That year, a group of physicians including Edward Tilt and Charles Locock formed the Obstetrical Society of London, a knowledge-promoting organization that
established gynecology and obstetrics as a professional discipline. With
the troubling rise in drastic surgeries for women's diseases, and the horrifying rates of maternal and infant mortality in England and Wales,
women's health, and lives, were perilously at stake. It was essential that
the discipline was regulated and good standards upheld. Brown was by
no means unqualified, and he did become a member of the Obstetrical
Society. But his naked ambition to perform controversial surgeries led
him, in 1858, to leave St. Mary's and set up on his own. In Notting Hill,
Brown opened the London Surgical Home for the Reception of Gentle-
women and Females of Respectability Suffering from Curable Surgical
Diseases. In the privacy of his fee-paying clinic, Brown advanced his
most radical cures—not for ovarian diseases, but for those hysteric and
nervous disorders that medicine claimed were epidemic among middle-
class girls and women.

In 1863, a twenty-year-old woman was admitted to Brown's "Home."
For two years her periods had been so heavy and painful that she couldn't
sleep. She was anxious and ill-tempered, which exasperated her mother.
Seeking solace, she courted the attention of men. What time she didn't
spend obsessing over her latest paramour, she devoted to long periods
of reading. Something had to be done. Brown examined her genitals
and found "evidence of prolonged peripheral excitement." She had inflicted her ills upon herself, he concluded, by indulging in the miserable
habit of masturbation. To cure her, he must remove the source of her
temptation.

Since founding the Home, Brown had "cured" many women this
way. Young girls, unmarried women, women who refused sex, women
who couldn't conceive, women who bled no longer. All were vulnerable
to hysteric and nervous illnesses if they were in possession of a clitoris.
To prepare the patient, Brown soaked a handkerchief with chloroform
and placed it over her face. When he was sure she was completely under,
he removed her glans with a snip of his scissors. He plugged the wound
with lint, bandaged her up, and applied one grain of opium to relieve

the pain. For a month afterward, she recovered at the Home in complete silence, with no visitors, no diverting activities, and only the blandest foods. After three months, Brown reported, her periods were normal. She no longer sought male attention; she was calm and placid and free of delusions. Within a year she married, and ten months later bore a healthy son. Brown considered his clitoridectomy a remarkable success.

In his 1866 book *On the Curability of Certain Forms of Insanity, Epilepsy, Catalepsy and Hysteria in Females,* Brown defined "hysteria" as a disease with a maddening array of symptoms, all of which began with "irritation" of the clitoris. Of course, his ignorance about the size and extent of the clitoris meant he fixated only on the visible glans. For him, the clitoris *was* the glans, and if women dared fiddle with it, they would induce paralysis, seizures, mental degeneration, blindness, mania, and, eventually, death. Women like the twenty-year-old appear on almost every page in lurid case studies. Apart from their age, marital status, and occupation, there is nothing about who those women were. There is no sense that they understood what would happen or had happened during and after his operations. Their feelings and voices are erased from his vainglorious tales of repair and recovery. But these women were clearly suffering from other diseases veiled by hysteria, like the abnormal menstrual bleeding and severe pain of endometriosis, the spinal irritations and temporary paralyses of multiple sclerosis, and the fittings and fainting of epilepsy.

Endometriosis and multiple sclerosis wouldn't be documented for decades, but epilepsy was well known and widely stigmatized. Convulsions and loss of consciousness, mostly affecting women, had been associated for centuries with lunacy, mania, and even demonic possession. Throughout the nineteenth century, epilepsy was a feminized disease thought to induce an "epileptic personality" inclined toward moral defects, violence, lewdness, nymphomania, and hyposexuality (no interest in sex). Epilepsy was deemed incurable, and it was often diagnosed in patients admitted to lunatic asylums across England. Many patients at the Home were young middle-class girls with epilepsy. Brown observed that many of them masturbated, which says far more about the trauma of his treatment and his perverted obsessions than it does about his medical "expertise." Nonetheless, he decided masturbation was both a cause and symptom of epilepsy, a disease provoked by the "mental emotion" women were "naturally prone" to. It was completely logical to Brown that "irritating" that fleshy, nerve-filled nub used up all the energy a woman's brain needed to function properly. Epilepsy was so dreadful and hopeless that clitoridectomy, Brown claimed, was a sufferer's only hope.

Contagion was an ever-present threat in Victorian London, the most populated city in the world. But it wasn't just epidemics like typhus and cholera that society dreaded. Lewd behaviors threatened the puritanical social order like a plague. Brown told parents they could tell if their daughter was masturbating because she would reject "the social influences of domestic life." If she was not stopped, she would lose all morality, be unfit for marriage, and turn, inevitably, to prostitution. Authors of popular home-health manuals encouraged parents to be vigilant for clues that their daughters had succumbed to "insidious contagion." Physician and surgeon Martin Larmont, in his widely published *Medical Adviser and Marriage Guide*, told awful stories of young masturbators left so hideously unwell they were cast out of polite society. Apart from damaging the digestion, circulation, nervous system, brain, senses, and appearance, masturbation, the author claimed, was a symptom of the disease of prostitution. By promoting the sanctity of marriage, parents could stamp out the loathsome habit, and the streets would no longer be filled with "wanton harlots and licentious profligates." Brown's horrific procedure probably seemed like a small sacrifice to readers of this material, terrified that their nervous daughters might be diddling themselves into a life of disrepute. Clitoridectomy wouldn't improve only the lives of sufferers, he insisted, but "the well-being of the whole human race." He recommended intervening as early as possible but drew the line at operating on girls younger than ten.

Brown was not the first or only man in his field to practice clitoridectomy. But the way he courted celebrity, in the eyes of London's more upstanding gynecologists, was decidedly ungentlemanly. To attract patients to the Home, he avidly promoted the dangers of masturbation and the benefits of his "cure." He made sure clergymen were aware of his "remedy" when faced with "distressing illnesses" in the women of their parish. In a city riddled with degeneracy and vice, the last thing the Obstetrical Society needed was Brown introducing the "dirty subject" and "serious medical work" of "Female masturbation" to family drawing rooms. In any case, Brown was hardly achieving his ambition of wiping out masturbation and sexual vice.

Prostitution was as visible in London as the necrotic sores and sunken bones of sailors with syphilis. As venereal diseases spread among the navy's sailors, who frequently visited sex workers, physicians and moralists wasted no time pointing the finger at "fallen women." Such a woman, according to gynecologist William Acton, was "a woman with half the woman gone . . . a social pest, carrying contamination and foulness to every quarter." Women were thought to have fewer symptoms and fatalities from venereal diseases than men, and, as had been the case in Paris, many believed sex workers were solely responsible for transmitting them. To control infection among the military, Parliament passed the Contagious Diseases Act in 1864. Moral "policemen" were tasked with registering all women known or rumored to be prostitutes. These men could force any woman to endure a humiliating and painful examination with a speculum. "The attitude they push into us first is so disgusting," recalled one "violated woman"; "they push them in, and they turn and twist them about; and if you cry out they stifle you with a towel over your face." If a woman was even suspected of having VD, she was sent to a lock hospital. The examination was supposed to be voluntary, but the "police" often used their authority to abuse underage and vulnerable girls and women. Those who didn't submit were sent to jail, so they seldom resisted.

While opposition to the Contagious Diseases Act was rising, Brown's practices were coming under increasing scrutiny. In 1866, a scathing review of his book appeared in the *British Medical Journal*. The authors were skeptical about Brown's motives and found his claims that clitoridectomy was safe and efficacious deeply suspect. The following year, the Obstetrical Society motioned to expel Brown. On April 3, members assembled "to hear, to judge, and to vote" on the resolution proposed by the secretary, Francis Seymour Haden. Haden began by underlining the ethical responsibilities of conducting medical care for women: "We are, in fact, the stronger, and they the weaker . . . They are not in a position to dispute anything we say to them, and we, therefore, may be said to have them at our mercy." By profiting from a "cure" with no basis in medical fact, Brown was nothing more than a quack. Haden refused to use the word "clitoridectomy": these women and girls had endured "disgraceful mutilation."

William Tyler Smith came forward to "defend women who have been or who are liable to be injured by the practices in question." He agreed that Brown's victims would be shamed for the rest of their lives for having a procedure that—to add insult to injury—their husbands or fathers had paid "100 or 200 guineas" for. Others brought up the crucial issue of consent. After describing how Brown butchered a patient's labia with a red-hot iron, Dr. Henry Oldham—who witnessed the operation—revealed that the patient "had no idea what had been done to her." "The nature of the operation had never been explained," said Oldham, "nor had she been asked if she would consent." The details were so harrowing that members pleaded, *Enough!*" Brown was expelled by a strong majority vote. He never practiced medicine again, and in 1873 he died after a series of strokes left him paralyzed.

On the streets of London, moral panic around sexual contagion thundered on. Even when middle-class wives contracted syphilis or gonorrhea, their husbands were never suspected of being carriers. Refined men were not thought capable of spreading these diseases, and besides, women's infectious sensibility meant this was easy to explain away. If a man's wife contracted VD because he'd been cavorting where he shouldn't, some physicians covered for them by diagnosing something completely different. Early feminist campaigners rallied against the injustices of punishing women for sexually transmitted diseases. In 1870, with the support of figures such as Florence Nightingale, the women's rights activist and social reformer Josephine Butler founded the Ladies National Association for the Repeal of the Contagious Diseases Act, which lobbied Parliament to end the violent, nonconsensual invasion of women's bodies in the name of disease control. The enforced examination of sex workers, to Butler, was medically endorsed "steel rape." In an 1870 letter, Butler wrote: "If all the male doctors in the world were to tell me with one voice that the Operation is painless, and two or three female prostitutes . . . were to whisper in my ear with sobs and shudders . . . that 'the pain is dreadful . . .' I should believe the female prostitutes . . . simply because I am a woman. I know my own make."

Born in 1828, Butler was the daughter of progressive parents who educated all ten of their children equally about social and political issues, including the abolition of slavery. Before Butler began her reform work, visiting women in workhouses and prisons, she suffered terribly with her mental and physical health. In 1864, her five-year-old daughter, Eva, died after falling down the stairs onto the stone hallway floor. Through her intense depression, Butler remained committed to helping women worse off than herself. While fighting against the act, which was not repealed until 1886, she wrote to the reformer Joseph Edmondson, "It is coming to be more and more a deadly fight on the part of us women for *our* bodies." The speculum represented the unchallenged stranglehold of male medical practices on the lives and liberties of all women. Physicians, and the moral "police," were free to intrude upon women's bodies because women were conditioned to submit to male authority. "If these doctors could be forced to keep their hateful hands off us," Butler wrote, "there would be an end to laws which protect vice, and to many other evils."

The Contagious Diseases Act demonized women who didn't obey the constraints of virtuous Victorian femininity. The medical attitudes circulating around the act were held by Brown, Hall, and all those who believed the voracious sexual impulses trembling in the minds and bodies of all women must, for the greater good, be cut cruelly down to size. Throughout the 1860s, English activists like Butler rallied against the social dogma and medical doctrine that women must limit their lives to domesticity and motherhood if their bodies—and society—were to remain pure, unsullied, and healthy. By the end of the decade, many debates about women's rights to education, political participation, and occupations outside of hearth and home had been brought to the fore.

Women were becoming empowered to speak and act against medicine's punishing myths. But with the rising urgency of the "Woman Question," physicians would concoct ever more onerous theories to justify women's entrapment within the narrow confines of the "separate sphere."

7

BLEEDING MAD

"We are human first, women secondarily," Josephine Butler wrote in 1869, in her editor's introduction to *Women's Work and Women's Culture*. This book of essays by educationalists and philosophers, reformers and suffragists, explored how nature and customs had come to define what it meant to be a woman in Victorian society. Nature decreed that women existed to reproduce, to nurture, and to mother. So it was customary for them to exist in the world only in the ways that obeyed their nature. To desire a life outside the "separate sphere"—the private domain of the home, the socially prescribed "women's place"—was an aberration. But for Butler and fellow progressives, custom repressed the "true nature" of women. Women possessed all the strength of character to pursue professions, participate in politics, and live independently. Expanding their lives and opportunities would not only benefit them—it would elevate all of society. Alongside essays about marriage, family life, suffrage, employment, and education, *Women's Work* featured "Medicine as a Profession for Women," a blistering argument for the importance of women doctors—then and throughout history—by English educator, activist, and physician Sophia Jex-Blake.

Medicine constantly reflected and enforced Victorian social ideals of womanhood and femininity, and as a rule, it was dominated by men. Men claimed knowledge about women's bodies, knowledge withheld from women personally as patients and professionally as aspiring physicians. Jex-Blake was one of the "Edinburgh Seven," the first women admitted to the University of Edinburgh to study medicine. The Seven fought tirelessly to be afforded the same level of medical education as their male counterparts, and they were met with fierce opposition before their entrance was granted in 1869. On November 18, 1870, the Seven were due to sit their anatomy exams. When they arrived at Surgeon's Hall, a crowd of protesters led by male students at the university—many of whom were drunk—blocked their entrance, bellowed abuse, and pelted the women with rubbish and mud. When they finally made it inside, with the help of janitorial staff and supportive students, their exam was interrupted once again by the protesters, who let the college's pet sheep loose in the hall. The despicable events of the Surgeon's Hall Riots were denounced in the press, and that day has come to symbolize women's valiant resistance to misogynistic opposition within the medical profession. A plaque with the dates of the riots, commemorating "Britain's First Female Medical Students," was hung outside Surgeon's Hall in 2015.

Jex-Blake became the first licensed woman physician in Scotland and one of the first in Britain. She passionately believed women's instincts and intelligence made them especially suited to medicine. And women doctors were urgently needed at a time when strict gender codes were preventing women from receiving the care and treatment they required. Jex-Blake observed that an "enormous amount of preventable suffering" arose because girls and women were fearful of revealing their intimate concerns to a man. Propriety dictated even what they could *say* about their own bodies. And male physicians could never truly sympathize with a woman's "state, both of mind and body." If women were valued, and listened to, as "human first" in the physician's office and the anatomy hall, then genuine understanding might replace the misconceptions and misbeliefs that had flourished in the gap between female shame and male superiority.

With the "Woman Question" now on the table, physicians were more insistent than ever that women were physically, intellectually, and temperamentally unsuited to life outside the separate sphere. Not only were women vulnerable to myriad illnesses and diseases, thanks to the whims of their reproductive organs, but the very nature of female biology meant that they were, by default, unwell—at least for a week of every month. There was no more obvious impediment to women's progress, according to many Victorian medical men, than menstruation. And for women themselves, there was no other aspect of their health that needed the humanity and compassion of female doctors more urgently.

In all its frequencies and flows, menstruation was never far from the thoughts of physicians of "women's diseases." Since gynecology had become more professionalized, theories about its impact on women's physical and mental health were particularly prominent. It's hard to know how Victorian women actually felt about menstruating. Periods were still shrouded in centuries-old secrecy, superstition, and taboo; few women would have reflected on an experience that instilled such shame. Most women endured their periods quietly and stoically, especially if they were working class or in service and had no other choice. But mid-late-nineteenth-century medical opinions were not based on the every-day experiences of most women. Physicians postulated theories based on severe pathologies observed in a minority of patients. Since they had little understanding of what was "normal," the myth that menstruation was an illness crystallized into medical and cultural lore. A popular euphemism for periods was, indeed, "unwell." Even in bestselling home-health manuals, a menstruating woman was instructed to strictly control her "conduct," lest she fall foul of "hysterics." Unless she judiciously avoided "trash" food, tight clothes, cold rooms, and bad thoughts, she would risk not only destroying her physical health and fertility but also losing her mind.

It was widely accepted that menstrual health could radically affect women's state of mind and vice versa. Medical ideas about the influence of menstrual pathologies on emotions, behaviors, and actions were even enshrined in law. Back in 1845, Martha Brixey, an eighteen-year-old nursery nanny, stood trial at the Old Bailey for murdering eight-month-old Robert Barry Ffinch. Brixey's mistress, Mrs. Ffinch, noted that Martha had been taking medicine for "some derangement to which some young women are subject." Martha wasn't pregnant, but her "constitutional functions" had stopped. She was beset by pains in her head and would plead with the other maids to let her leave the house. On the morning of Sunday, May 5, Mr. and Mrs. Ffinch were in the dining room when Brixey ran in, crying, "Will you forgive me? Oh, sir, I am a murderer! I have cut the baby's throat!" They found their child in his cot, covered in blood, with one of the table knives lying across him. In court on May 12, John Burton, the Ffinch's physician, was asked if Brixey's condition could affect her mind. Yes, he replied; young women were vulnerable to "violent fits of passion" when their "actions of nature" were suspended. Brixey was found not guilty on grounds of "menstrual insanity."

Physicians had a lot to say about menstruation, but they were woefully misguided about what it actually was. During the early 1800s, many thought that ovulation was triggered by intercourse and that menstrual blood was an expulsion of nutrients stored up for pregnancy. By the 1850s, medicine broadly understood that the ovaries, rather than the uterus, triggered menstruation. It was also acknowledged that an ovum wasn't coaxed out of its hiding place by the ever-helpful penis but was in fact released spontaneously whether there was a man around or not. Although gynecologists were hazy on the details, the so-called ovular theory of menstruation became popular from then on. The ovaries replaced the uterus as the epicenter of women's fertile and sexual energies and impulses.

In 1851, Edward Tilt proposed that disorders of the ovaries, which he termed "ovaritis," were caused by having sex either too often or not often enough. He referred to autopsy findings by Dr. Henry Oldham— who testified to Brown's barbarism—which suggested "the ovaries of prostitutes are seldom without morbid lesions." Tilt, of course, blamed these "lesions" entirely on women sex workers' excessive sexual activity. It didn't occur to him that poverty, living conditions, lack of access to medical care, or anything other than female voracity might be the cause. If "ordinary" women weren't receiving enough sexual stimuli (from their husbands, naturally), ovaritis could activate a "cerebrospinal" sympathy manifesting in hysteric symptoms. In addition to a dearth or surfeit of sex, causes of "ovarian irritation" were said to include childhood illnesses, horseback riding, and taking train journeys while menstruating. Women prone to nervousness were claimed to be most vulnerable, as were girls with long eyelashes. But some causes were neither physical nor "constitutional." The disease often arose from "moral causes" or "excitements," which exaggerated "the impulse of unsatisfied desires." He believed women could overexcite their ovaries by looking at books and pictures, having conversations, listening to music, and enjoying a social life. For unmarried women and girls, the delights of literature could even cause an orgasm. If the patient continued to get overexcited by reading, she would irritate her ovaries so much that she would inevitably turn hysteric.

Over the next decades, debates intensified about whether hysteria originated in the nervous system or the reproductive organs. For the more evolved Thomas King Chambers, senior physician and lecturer at St. Mary's, associating hysteria with the uterus was embarrassingly old hat. "Will you please forget once and for all that hysteria derived from the Greek?" he urged his students in 1861. "It is no truer to say that women have hysteria because they have wombs than that men are gouty because they have beards." Chambers viewed hysteria as a mental illness that affected the organs associated with "pain and pleasure"—the heart, lungs, and stomach. Its underlying causes could be understood only by actually listening to patients and observing their symptoms, rather than reducing them to wombs on legs. Unwell women were suffering because almost any illness they had could be explained away by the nebulous medical myth of hysteria. There was no defined classification of "hysteria," no confirmed diagnostic proof. Genuine understanding about women's bodies and minds had been obscured for centuries by unseemly superstitions about female sexuality and the reproductive organs. Physicians treating women with symptoms they interpreted as "hysteric" were coming up against the heady combination of their own ignorance *and* their moral guilt. No wonder, Chambers remarked, that so many were "disposed rather to punish than to cure the patient that has thwarted them."

Chambers noted that the many symptoms labeled hysteric—from unexplained pain, vomiting, and catalepsy to palpitations, crying fits,

and convulsions—often followed some shock, fright, or emotional misery. One of his patients was a seventeen-year-old nursery maid rushed
to St. Mary's with muscle pain, leg paralysis, drenching sweats, and a
racing heart. After four days her "history oozed out in driblets" as she
chatted with a "motherly old woman in the next bed." She had been in
service since she was twelve. Sixteen months earlier, she returned home
to discover her beloved father had died. Her family hadn't thought to
tell her. Her intense grief meant that she wasn't able to perform her
work duties, so she was fired. She started having what would now be
understood as anxiety attacks: racing pulse, uncontrollable bouts of
laughing and crying, and "depressed spirits." Her periods had stopped,
but when she started to bleed again it made no difference to her illness.
Chambers diagnosed "hysteria arising from a distinctly mental cause
and exhibiting itself in mostly mental symptoms." He wasn't insinuating
that his patient's pain was all in her head. Rather, he acknowledged that
her illness was an intricate concert between mind and body. The severity
of her symptoms proved how powerfully a woman's emotional experiences could affect her physical health.

Chambers knew "hysteria" had much more to do with "deficiency of
life" than the precarities of female biology. His ideal treatment was a
complete change of scene. For poor women, a stay in the hospital meant
they could recover "without being perpetually subjected . . . to the influences which originated the disease." Well-off women might recuperate
at the countryside or by the sea. But daughters and wives of "farmers,
shopkeepers, curates, and the like" were neither wealthy nor destitute
enough to afford a convalescent minibreak. Suggesting that class and
circumstances played a role in hysteria was radical, not least because it
threw a spanner in the works of the hysteria industrial complex. Gentle-
men gynecologists were making money hand over fist by treating girls
and women whose families could afford spurious "treatments" for tenu-
ous diagnoses. By holding fast to hysteria as a disease of the reproductive organs "most common in the upper classes of the civilized races,"
men like Tilt were free to spill nonsense that "pampering" the imagination and intellect excited the ovaries. It didn't matter if menstruation
wasn't disordered. Tilt believed the ovaries had such a "poisonous"

influence on the nervous system that simply having a period could ignite hysteria in any predisposed young women. And this meant those "in whom emotion is intensified, at the expense of reason and self-control, by injudicious training in childhood, and the subsequent pampering that ill-fits them for the trials of life." So, any woman who menstruated would become hysteric if her interests, hobbies, and thoughts hadn't been controlled from childhood.

From the mid-1860s, new theories about the relationship between the ovaries and nervous system rejuvenated gynecological theories of hysteria. In 1865, German physiologist Eduard Friedrich Wilhelm Pflüger proposed that menstruation had a neurological cause. According to his hypothesis, the graafian follicle, as it prepared to release the ovum, stimulated nerve impulses in the ovaries that reflexively triggered ovulation and menstruation. Yes, he believed these events happened at the same time. Tilt was a huge fan of these "scientific" reflex theories, as were many American physicians who also believed female biology made women insane. Since menstruation was an involuntary process, women were thought to have no control over its impact on their nervous systems.

The primacy of the ovaries in theories about female insanity were dynamite for scalpel-happy gynecologists. Brown and other English surgeons had pushed ovariotomy as a last resort for cysts and tumors. No one was using surgical measures—yet—to treat menstrual disorders and the nervous symptoms they were thought to cause. Then, on August 17, 1872, twenty-three-year-old Julia Omberg, from the city of Rome in Georgia's Florida County, lay down on her kitchen table, got knocked out with chloroform, and had both her ovaries removed by a gynecologist and former Civil War surgeon named Robert Battey. Assisted by three other physicians, Battey dilated Omberg's cervix with the kind of speculum invented by James Marion Sims, made an incision in her "vaginal cul-de-sac" (pouch of Douglas), pulled down each ovary with forceps, secured them with ligatures, and removed them using *écrasement*, surgical parlance for "crushing."

Battey had been Omberg's physician since she was sixteen. He described her as a "bashful, sensitive and retiring girl" whose ill health made her an invalid. Her periods were nonexistent, and her body and mind were exhausted from "efforts at menstruation." By eighteen, she was so unwell that marriage was out of the question. When Battey first suggested removing her ovaries, she apparently embraced this "glimmering flash of light across the dark and portentous sky which had long overshadowed her life." During surgery, her friends and family were waiting outside, ready to lynch Battey if she died under his hands. She survived the operation and lived, in good health, to the age of eighty.

Battey considered himself quite the revolutionary, but he was by no means the first surgeon to practice and promote ovariotomies. His fervor was inspired by meeting the respected English gynecological surgeon Thomas Spencer Wells while on a military tour in 1859. Having weathered the medical and moral storm in the 1840s and 1850s, Wells pioneered safer ovariotomies for life-threatening tumors and cysts while working at London's Samaritan Free Hospital for Women. While Wells wanted to relieve women's suffering and save their lives, other advocates were not so altruistic, or selective, when justifying this drastic intervention. Wells regarded his ovariotomy as a "triumph" over "opposition of all kinds," and he feared its benefits would be ruined by "rash, inconsistent, thoughtless partisans, whose failures do not reflect so much discredit on themselves as on the operation which they have badly performed in unsuitable cases."

Battey was exactly the kind of "zealous but injudicious advocate" Wells feared. But Omberg's survival cemented Battey's perception of himself as a Columbus of the ovaries, and he went on to perform his "normal ovariotomy" on many women throughout the 1870s. Most were private patients, age thirty or younger, who were burdened by some "grave disease which is either destructive to life or . . . health and happiness . . . and which we may reasonably expect to remove by effecting the change of life." In 1873, Battey announced to the Georgia Medical Association that he had carved "out a new pathway through consecrated ground, upon which the foot of man has not dared wittingly to tread." What was more, he had "invaded the hidden recesses of the female organism and snatched from its appointed seat a glandular body, whose mysterious and wonderful functions are of the highest interest to the human race." The power of ovarian nerves to cause so many physical—and psychological—illnesses was reason enough to rid women of them. But many English surgeons objected to childbearing women being "castrated" and "unsexed" by some two-bit surgery made fashionable by an American upstart. They were also slightly concerned about the "hazardous" nature of the operation. For detractors, these were reasons enough to shut it down; but for advocates, this meant the operation had to keep being done until it was perfected.

Battey exalted the miraculous effects of his operation, at least for patients who survived. He talked about women "bounding . . . into perfect health and comfort" after his operations; others were "bright and cheerful" and "ever trying to cultivate the grace of thankfulness." The eagerness of patients was a shrewd marketing strategy for such surgeries throughout the 1880s. For opponents of ovariotomy, women's enthusiasm proved the operation was nothing but a trendy fad. Regardless of whether women really did yearn to have their healthy ovaries ripped out, stories of pleading willingness and bountiful recovery veiled the sinister enforcement of the operation on disempowered women during the 1880s and 1890s in public hospitals in Britain and asylums across America.

In 1885, a twenty-nine-year-old woman diagnosed with nymphomania and "hystero-epilepsy" at the clinic for Mental and Nervous Diseases in Philadelphia Hospital gave a rare insight into what it was like to endure gynecological surgeries for mental illness. At the beginning of a lecture, her neurologist, Charles K. Mills, brought her into the hall so that his students could "note her appearance." After he sent her out, he explained that she had pleaded to be sent to an asylum, but Mills persuaded her to undergo treatment at the hospital. He then read out her history, written in her own words. She started having sexual feelings at the age of six, but until she was removed from school at age twelve, her physical health was good. At thirteen, she started her period but "was taught nothing of the laws of my being." She didn't understand how babies were made, and impure thoughts obsessed her: "I was guilty of immorality before I knew what it meant." She started masturbating and soon suffered pain in her head, heart, and uterus. Medicines did nothing to calm the convulsions that shook her every nerve. Her clitoris glans was removed, but to her doctor's amazement it grew back. Her labia were then sewn shut, but she was relieved of her symptoms for only six weeks. "I tormented the doctors to operate again," she said, "but they were afraid it would kill me."

In 1881, she trained to be a nurse. For seven months she was untroubled by her nymphomania. But when she was forced to give up work, it crept back. Her ovaries were removed, but her nervous system, "craving the stimulation it was accustomed to," wouldn't be quieted. The surgery did nothing to abate her sexual feelings, or her spasms, screaming fits, and loss of speech. When she felt weak or excited, her symptoms forged forth; music made her unbearably tense. At night, consumed by the urge to "shake [her] family in their sleep," she calmed herself by placing a wet towel over her head. All she could do was pray to God for help.

Mills encouraged his intelligent "nervous" patients to write their own histories, because "more light is thrown upon the case than by an ordinary study." Addressing the fact that clitoridectomy and ovariotomy did nothing to help his patient, Mills concluded that "operative procedures" offered no "radical cure" in cases "intrinsically nervous or mental in their nature." This was an incredibly forward-thinking statement in an era when the ovaries were the principal seat of female sexual maladies. Mills was acknowledging that women had independent brains, and that their thoughts, feelings, and desires were not governed by their reproductive organs. But even though his patient explained that her troubles began when she left school and were relieved when she trained as a nurse, Mills didn't make any connection between the frustrations of her life and her "nymphomania." Still, by respecting and valuing his patient's voice and experiences, Mills was trying to shatter those punitive myths that were condemning women to ovariotomists' tables.

8

REST AND RESISTANCE

Since the middle of the nineteenth century, progressive campaigners in America had been challenging the ideology that a woman's place in society was defined by her reproductive biology. The assumption that women were obliged to limit their existence because their "dominant function" was to bear and raise children was, as in England, enshrined in law and embedded in culture. On July 19, 1848, debates about women's opportunities and liberties galvanized into a recognized national movement. Three hundred women gathered at the Wesleyan Chapel in the town of Seneca Falls, New York, for a convention on women's social, civil, political, and religious rights. Organized by a group of abolitionists and social reformers including Elizabeth Cady Stanton and Lucretia Mott, Seneca Falls was a call to arms against the many "customs" that decreed women should be subservient to men. The first day was exclusively for women, but men were invited to join the discussions on the second day. One was Frederick Douglass, the leading abolitionist, lecturer, and political activist. Douglass was born into slavery in 1818, on a plantation in Talbot, Maryland, and he escaped to freedom in 1838. He was a leading member of the antislavery movement and in 1847 launched the abolitionist newsletter *The North Star*. Douglass was a dedicated and vocal supporter of women's equal rights. "We hold women to be justly entitled to all we claim for men," he wrote in an editorial on the convention in *The North Star*. "All that distinguishes man as an intelligent and accountable being, is equally true of women." Douglass's was the only Black voice onstage or in the audience at Seneca Falls.

"The history of mankind is a history of repeated injuries and usurpations on the part of man toward woman," declared Elizabeth Cady Stanton on the morning of July 20. Stanton was reading from the *Declaration of Sentiments and Grievances*, a document modeled on the US Declaration of Independence, which stated the "candid facts" of man's "establishment of an absolute tyranny" over woman. The document, signed by one hundred delegates—sixty-eight women and thirty-two men, including Douglass—was published shortly after the conference by Douglass's *North Star* press in Rochester, New York. The *Declaration* began by stating that under the Constitution, and God, "men and women are created equal." All women had the unquestionable human right to "life, liberty, and the pursuit of happiness." But systems of power and governance, enforced by men over centuries, had robbed women of those rights. When married, women became men's legal property. Man had made woman entirely beholden to him by denying her economic independence. He imposed horrendous double standards around moral codes and behaviors. And he had also decreed that her "sphere of action" should be entirely limited to the home. He had closed off all "avenues" to "honorable professions," including medicine, and, most egregiously, had "denied her the facilities for a thorough education."

Equal education had been key to social reform debates since Mary Wollstonecraft proposed that boys and girls should be schooled together. For Stanton and many others who lobbied for equality, education—especially further and higher education—was a crucial battleground. They were demanding that women have access to exactly the same institutions and academic programs as men. But apart from Oberlin in Ohio, which admitted women in 1833 and awarded its first bachelor's degrees in 1841, no US college permitted women to be educated alongside men and to the same level.

In the spirit of Seneca Falls, a series of women's rights conventions were organized across the United States. Alongside debates about suffrage, political participation, marriage laws, employment, equal pay, and the Declaration of Sentiments, women's college education was high on the agenda. In the years before the Civil War, some incredible strides were made for women's coeducation, at both the secondary and collegiate levels. By 1860, many private colleges had followed Oberlin's example and thrown their doors open to women, including Hillsdale in Michigan, Westminster in Pennsylvania, and Alfred University in New York. In 1862, Mary Jane Patterson, a graduate of Oberlin, became one of the first Black women in the United States to be awarded a bachelor of arts degree after completing the same studies, over four years, as male students. She went on to become principal of the Preparatory High School for Colored Youth in Washington, DC, which became Dunbar High School, one of the most important academic institutions for Black students during the first half of the twentieth century. Patterson spent her teaching career pioneering education opportunities for Black women.

After the Civil War, as the higher education system became more structured and professionalized, a swathe of public and state universities, including Michigan State, Kansas State, and the University of Wisconsin–Madison, started offering coed degree study. The opportunity for women to study alongside men was gradually becoming a reality. But to those ever-lurking opponents of gender equality, this monumental shift in education culture didn't change their opinion that women's minds—and bodies—were naturally domestic and fundamentally defective. They believed that women's basic biology would prevent them from attaining male standards of academic excellence. As had been the case in England, where arguments about women's physiological inferiority were trotted out whenever the "Woman Question" was raised, anti-feminist physicians in America took it upon themselves to warn the public of the perilous dangers of coeducation.

The embers of dissent around equal education were stoked ferociously in 1872 after Edward Hammond Clarke, a respected Boston physician, gave a lecture on the subject to the New England Women's Club (NEWC). Clarke's "Sex in Education; or, a Fair Chance for Girls," was meant to enlighten the NEWC on coeducation, that vital cornerstone of women's liberation. He was addressing progressive club women, for whom this issue was hugely important. And he certainly knew his audience when he declared that "whatever a woman can do, she has a right to do . . . the relation of the sexes is one of equality, not of better or worse, or higher or lower." But they would have balked at the about-face that followed: just because women *can*, doesn't mean they *should*. Clarke couldn't stymie national progress. But he could counsel women against pursuing college education by telling cautionary tales about female patients made ill, mad, and infertile by the rigors of study.

Clarke wasn't against educating girls and young women per se, but he vehemently opposed coeducation that didn't respect their "special" physiological burdens. In 1873, he published an extended version of his lecture, written for popular rather than medical readers, in which he argued that a fair education for girls involved limited intellectual labor and allowed them to sleep most of the time. "Victims" of "modern" education, he claimed, were "pathological specimens" haunting the country's classrooms and colleges. Miss A was one of Clarke's "living illustrations." When she entered seminary school at fifteen, she was bright and healthy. But she was so anxious to do well that she ignored the "periodical tides of her organization." She stood up to recite, hunched over her books, and soon her periods became extraordinarily heavy. She graduated with a stunning report but was left aching, bleeding, and convulsing. Clarke diagnosed menorrhagia-induced Saint Vitus's dance, a disease in which the muscles of the hands, feet, and face twitch uncontrollably. The treatment? No study whatsoever, and rest, rest, and more rest.

When she turned nineteen, Miss A didn't want to rest anymore; she wanted to go to college. According to Clarke, she graduated sicker than ever; her periods stopped, and her reproductive organs were underdeveloped. "Doubtless the evils of her education will affect her whole life," he declared. "Nature punishes disobedience." Clarke wasn't really concerned about protecting young women from incurable diseases. His fear, shared by many anti-feminist physicians, was that education would lead middle-class women to abandon "the true womanly standard." In his dystopian vision, the country would soon be overrun by wasted armies of infertile spinsters. Decent men would be forced to ship in wives "who are to be mothers in our republic" from "trans-atlantic homes."

Clarke's "brief monograph," by the standards of the time, went viral. It went into its second printing a week after publication and gained legions of admirers on both sides of the Atlantic. One was Henry Maudsley, the British psychiatrist who founded the eponymous hospital in London. Furiously opposed to professional and educational equality, Maudsley wrote his own diatribe on the "baneful effects upon female health" of "excessive educational strain" for *Popular Science Monthly* in 1874. His argument was basically a regurgitation of Clarke's with less zombie apocalypse and more wombs for brains. He believed that, from puberty, a young woman's body is entirely geared toward motherhood, and that her mind is fashioned only for soft, yielding, nourishing tasks. Maudsley also subscribed to the popular notion that the ovaries were in sympathy with the brain. Women were thought to only have enough energy to serve one or the other: "When Nature spends in one direction, she must economize in another direction," Maudsley declared. For a young woman predisposed to some vague nervous illness, the "constitutional drain" of menstruation meant that she was unable to withstand "the enemy that was lurking." Pile on the pressures of schooling and she would be riddled for life with "a variety of troublesome and serious disorders" including infertility.

For Maudsley, it was manifestly unwise and dangerously unhealthy for women to "contend on equal terms with men" in any area of life. Any person who insisted that the difference between the sexes was socially constructed—and not biologically determined—was ignoring the irrefutable facts of women's "special functions." Advocates of women's equality who wanted to "throw open to them fields of activity from which they are now excluded" were "zealous fanatics." Maudsley's thinly veiled issue was with women becoming doctors. At the time, the Medical Act in England still forbade women from obtaining licenses to practice medicine. Elizabeth Garrett Anderson was the country's only licensed female doctor. Born in 1836, Garrett Anderson obtained a legitimate medical education amid a culture of vehement opposition from the male medical establishment. She worked as a surgical nurse at Middlesex Hospital, and although she was refused entry to study medicine, she was permitted to study apothecary. She also received private tuition in anatomy and physiology while continuing to work as a nurse. Despite leaving the hospital with qualifications, including in chemistry, she was refused entry to many medical schools in England and Scotland because she was a woman.

In 1862, Garrett Anderson was admitted to the Worshipful Society of Apothecaries, which at the time did not discriminate on the basis of gender. She gained her medical license after passing the society's examinations in 1865, before becoming the first woman to obtain a medical degree from the prestigious École de médecine at the University of Paris, in 1870. By the time Maudsley's article was published, Garrett Anderson was the first woman member of the British Medical Association. She was also setting up the London School of Medicine for Women, the first institution in England to train women doctors, in collaboration with Sophia Jex-Blake; Elizabeth Blackwell, the first female physician to obtain a medical degree in the United States; and Elizabeth's sister Emily Blackwell, the third to do the same.

In 1874, Garrett Anderson wrote a brilliant response to Maudsley for the progressive magazine *Fortnightly Review*. She saw not a grain of truth in the notion that menstruation impaired "nervous and physical force" so dramatically that it was "useless for women . . . to pursue careers side-by-side with men." As a woman, and a physician of women, she rejected his claim that "active work of the mind or body" sent periods haywire. The nervous maladies Maudsley warned of were caused by "the depressing influence" of relinquishing "adequate mental interest and occupations" for marriage and motherhood. Real thought, genuine interest, and "solid intellectual work" were the cure, not the cause. Garrett Anderson also pointed out that Maudsley's rant featured no actual clinical evidence, and most of his opinions were cribbed from Clarke's exaggerated case studies. She also astutely observed that both men based their arguments on middle-class girls who had access to education. They both swerved the fact that women working in factories and service were able to perform manual labor while menstruating "as a rule, without ill effects." But conveniently, these women didn't have the option to pursue lives of the mind or strive for professional parity.

The strength of response to these pseudomedical tirades was

unprecedented. In 1874, Julia Ward Howe compiled essays by reformists and educators into the book *Sex and Education: A Reply to Dr. E. H. Clarke's "Sex in Education."* Howe objected to Clarke's flagrant marshaling of alternative facts: "No woman could publish . . . speculations concerning the special physical economy of the other sex . . . without incurring the gravest rebuke for insolence and immodesty." Like Garrett Anderson, Howe knew the social conditions that befit middle-class girls for domesticity were the root cause of ill health. Girls were confined to the home, while boys played outside; young women were laced into limb-paralyzing dresses, yet boys' clothes let them move freely; boys ventured into adolescence with the "healthful hope" of turning their interests into professions, whereas girls embarked on womanhood with the "dispiriting prospect of a secondary and derivative existence." By consulting professors at coed colleges, Howe revealed that menstrual ill health was incredibly scarce. In fact, the general health of many women students improved during their studies. All the authors in Howe's book knew that Clarke's real motivation was to maintain the separate sphere by appealing to age-old superstitions that illness was a punishment for female ambition. "Open the doors of your colleges to women, and you will accomplish the ruin of the Commonwealth," Howe wrote, summing up Clarke's "prognosis": "Disease—already, according to him, the rule among them—will become without exception."

That year, Eliza Bisbee Duffey, an expert on women's health and a fierce advocate for equality, also debunked Clarke's myopic propaganda. Most of Clarke's "living illustrations" became desperately unwell *after* finishing their studies: "They found nothing in this life to satisfy their mental needs. No career was open to them. Their energies were forced back upon themselves, and they pined and became invalids because they had *nothing else to do*." As a woman who had forged for herself a life denied to so many, Duffey understood how it would have felt to have her thoughts stifled, her ambitions restricted. She spoke to and from experiences Clarke knew nothing about—what it meant to live as a woman, to inhabit a female body. Periods happen to the body, not the brain. But until medicine understood and accepted this basic fact, women would be forced to yield every month to "imagined" weaknesses.

"Let the healthy women of America tell the Doctor better than this," Duffy implored.

Mary Putnam Jacobi, the pioneering physician, scientist, and medical teacher, enabled women to do just that. From childhood, she had longed to become a doctor. When she was nine, she found a dead rat and considered dissecting it so she could study its heart, but "courage failed" her. Her father, George Palmer Putnam, was a renowned book publisher who encouraged his daughter to write; in her early teens she had a short story published in *The Atlantic*. But he was less keen on her ambitions to become a doctor. Undeterred by his offer of money in return for her relinquishing her dream, Putnam Jacobi left home to study and train at the Woman's Medical College of Pennsylvania, the second institution in the world to award women medical degrees. In 1871, she became the second woman, after Garrett Anderson, to graduate the École de médecine. After being appointed professor at the newly established Women's Medical College at the New York Infirmary, and through her presidency of the Women's Medical Association of New York City from 1874, she campaigned for medical schools across the country to extend admission to women. In 1875, in response to the furor around Clarke's thesis, Harvard University's revered Boylston Medical Prize essay committee invited responses to the question of whether women required "mental and bodily rest during menstruation." Putnam Jacobi submitted an essay for the prize, and, unlike Clarke, she based her argument on original clinical research.

Putnam Jacobi saw how menstruation had become wildly over-pathologized in male gynecological literature. Where in past centuries menstrual blood was seen as an excess of vital forces, now it was a draining and "constantly returning debility . . . demanding rest as decidedly as a fracture or a paralysis." Putnam Jacobi analyzed questionnaires completed anonymously by women, mostly patients at the New York Infirmary, about their experiences of menstruating—blood flow, pain, energy levels, and so on—as well as their education history, occupations, physical activities, and general health. She found that mental exertion had little, if any, impact on menstrual health, and the female brain did not become defective during menstruation. Putnam Jacobi won the Boylston Medical Prize, the first woman to do so.

By 1876, Putnam Jacobi had extended her research to 268 women from a range of classes, backgrounds, occupations, and education levels. She also made experimental analyses of participants' physiological changes before, during, and after menstruation by taking urine tests, mapping body temperatures, and charting pulse rates using an early blood-pressure tracing device called a sphygmograph. The week before menstruation, for most women, was a "period of increased vigor and . . . increased nervo-muscular strength," where the "nerve-force" needed to support normal, painless periods was established. The idea that women suffered a kind of nervous breakdown during their periods was, in other words, a fiction. Unless a woman had to rest because her cramps were so intense, "the habit of periodical rest" could "easily become injurious." And if she was in extreme pain, she probably had an underlying gyne-cological disorder, not some spurious nerve derangement. By far the most ubiquitous cause of "disordered and painful menstruation" was "feeble muscular exercise." "There is nothing in the nature of menstrua-tion to imply the necessity, or even the desirability, of rest, for women whose nutrition is really normal," Putnam Jacobi concluded.

In 1877, Putnam Jacobi published *The Question of Rest for Women Dur-ing Menstruation*. By writing about a subject deemed beyond the knowl-edge of women, based on their thoughts and feelings about their lives and bodies, Putnam Jacobi was a revolutionary. She had gained acclaim for research that demystified punitive theories about female physiology. And she had done this as a well-respected physician defending women's right to pursue medical education. The myth of menstrual incapacity was so ingrained that it was regularly touted in arguments against women becoming doctors. A few years earlier, Edward Tilt, then president of London's Obstetrical Society, praised members' almost unanimous deci-sion not to admit female physicians because they were manifestly unfit "to bear the physical fatigue and mental anxieties of obstetrical practice at menstrual periods."

It is infuriating that male gatekeepers of obstetrics and gynecology even entertained the idea that menstruation made women unfit to care for other women. In truth, the men parroting this nonsense were hell-bent on keeping women out of their "hallowed discipline." But the grip of medical misogyny was beginning, at last, to loosen. Putnam Jacobi's myth-busting investigation was a triumph of rational science over sexist speculation, and it coincided with some monumental strides for women in medicine. In 1876, Parliament passed the Enabling Act, which allowed all medical associations in Britain to license qualified physicians regardless of their gender. That same year the American Medical Association admitted its first woman member, Sarah Hackett Stevenson, the Illinois physician who went on to be the first woman appointed to the state's Board of Health. But neither social progress nor scientific objectivity could disarm men who insisted that women, and their pesky thoughts and feelings, should be confined to the kitchen.

Earlier in the 1870s, an American neurologist named Silas Weir Mitchell had been busily concocting theories about the threat intellectual activities posed to "future womanly usefulness." Mitchell thought coeducation ridiculous, and the possibility of girls receiving "masculine" education before the age of seventeen appalled him. "Nervous maladies," in his opinion, were so endemic among American girls and women that even without education they were "physically unfit" to fulfill their duties as wives and mothers.

While working as a surgeon during the Civil War, Mitchell observed how nerve pain caused by bullet wounds exhausted the minds and bodies of soldiers, making them near hysterical. He devised a treatment of bed rest, a fat-heavy diet, massage, and electric muscle stimulation to restore depleted nerves. After the war, Mitchell suffered a breakdown and diagnosed himself with "neurasthenia," a term made popular by American neurologist George Miller Beard in 1869 for nervous exhaustion exacerbated by the stresses of modern living. Although "neurasthenia" could affect both men and women, its causes were decidedly gendered. Men developed the condition by working too hard, while in women it was usually linked to domestic and family pressures, or the inevitable fallout of studying too hard when they should have been obeying the limits of their biological destiny. Mitchell treated his own bouts of neurasthenia, or "a rather nervous temperament," as he put it, with "rest and recreation" in the 1860s and 1870s. But although he recognized that men and women alike benefited from physical rest to "cure" their addled minds and nerves, his fundamental belief in women's physiological, mental, and social inferiority meant that his proposed treatment for them was more moral conditioning than medical care. After Mitchell turned his attentions to women's nervous illnesses in 1873, he promoted his infamous "rest cure" as a two-birds-with-one-stone remedy for improving the delicate female constitution and making women toe the domestic line.

Mitchell insisted that women with nervous exhaustion and "hysteric" symptoms—especially if they were young, thin, and anemic—should be kept in bed for about two months, fed rich foods including raw beef soup and four pints of milk a day, massaged regularly, given electrotherapy, and forbidden any activity whatsoever apart from teeth cleaning. "Nothing is more common in practice," he wrote in 1877, "than to see a young woman who falls below the health standard, and is tired all the time, by and by has a tender spine, and soon or late enacts the whole varied drama of hysteria." For Mitchell, hysteria was nothing more than a litany of complaints dreamed up by pampered middle-class girls to perplex physicians and garner sympathy. His methods were designed to break an unwell woman's resolve and make her snap out of her attention-seeking ways. "To cure such a case," he advised, "you must morally alter as well as physically amend."

Miss B, a "sturdy, handsome girl," age sixteen, suffered convulsions, stomach problems, and limb paralysis before she entered Mitchell's "care." He considered her "a child who to be made well had to be calmly and firmly ruled." Other girls apparently loved to play the good patient because they were flattered by Mitchell's attention. Not Miss B. She was isolated at the Philadelphia Infirmary for Nervous Diseases, where Mitchell was lead physician, with one nurse to attend her. She was banned from using her hands for any reason, even to feed herself. She loved to knit, sew, and read, but all were forbidden. She hated milk and vomited after being made to drink it. "One or two scoldings, some show of disgust, and the promise that she would soon feed herself if she obeyed my wishes, helped us through this," Mitchell wrote. He was not above force-feeding patients through the nose or rectum if they refused to eat. After a year of rest cure, Miss B was so weak she could barely walk with crutches. "This is what it means to treat hysteria," he wrote. "There is no shortcut, no royal road." Mitchell's medical "expertise" consisted of humiliating and abusing girls and women. But his methods were deemed so effective that his popularity and eminence spread across Britain and America.

In 1892, Charlotte Perkins Gilman brought the rest cure to public attention through a short story in *The New England Magazine*. "The Yellow Wallpaper" is about a woman with severe depression whose mental health deteriorates further after she is confined by her physician husband to a gaudily wallpapered bedroom. For three months she is made to rest and abstain from all intellectual and creative activity. Her husband thinks nothing is wrong with her, save a "slight hysterical tendency." "Bless her little heart!" he exclaims. "She shall be as sick as she pleases!" "The Yellow Wallpaper" reflected Gilman's views about the deleterious effects of marriage on women's bodies and minds. And it was inspired by her own experience of being subjected to the rest cure in 1887 by Mitchell himself.

After the birth of her daughter Katherine, in 1885, Gilman suffered "a growing melancholia . . . that consists of every painful mental sensation . . . utter weakness" and "a steady brain-ache that fills the conscious mind with crowding images of distress." She couldn't read, write, paint, talk, or listen. Pain consumed her mind. She held and nursed her daughter but couldn't feel love. When Katherine was five months old, Gilman left her with her mother and a nurse and traveled from her home in Connecticut to visit friends in California. On returning home, the "dark fog rose again." Her mother's friend gave her $100 to "go away somewhere and get cured."

Gilman had heard of Mitchell—"the greatest nerve specialist in the country"—and wrote to him explaining how desperately she needed help. "I am a teacher by instinct and profession," she wrote. "I am a reader and thinker. I can do some good work for the world if I live. I cannot bear to . . . linger on this wretched invalid existence . . . There is something the matter with my head. No one here knows or believes or cares . . . but you will know." Mitchell treated Gilman with the rest cure at the Philadelphia Infirmary, which she found "agreeable enough." After a month he found nothing wrong with her. He sent her home with this prescription: "Live as domestic a life as possible. Have your child with you all the time . . . Lie down an hour after each meal. Have but two hours intellectual life a day. And never touch pen, brush or pencil as long as you live."

Gilman obeyed Mitchell's instructions for months. But soon she felt "perilously close to losing [her] mind." "The mental agony grew so unbearable that I would sit blankly moving my head from side to side—to get out from under the pain," she wrote. "Not physical pain . . . just mental torment, and so heavy in its nightmare gloom." In the fall of 1887, she separated from her "devoted" and "loving" husband. "It was not a choice between going and staying, but between going, sane, and staying, insane." Over the next years she continued to write and lecture, but she was exhausted by her "wilted nerves." "To do anything . . . is incredible effort, as if trying to rise and walk under a prostrate circus tent, or wade in glue." Her friends didn't believe she was unwell because she seemed so capable; but how could they understand what she might have achieved if she hadn't been so broken?

In "The Yellow Wallpaper," the narrator's husband threatens to take her to Mitchell if she doesn't "pick up faster." After the story was published, Gilman sent a copy to Mitchell, but he never responded. It wasn't until 1902, when Gilman met Mary Putnam Jacobi, that she began to recover. Putnam Jacobi had developed a groundbreaking theory that hysteria, which she saw as a disorder of the nervous system, should be treated by stimulating patients' senses and intellects and not by diminishing them with constant rest. Where Mitchell dismissed the reality and severity of Gilman's mental illness, Putnam Jacobi listened, and believed her.

At the time, Gilman's depression was so severe that she found it impossible to write. Over several months, Putnam Jacobi prescribed tasks to gradually restore her brain's "capacity for action." First, she built structures with kindergarten blocks; she read; within a few months she could write a little. "All this intelligent care helped me much," she reflected in her memoir, in 1935. Years later, in an article titled "Why I Wrote 'The Yellow Wallpaper,'" she explained that she wanted to reach wives and mothers who were vulnerable to punishing medical interventions, and to empower them to challenge their male physicians. "It was not intended to drive people crazy," she wrote, "but to save people from being driven crazy, and it worked." The rest cure had sent Gilman "so near the borderline of utter mental ruin that [she] could see over." Her healing came from the "joy and growth and service" of writing, where she regained "some measure of power." Today "The Yellow Wallpaper" is one of the most important and widely read texts for feminists arguing against medicine's control over women's bodies and minds.

Mitchell's attitudes toward women and his treatments were horrendous. His rest cure became popular because it offered a solution to a problem that medicine itself had created. In his twisted way, Mitchell rightly questioned the validity of hysteria. By the late mid-nineteenth century, it had evolved into a spurious diagnosis for almost all pathologies of women's bodies and minds. Mitchell described hysteria as "the nosological limbo of all unnamed female maladies" and argued that it should "be called mysteria for all its name teaches us of the host of morbid states . . . crowded within its hazy boundaries." For a few years, gynecologists and physicians, especially in Britain, had been admitting that the term had become as unruly and undefined as the women it was meant to pathologize. In 1866, surgeon and anatomist Frederick Carpenter Skey announced that diagnosing "hysteria" was like trying to discern an "object floating in the sky . . . or an early star in the evening." A few years later, Edward Tilt declared that hysteria had become a "'will-o-the-wisp,' misdirecting . . . attention from the real cause of nervous symptoms."

Hysteria was losing its legitimacy as a diagnosis for physiological disorders, but this didn't mean that the term was consigned to the historical wastebasket. Over hundreds of years, it had become a shorthand for aberrations of idealized femininity. "Hysteric" women defied their maternal destiny; they had designs on a life outside the separate sphere; they desired sex, courted attention, and feigned illnesses for sympathy. They were erratic, deviant, deceptive, and devious. By the later decades of the 1800s, "hysteria" was synonymous with deranged feminine behaviors and emotions. It's no surprise that emerging mind and nerve doctors—alienists and neurologists—were eager to pin down that amorphous object and define it on their own terms.

In the 1870s, Jean-Martin Charcot, head neurologist of Paris's notorious Salpêtrière hospital asylum, became determined to solve the riddle of hysteria. Through experiments on young women patients, he constructed a theory that symptoms labeled "hysteric"—convulsions, delirium, ovarian pain, palpitations, paralysis, choking, and others—were rooted in emotional traumas that could be awoken under hypnosis. Soundly denounced as quackery by most of the medical establishment, hypnotism had been used on women as a supposed cure for mysterious ailments since the eighteenth century. For Charcot, hypnotism was a legitimate technique for demonstrating the dramatic symptoms of what he called *la grande hystérie*. During the 1880s, in his famous Tuesday-morning lectures at the Salpêtrière, his hysteric "queens," as they became known, were made to swoon, thrust, pose, and contort in front of an audience of men from Paris's scientific, artistic, and literary coteries. One of the men who witnessed these pathological peepshows was Sigmund Freud, who was heavily influenced by Charcot's theories in his famous and influential psychoanalytic studies of female hysteria and its roots in the unconscious.

Charcot and Freud claimed they were rescuing hysteria from misapprehension and obscurity with these new definitions. But in reality they were reinforcing long-held ideas that women's unexplained, mysterious physical symptoms were all in the mind. They were doing what women's physicians had always done: interpreting disorders that confounded understanding according to their invented theories—and not by listening to, believing, or trusting women. Hysteria, and all its associated symptoms, was now a mental illness invented by mind doctors seeking to master and control the forces of femininity. These new definitions were not based on class and wealth; Charcot, especially, used poor women who had been abused and exploited as specimens to manipulate and extract knowledge from. By forcing them to "perform" hysteria on his stage and in clinical photographs, he created a spectacle of hysterical femininity, in which vulnerable women were under the spell of the master clinician. "Hysterical" women had lost control; they were out of control—hypersexual, enthralled by fantasies, possessed, mad. Unbuckled from the body, hysteria had become a cultural leitmotif for feminine temperament unbound, untamed, and unbidden.

As the end of the nineteenth century beckoned, hysteria would begin, at long last, to be dismantled as a diagnosis for any and all "female" pathologies that physicians failed to understand. Gradually, new medical knowledge, diagnostic techniques, medications, and therapies would reveal what was lurking beneath those ingrained layers of misconception, misapprehension, and misunderstanding. But as evidence-based medical knowledge was layered upon misbeliefs, women would become subject to a whole new spectrum of mystifications. The world was changing, but women were still subjugated by centuries of mythmaking about their defective and inferior female biology. As the twentieth century ushered forth, women faced an intense battle to claim control of their bodies, minds, and lives from the grip of medical oppression.

PART TWO

LATE NINETEENTH CENTURY–1940s

9

SUFFRAGE AND SUPPRESSION

In 1851, Harriet Taylor Mill, the English philosopher and women's rights advocate, was writing an essay about the "organized agitation on a new question" that had recently "arisen in the United States." She was eager to inform readers in England about the Seneca Falls Convention, which she saw as the first "public manifestation" of a political movement "not merely *for* women, but *by* them." Born in 1807 to an obstetric surgeon and his wife, Taylor Mill was educated at home and loved to write poetry. She married her first husband, thirty-nine-year-old John Taylor, when she was just eighteen, and within a few years had three children. While pregnant with Helen, her third child, Taylor Mill published essays, poems, and book reviews, and her interest in social reform and women's rights bloomed. Around this time, she met, and became close with, John Stuart Mill, the English philosopher, sociologist, Liberal Party politician, and ardent supporter of women's equality. Their relationship was an intimate meeting of minds; they exchanged impassioned letters about the stifling conditions of marriage and the diminishment of women's social, legal, and political rights. The couple's affair, by the standards of the time, was a scandalous rebuke of convention. For a while, Taylor Mill separated from her husband and continued her relationship with Stuart Mill. After John Taylor died of cancer in 1849, Taylor Mill's own health started to deteriorate. She temporarily lost the use of her legs, contracted tuberculosis, and had "nervous disorders." But through it all, this unwell woman was a radical thinker and trailblazing reformist who continually questioned Victorian society's hypocritical hold over women's rights to think, act, and love on their own terms.

Taylor Mill eventually married Stuart Mill in 1851, the year her essay "Enfranchisement of Women" was published in the *Westminster and Foreign Quarterly Review*. The "question" that had arisen in the United States was exceptionally important to Taylor Mill and her new husband. It was the question of "the enfranchisement of women; their admission, in law and in fact, to equality in all rights, political, civil and social, with the male citizens of the community." Right at the top of "the history of repeated injuries and usurpations on the part of man toward woman" laid out in the *Declaration of Sentiments* was the denial of women's "inalienable right to elective franchise"—her right to vote, her suffrage. In her essay, Taylor Mill explained that she hadn't read the proceedings from Seneca Falls published by Frederick Douglass's *North Star* press. But she had studied those of the National Women's Rights Convention, held in Worcester, Massachusetts, in 1850. The demands made there were nothing less than complete equality in education, employment, and the "formation and administration of laws." Taylor Mill was imploring radicals in Britain to rise up and make the same demands.

"Women have never had equal rights with men," she wrote. Custom alone dictated that women were "legally inferior." The belief that women were physically and mentally weak had warranted their subjection and barred their inclusion in political and civil affairs. Those "many persons" who still alleged that women's "field of action" should be restricted argued that "the pursuits from which women are excluded are *unfeminine*." A woman's place, they maintained, was not in "politics or publicity, but private and domestic life." Taylor Mill, a woman with fierce intellectual ambitions who chose for herself how she would live, faced the criticism that was always waged against women who dared to question and resist the doctrine of the "separate sphere." And in her writings, she resolutely rejected such misogynistic myths. It was up to the individual, she insisted, to decide what her "proper sphere" was. In the past, women had "shown fitness for the highest social functions exactly in proportion as they have been admitted to them." Those "persons" who hammered on about "natural" domestic femininity asserted nothing but their "great ignorance of life and history."

The suffrage movement was the most important struggle for the expansion of women's rights in history. And from the very beginning, women's need to regain control of their bodies from society's—and medicine's—pernicious constraints was at the center of this struggle. For early advocates like Taylor Mill, Seneca Falls represented the inauguration of this movement. But women's suffrage emerged and advanced against a complex backdrop of heroism and division, collective force, and splintered factions. Despite the fact that Frederick Douglass was instrumental in galvanizing support for suffrage at Seneca Falls, white suffragists, namely Elizabeth Cady Stanton, failed to integrate and represent the needs and voices of Black women in the *Declaration of Sentiments*. Black leaders of the abolitionist movement across the United States had been organizing and campaigning for Black people to be afforded the same rights as whites for years before Seneca Falls.

In 1851, at the women's rights convention in Akron, Ohio, Sojourner Truth, the lecturer and abolitionist, stood up and declared, "I am a woman's rights." Truth's speech, known as "Ain't I a Woman?," is one of history's most important articulations of women's and civil rights. Truth was born into slavery. She gained her freedom in 1828. As the only slave-born representative at the convention, she spoke powerfully to the fact that rights for women had to mean rights for *all* women. Truth's "women's rights" were there in her muscles, which could "do as much work as any man"; in her strength to reap, husk, plow, chop, and mow; in her appetite, her "pint-full" intellect. Her "women's rights" were a truth of her being and a reality of her body. Truth's speech was incredibly inspiring to Black women and antislavery and suffrage activists. In May 1867, she gave a rousing speech at the first anniversary of the American Equal Rights Association, an organization formed at the Worcester convention to "secure Equal Rights to all American citizens, especially the right of suffrage, irrespective of race, color or sex." In the years following the end of the Civil War and the ratification of the Thirteenth Amendment to outlaw slavery, important campaigns to extend the civil and voting rights of emancipated men left women questioning the inclusion of their rights in constitutional changes. "There is a great stir about colored men getting their rights, but not a word about the colored women," proclaimed Truth. "And if colored men get their rights, and not colored women theirs . . . I suppose I am about the only colored woman that goes about to speak for the rights of the colored women. I want to keep the thing stirring, now that the ice is cracked."

In 1869, the Fifteenth Amendment was passed, granting voting rights to men regardless of "race, color or previous condition of servitude." Stanton had famously announced that she would "cut off this right arm of mine before I will ever work or demand the ballot for the Negro and not the woman." Others shared her opinions, and, incensed at the denial of women's elective franchise in the amendment, the groups splintered until 1889, when they re-formed as the National American Woman Suffrage Association, which focused solely on achieving women's voting rights. As the cultural critic Evette Dionne writes, "There was no commitment to ending discrimination, poverty, lynching, or any of the other urgent issues that mattered to black women." In suffrage associations and women's clubs, Black activists, writers, and educators, including Ida B. Wells-Barnett and Mary Church Terrell, contributed to the fight for women's suffrage alongside the expansion and protection of the civil and social rights of Black people, rights that had been cast aside by the movement's dominant white leaders.

Sadly, Harriet Taylor Mill did not live to see the progression of the campaign she galvanized. She died in Avignon, France, in 1858, of respiratory failure caused by a mysterious illness. As women's suffrage campaigns were crystallizing in the United States, the debates that Taylor Mill had brought to the fore in Britain were also growing into a national movement. Support, at political and grassroots levels, was swelling. Women's suffrage groups formed in London, Manchester, and Edinburgh, and in November 1867 the scientist and activist Lydia Becker formed the National Society for Women's Suffrage, the foundational organization of the British movement. But as campaigns for women's enfranchisement gained public and political attention, detractors started loudly voicing their objections. Women's suffrage was not just a campaign for equal voting rights and political participation. Suffragists were fighting against all the conditions and circumstances that limited women's lives and freedoms. And that meant all the sexist ideologies behind society's insistence that women should limit their lives, ambitions, and desires to the "separate sphere" of marriage and motherhood. And these ideologies had been consistently reflected, validated, and justified by medicine. While women were striving to overturn the disempowering limitations imposed on their bodies and minds for centuries, anti-feminist medical men were using their knowledge as weapons to uphold those limitations.

When Stuart Mill published his famous work *The Subjection of Women* in 1869, he argued that women's "legal subordination" was based on entirely false assumptions about mental acuity, nervous constitution, and biological purpose. Borrowing from his wife Taylor Mill's essay, he explained that there was nothing "natural" about the medical lore of female inferiority. But for men like the influential neurologist, psychologist, and asylum physician James Crichton-Browne—whose whole career was based on upholding male physiological and psychological supremacy— ideas like Stuart Mill's were laughable fictions. Crichton-Browne was heavily invested in Charles Darwin's theories of the evolutionary bases of sex differences. They were friends and collaborators who corresponded while Darwin was writing *Descent of Man, and Selection in Relation to Sex* (1871). For Crichton-Browne, Darwin's theories were irrefutable proof of women's mental and physical inferiority, and also their hereditary susceptibility to insanity, hysteria, and other diseases of the mind. How could the Mills claim the subjection of women was cultural and social when Darwin proved it was not only innate but also essential for the perpetuation and survival of the human race?

"The bodily differences between men and women which underlie their intellectual disparities are universal and intimate, and involve every organ and tissue," declared Crichton-Browne. Female human animals, the Darwinists believed, were anabolic, which meant their metabolism was directed toward nurture and nourishment. Every cell of the female body reflected the most idealized feminine traits—"woman is more receptive, tranquil, affectionate . . . patient, trustful, compassionate, and timid." Male creatures were katabolic—active and energetic—so they were biologically fitted for bravery, passion, independence, intellect, and "originality." Darwinism conceded that women were more intuitive and perceptive than men. But these qualities were also indications of females' lower position on the evolutionary ladder, because they were "character-istic of . . . a lower state of civilization." And the proof of these inviola-ble gender differences, for Crichton-Browne, was in the postmortem pudding.

After supervising more than four hundred autopsies at the West Rid-ing Pauper Lunatic Asylum in Wakefield, Yorkshire during the 1860s and 1870s, Crichton-Browne concluded that not only was the female brain smaller and lighter, but its gray matter—the region of cells involved in decision making, memory, self-control, speech, and sensory perception—was of a "lower specific gravity." Women were protected from "male" degenerative brain diseases by their "anabolic habit" and "tranquil and sheltered lives." But "if all this is to be altered" by allowing them to "struggle for life on equal terms with men," they would sacrifice their immunity to the most destructive forms of insanity. Suffrage was exactly the kind of "alteration" Crichton-Browne was sure would cause incalculable injuries to women's taxed bodies and diminished little minds. Women were already vulnerable to "functional" nervous disorders aplenty if they even entertained thoughts of a life beyond the "narrow sphere." Imagine what "unfortunate results" would ensue if their desire for political parity were actually indulged? If a woman tried to exceed her feminine destiny, her mind—and body—would inevitably collapse under its own rebellious weight.

In January 1878, Senator Aaron Sargent proposed extending suffrage through the so-called Susan B. Anthony Amendment. A petition of thirty thousand signatures gathered by suffrage societies was then pre-sented to the Senate Committee on Privileges and Elections that June. But the committee decided to "indefinitely postpone" the issue, because "it would be unjust, unwise, and impolitic" to impose such burdens on "the great mass of women . . . who do not wish for it, to gratify the few that do." Women could already vote in the territories of Wyoming, Utah, and Washington. On January 25, 1887, the year after the Select

Committee on Woman Suffrage was formed, the amendment was finally debated. Opponents trotted out the same old arguments about the "female sex" existing to make the "home sweet and pure." Female "emotionality" was at odds with the logic required in public affairs; women should be content in the "jurisdiction" of wife and mother; who would feed the babies when they were out at the ballots?—and so on and so on. Senator Joseph Dolph of Oregon thought "sex distinction" was the least defensible argument against votes for women: "God speed the day when . . . women shall stand before the law freed from the last shackle which has been riveted on her by tyranny and the last disability that has been imposed upon her by ignorance." The Senate also considered statements from members of the National Women's Suffrage Association heard by the Select Committee back in 1884. They spoke of the support within their communities and countered accusations that suffragists were all unhappy wives and dissatisfied mothers. Mary Seymour Howell, a leading New York activist, spoke passionately about how important the vote was for all women, from the "married" to the "fallen." Those who claimed not to want suffrage, she said, were being kept in the dark about how diminished their social and civic rights actually were. The senators submitted their votes, but the amendment was defeated. The fight for women's right to be heard continued.

In 1894, Mary Putnam Jacobi, the heroic detractor of medical misogyny, published her book *Common Sense Applied to Woman Suffrage*, in which she skewered the fallacious arguments of the anti-suffragists, or "antis," while explaining why women urgently needed the vote. How could anyone still claim that women were suited only to domesticity—the 1880 census had shown that over 2.5 million were already in employment. Who could deny that they were contributing to the "wealth of the state"? And surely no one really believed that subordination was for their benefit and protection? The Married Women's Property acts, passed in the US and UK, meant women's independent citizenship was legally enshrined. Women could now receive higher education equal to that of men; they had the same rights to practice in the medical profession as men.

Putnam Jacobi saw Seneca Falls as the beginning of a revolution, not only toward women's suffrage but against dominant medical and social justifications for all their diminished rights. "Until to-day," she wrote, "the incapacity of women for the suffrage was attributed, not merely to their deficiency in physical force, but to the profound mental and moral inferiority of her entire nature." This antiquated belief, cemented into "Canon Law" by "Adam's seduction by Eve" had been a very efficient patriarchal-control measure. But its force, thankfully, was waning. With withering precision, Putnam Jacobi attacked some loathsome antis, including British historian Goldwin Smith. She quipped that his influential 1875 article "Female Suffrage" was "a wonderful collection of unrelated parts." Smith saw suffrage campaigns as a callous conspiracy to destroy "relations between the sexes" and bring about "national emasculation." Smith, by the way, thought "wife-beating" was an acceptable response to "husband-nagging." He also thought marriage restrained men from acting on their most forceful "passions"; so if women got the vote, it would be their own fault when "surplus" unmarried men turned into rapists.

Men like Smith had become "accustomed" to seeing women as "sex, and nothing else." Suffrage was forcing them to face the inconvenient truth that women were human people and not baby-making serfs. The antis couldn't, or wouldn't, accept that women could marry, bear children, work, and have a say in politics. The "differentiation of the sexes," Putnam Jacobi observed, was "merely . . . the permanent maintenance of such inequality of horizon and opportunity as shall always leave women at some disadvantage." Men who opposed suffrage *delighted* in keeping women at a disadvantage. "All the feminine charm, all the womanly grace . . . that from the beginning of time men have been ascribing to women, does not lie in them, but outside of them," she wrote. "It is not a potency, it is a situation; it is not a natural force, it is a political contrivance; it has not been celebrated in poetry and song because men love women, but only because men love to order women around! What a mournful disillusion!"

No matter how intelligently Putnam Jacobi and others called them out, the antis didn't waver. Anti-suffrage women were among the most zealous parrots of these views. In 1899, the New York State Association

Opposed to Woman Suffrage told the International Congress of Women that no "possible future conditions can ever alter the physiological differences between the sexes." "Once the incontrovertible and unalterable fact of physical limitation is faced . . . all the plausible arguments about this question of the suffrage . . . fall away." That year, the Massachusetts Association Opposed to the Further Extension of Suffrage to Women included a reprint of an egregious piece of internalized misogyny called "Nature's Stern Barrier," by journalist and poet Katherine E. Conway, in the new periodical *The Remonstrance*. "We never can have the physical strength of men," she insisted. Women's "mental outlook," "personal feelings," and "over-sensitive consciences" were an impediment to political progress. Female "partisanship is . . . intense and exhausting," and the "strenuous business" of "direct participation . . . will of a certainty injure women."

In July 1908, the British Women's National Anti-suffrage League launched the *Anti-suffrage Review*. The first issue announced that women of "sound mind" did not want the duty of voting: "Have not the spectacles of the last few weeks shown conclusively that women are not fit for the ordinary struggles of politics, and are degraded by it? Their nerves are of a different tension from men's." On June 21, thirty thousand suffragists marched through London's Hyde Park in seven processions. Organized by Emmeline Pankhurst, who founded the national Women's Social and Political Union (WSPU) in Manchester in 1903 with her daughters Christabel and Sylvia, "Women's Sunday" was the was the largest women's political rally the country had ever seen. By the end of the nineteenth century, some were allowed to vote in county and borough council elections. The National Union of Women's Suffrage Societies, formed by Millicent Fawcett, had united suffragist organizations across the country. But peaceful campaigns had led to only so much change.

The WSPU called for direct action in the fight for political equality for all women, regardless of social class, marital status, or occupation. Famously, its motto was "Deeds, not words." But the new prime minister, Herbert Henry Asquith, strongly objected. Asquith had challenged the women of Britain to prove they wanted the vote, and "Women's

Sunday" was their answering cry. A reform bill had been debated but not passed in 1905. Angered by being so near but yet so far, the WSPU began campaigns of civil disobedience—protesting, heckling, and lobbying—in 1906. Soon, WSPU members were chaining themselves to the railings of government buildings. After a protest outside Asquith's house in June, three suffragists were detained in London's Holloway Prison. As the WSPU's activism escalated over the next two years, so did the number of suffragists being locked up. By 1908, around three hundred had been imprisoned for acts of protest.

On December 5, 1908, while Emmeline and Christabel Pankhurst were confined in Holloway, a group of WSPU members attended a meeting of the Women's Liberal Foundation at London's Albert Hall. Chancellor of the Exchequer David Lloyd George—who was in favor of votes for women—was giving a speech. The WSPU were eager to hear his "definite pledge . . . of immediate action in the matter." All they heard were "sympathetic" and "hollow" declarations that a reform bill would be debated soon. For the WSPU this was "the last insult." They "had asked for bread, and the Chancellor . . . offered them a stone." Women seated near the speakers' platform stood up and removed their cloaks to reveal prison garb. Three hundred Liberal Party stewards were installed in the hall, and policemen lined the corridors. To defend herself against the assaults frequently meted out by male stewards, Helen Ogston had a dog whip hidden in her clothing. She was the first to raise her voice and was immediately set upon "with great violence." She struck her whip at the worst offender before being dragged into the corridor, where she was rescued by a Liberal woman doctor. Dissent mounted in the hall. Women chanted, "Deeds not words. Deeds not words." Each time George tried to speak, he was drowned out by more shouts. More suffragists were roughly hustled out. When George proclaimed, "If Queen Elizabeth . . . had been born today," one retorted, "She would have been in Holloway Prison!"

Two days later, the WSPU newspaper *Votes for Women* reported on the stewards' "excessive violence and brutality." "Women were seized, flung down . . . or dragged out, and pommelled . . . when they were perfectly powerless to resist." Some were sexually assaulted once they

were in the corridors and "outside the control of public opinion." Anger
from both sides of the political fence filled the newspapers. Whether one
was for or against votes for women, the spectacle of violence against
them—in front of a representative of the British government—was scandalous. "Brutality was witnessed by so many spectators that there is now
no attempt at denial," *Votes for Women* stated. The suffragists' bodies were
now the battleground in this most inflammatory ideological war. For the
WSPU, women's willingness to face violence showed the "strongest de-
termination to make their protest against injustice heard."

The week after the meeting, a drawing of Ogston's self-defense
graced the *London Illustrated News*. "The Woman with the Whip"
symbolized the extremity of the WSPU's "militancy," and the British
and American press responded vividly. The "coarse" and "unchival-
rous" stewards were deplored. But these "shrieking women" and "silly
viragos" proved that women were "wholly incapable of governing themselves," let alone governing others. According to *The Globe*, their behavior demonstrated that women were pathologically incapable of keeping
a lid on their emotions. Give women like these the vote and the "whole
of politics" would be confused "by an injection of hysteria." Crying
"hysteria" was a provocative way of belittling the campaigners and un-
dermining the seriousness of the cause. These women were not trying
to bring about social and political change, critics charged; they were a
coven of hysterics who had lost control of their bodies and minds. *The
Globe* remarked that recent events were enough "to make the thoughtful
wonder whether the abolition of the branks and the cucking-stool may
not have been somewhat premature." Quipping about bringing back
methods of torture reserved for angry women in medieval times was,
apparently, completely warranted. "The ducking-stool and a nice deep
pool were our fore-fathers plan for a scold. Could I have my way, each
Suffragette to-day, should 'take the chair' and find the water cold," chimed
a rhyme on an anti-suffrage postcard. The suffragists were the modern-
day scolds, the disorderly hags, the deviant witches.

On December 11, 1908, *The Times* ran an editorial containing a "diagnosis" of the WSPU's "hysteric morbidity": "One does not need to be
against women suffrage to see that some of the more violent partisans

of the cause are suffering from hysteria. We use the word not with any scientific precision, but because it is the name most commonly given to a kind of enthusiasm that has degenerated into habitual nervous excitement." They were obviously emotionally stressed and had taken leave of their faculties. Their herd mentality proved they were weak-minded and imitative. They had caught hysteria from other "extremists"—and "once spread it is very difficult to control." They were clearly concerned only with indulging their insatiable passions—no matter how immoral. The *New York Times* thought the article, titled "Hysterical Excitement," was "the most interesting contribution to the current literature of the question."

Until 1908, the antis' connection between suffrage and women's health was vague and abstracted. They peddled pseudomedical, Darwinian notions about the terrible consequences of women transgressing nature's boundaries. But in September 1909, the extent to which women would suffer for suffrage was thrown into harrowing relief. Mary Leigh, a working-class teacher and WSPU member from Manchester, was sentenced to two weeks in Birmingham's Winson Green Prison after protesting her exclusion from a meeting at Bingley Hall where Asquith was speaking. Leigh and two others climbed onto the roof, pulled tiles up with hand axes, and flung them at policemen and Asquith's car. In prison Leigh went on a hunger strike, like others before her, to protest being treated as a criminal and not a political prisoner. Fasting suffragists had usually been released to preserve their health. But as more went on hunger strikes while serving short sentences, wardens worried other prisoners would adopt the tactic. The government was also adamant that the suffragists would not be praised as martyrs. In September 1909, Home Secretary Herbert Gladstone authorized prison doctors to forcibly feed any suffragist refusing food.

One afternoon, two wardresses and doctors entered Leigh's cell. The wardresses held her down while one doctor inserted a rubber tube up her nose and down her throat. The other poured milk down the tube through a funnel. "The sensation is most painful," she told her solicitor. "The drums of the ears seem to be bursting and there is a horrible pain in the throat and the breast. The tube is pushed down 20 inches." When it was over, Leigh was sprinkled with cologne and locked in a punishment cell. She was subjected to this ordeal many times.

The suffragist community, members of the medical profession, and the public were shocked that such procedures were being inflicted on women. *Votes for Women* published statements from sympathetic doctors about its dangers, especially for those with underlying health problems like lung weakness, heart disease, digestive disorders, and bronchial complaints. Responding to letters about "fasting prisoners" in the *British Medical Journal*, Louisa Garrett Anderson, the pioneering physician, surgeon, and suffragist, and daughter of Elizabeth, decried "forced feeding" as an "experiment" being performed on already unwell women for the purpose of political posturing. One Dr. Roberts feared suffragists would be driven insane by such "revolting torture" and "official cruelty." Mary Richardson, the Canadian-born suffragist, was one of scores of women forcibly fed before the beginnings of World War I when the WSPU suspended its campaigns. While serving six months in Holloway for an arson attack, she endured the "operation" of nasal feeding by the prison physician, Dr. Pearson, thirty times. A representative from the Home Office assessed her case and decided she should be fed down the throat. Richardson refused, so Pearson pulled her teeth apart and inserted a screwed steel gag to force her mouth wide open. "I cried out at his cruelty . . . I was almost driven mad by it."

Pearson claimed Richardson was in a "dangerous state of mind." She stated that he punished her by instructing wardresses to refuse to open her cell and to shout at her as if she were "a lunatic." She also said she was given "curious mixtures" before her feedings. When she asked Pearson what the foul-smelling stuff was, he replied, "That's my business." Richardson was convinced she was being dosed with bromide, a sedative and anticonvulsant. In her statement, she warned that unwitting drugging was becoming a frighteningly common tactic. "Mr. McKenna [Reginald McKenna, then home secretary] knows that to even temporarily check the Suffragette defiance of physical torture he must introduce something to deaden the minds of his defiant prisoners."

Richardson had been imprisoned before. She had gained a reputation as one of WSPU's most militant members. After a previous sentence, she swore an affidavit that Pearson said he would starve her until she was "a skeleton and a nervous and mental wreck." He also threatened to send her "to an institution where they look after nervous wrecks" if she reoffended. In the House of Commons, the Liberal MP Josiah Wedgwood asked McKenna if there would be any inquiry into Richardson's allegations. McKenna said her statements were "wholly inaccurate." Pearson had simply warned her of the "mischief she might do to herself, physically and mentally, by refusing food." He was responding as any caring doctor should to a patient hell-bent on injuring herself. Richardson's allegations were dismissed given the conflict of evidence.

McKenna endorsed "artificial feeding," as he coolly referred to it, as a therapeutic measure to save the lives of suicidal suffragists. The practice, he said, was "unattended by danger and pain" and presented no danger to life unless it was met with "violent resistance." This is chillingly reminiscent of prominent English gynecologist Robert Lawson-Tait's infamous assumption that "no man can affect a felonious purpose on a woman in possession of her senses without her consent" because "you cannot thread a moving needle." He was implying, despicably, that rape was impossible if women submitted, and that if a woman claimed she was raped, she must have submitted. The violation, the assault, was not in the action but in the resistance to it. McKenna, similarly, was suggesting that women's refusal to submit to a horrific abuse of their bodies was the cause of their suffering. This assessment is particularly sickening, because some suffrage prisoners were force-fed through the rectum and vagina.

For centuries, many medical "cures" for women's apparent deviancy and defiance had been punishments masquerading as therapies. Force-feeding was not a health-preservation measure; it was an unremittingly cruel tactic to break women's resolve, to weaken their will, and to make them submit. Women's suffrage, according to many physicians, was already a destructive illness, a dangerous pathology. By virtue of their intent to upset male supremacy, these women were displaying all the traits of mental breakdown, insane possession, and hysteria. Over the past three decades, hysteria evolved from a clinical speculation into a gendered slur. Those suffragists who fought back against the horrors of the feeding tube were resisting all the social forces that for too long had justified medicine's attempts to diminish women's lives and control their bodies.

10

BIRTH CONTROL

Throughout the suffrage movement, women rose up against medicine's complicity in the social control and limitation of women's lives and rights. Force-feeding, like so many punishments meted out to women "for their own good," was just one of the ways that male-dominated medicine continued to establish dominance over women's bodies and minds. In the delivery room, where women performed their sacred duty of bringing new life into the world, women were still suffering because of medicine's misogynistic insistence on the necessity of pain. Back in 1871, Elizabeth Cady Stanton condemned the "sufferings of maternity" in a speech titled "On Marriage and Divorce" at a women's rights convention in San Francisco. The "torture of bearing children" was a punishment forced on women in a society that held the female sex responsible for all the world's sin. Medicine then claimed that obeying the "natural law" of childbearing was the only way for women to obtain "health and happiness." The passage from the book of Genesis that women "in sorrow . . . shall bring forth children" still dominated perceptions that pain was women's lot in life.

It had been possible for women to receive pain relief during labor since the mid-nineteenth century, when James Young Simpson pioneered "blessed chloroform." But obstetric anesthesia was not routine. By the early 1900s, most women still gave birth at home, assisted by midwives and family members. Inhalation anesthetics like chloroform, and also ether and nitrous oxide, were available only from a physician.

Even if a woman could afford to be attended by a general practitioner or obstetrician, she would be offered anesthetics only if he was able—and willing—to administer them. Many physicians had doubts about safety and efficacy; others denounced narcotic intervention in the "natural" process of childbirth on moral and religious grounds. Aside from beliefs that anesthetics were dangerous, time-wasting, and likely to drive women erotically insane, most physicians still felt that *they* should be the judges of the pain of childbirth. Attitudes such as those perpetuated by Charles Meigs, that labor pains were physiologically essential *and* not nearly as severe as women claimed, had dominated arguments against obstetric pain relief for decades.

Challenging the necessity and inevitability of pain became an important part of women's struggle for freedom from social and medical mystifications. And these debates continue today, though most obstetricians and midwives aren't insisting that women must endure labor pain as a God-given punishment. But many who give birth in hospitals and maternity facilities still find that their decisions and needs, especially around anesthetic and analgesic interventions—such as epidural spinal blocks and opioid pain relief—are delayed, ignored, trivialized, or denied. Pervasive myths still circulate around the benefits of so-called natural and normal births, leading many women who are permitted pain relief to internalize the false idea that they have failed in some way—as women and as mothers. In the early 1900s, for women who were committed to the suffrage agenda but also wanted children, wresting back control of childbirth was a way to establish their rights to be in charge of their own bodies and medical experiences. And the motivations behind these burgeoning campaigns—affording women the respect and dignity of body autonomy and informed medical choice—are just as urgent today.

Another way of giving birth, in a place where women's pain was taken seriously enough to alleviate it, was being developed in the early 1900s, at the Frauenklinik, the women's hospital of the State University in Freiburg, a city on the edge of the Black Forest in Baden, Germany. Two obstetricians were perfecting a birth method in which women's pain would miraculously float away. And the realization that a birth experience like this was possible was, for many women, a revelation. Over the next decade, the efforts of women patients and women's rights activists would change not only women's experiences and perceptions of pain, but the medical and social culture of reproduction and motherhood.

In 1913, an American suffragist and writer named Mary Sumner Boyd traveled from New York to Freiburg to experience this wondrous new pain-free labor. Headed by the leading obstetric physician Bernhard Krönig and his assistant Karl Gauss, the Frauenklinik was then the only place in the world where women were able to give birth during *Dämmerschlaf,* or "twilight sleep." When Boyd felt the pangs of her first contraction, she was injected with a combination of morphine and scopolamine—a psychoactive derived from nightshade plants. She started to feel drowsy. A second injection of scopolamine plunged her into "clouded consciousness."

When she awoke, her washed, fed, swaddled newborn was brought to her by a nurse. She felt as if she had been slumbering peacefully, but in reality she had lain on her back as an obstetrician and a nurse guided her through her labor. She responded willingly to their instructions; pushing when asked to push, panting when told to hold back. She delivered her baby with her own muscles. Her body endured all the pain of this incredible effort. But her mind couldn't recall a thing. Scopolamine acted as an amnesiac, wiping away the memory of pain. Recovering in her private room overlooking the mountains, she marveled at the miracle of her "painless child."

Boyd hadn't been instructed to undergo *Dämmerschlaf* by her physician or her husband. She'd found out about it from New York society women who had given birth at the Frauenklinik and rhapsodized about their experiences. Krönig and Gauss had given *Dämmerschlaf* to the women of Freiburg since 1906, and affluent women from Russia, India, and South Africa had made the painless pilgrimage. Boyd's friend, Mrs. Temple Emmett, was the first American to "brave the Dämmerschlaf." She happened to be in Freiburg while she was pregnant and made arrangements to have her baby at the Frauenklinik. But her experience was not a tranquil dream. Her early contractions were agonizing, and her first morphine hit was no match for the "violence of the pains." She recalled "being bound and helpless." During *Dämmerschlaf*, women remained on their backs with their legs hoisted into stirrups, and often their wrists were restrained. Balls of oil-soaked cotton wool were placed in their ears. When babies were born, their cries were muffled with a cloth. The soundproof room with double-padded doors was kept dark, save for the soft green glow of the *Dämmerschlaf* lamp. Krönig insisted that "shielding" women from all "mental and physical stimulation" was essential for maintaining the delicate state of "clouded consciousness." All these "preparations" happened after they were "put to sleep."

At one point, Mrs. Emmett was woken by a bright examination lamp. The nurse quickly placed a thick gauze mask over her face. Bound to her bed and deprived of her senses, she received her second scopolamine injection and "went immediately into a perfect Dämmerschlaf." She remembered nothing more of her labor. Her ordeal sounds, at the very least, frightening and disorienting. But her relief at being released from pain and fear convinced her to submit to sleep for her second and third babies. Both times she received scopolamine before her pains began, and she retained "not a trace of a memory."

Since 1900, scopolamine had been used occasionally as a surgical anesthetic, but this chemically precarious drug could be extremely dangerous. The idea that scopolamine might be combined with morphine as an obstetric pain reliever was first proposed by Richard von Steinbüchel, a doctor at Freiburg University. The dose to relieve laboring women was much smaller than that needed during surgeries, so Steinbüchel was confident it posed no risks to mother or baby. Krönig and Gauss furthered Steinbüchel's work by concocting a perfectly balanced dose that ensured the "complete *forgetfulness* of the course of birth" by removing the mental perception of pain. In the semicomatose state, "external impressions glide off" because scopolamine disturbed "the circulation of such a kind that the pain perceived by the nerves is not felt by the woman, or in any case it disappears . . . soon from the memory." Since the success of *Dämmerschlaf* depended on how little women could remember, Krönig and Gauss devised a test to ensure the amnesiac properties of their magical elixir. After the second injection, their patient was shown an object. Half an hour later she was shown it again and asked if she recognized it. If she did, she was given an additional dose. Otherwise no "repetition of the dose should be given until memory exists."

It wasn't only the promise of relief from pain that convinced women to submit to such medically controlled births. In 1908, Krönig claimed that his scopolamine-morphine dose had "no unfavorable influence" if it was administered by an obstetrician who supervised the entire labor. Urine tests on newborns suggested that scopolamine was passed to them in quantities too small to be harmful. Sometimes, babies were born struggling for breath. This was only temporary, Krönig assured, and nothing that a brisk massage from a nurse wouldn't cure. Of the 1,500 *Dämmerschlaf* births recorded, only one woman died. Of course, this had *nothing* to do with the drugs she received. Her pelvis was apparently too narrow. Her husband refused to consent to a cesarean section. She bled to death after her uterus ruptured.

Despite these haunting risks, the Frauenklinik still boasted mortality rates that were unbelievably small compared with those in the United States. Even though childbirth was becoming more medicalized—at least for women who could afford it—it wasn't any less perilous. Maternal deaths in the United States were among the highest in the world. The US census of 1910 identified the "puerperal state" as the leading cause of death in women between the ages of twenty and thirty-nine. An astounding 45.5 percent of all women's deaths between twenty and twenty-nine occurred either during childbirth or within six weeks afterward. Childbirth was more of a danger than accidents, cancers, diabetes, heart diseases, congenital defects, and contagious illnesses. The second most common cause of death in women of these age groups was suicide. Protracted labors often left women with perineal tears and lacerations in their cervixes and vaginal tissues, which could lead to fistulas and uterine prolapses. Women were also at risk of infections and fatal sepsis if they hemorrhaged after delivery. Over the last decades of the nineteenth century, forceps had become increasingly popular. But if this instrument was wielded by inexpert hands, the consequences for both mother and baby were terrible. Whether a woman deserved pain relief before the metal tongs were forced into her birth canal was left to the physician's discretion.

"Happy mothers," Stanton had declared, could never be made out of "sick women" haunted by the "dark shadows" cast over "the best part of their lives." Women's homes had become hospitals, since they were left with no choice but to deliver multiple children and raise them while depleted of "health and happiness." The dangers of delivery, the horrors of its aftermath, and the inevitability of torturous pain instilled fear into women's hearts. From the late 1800s, obstetricians who supported anesthetics argued that the drugs relieved "insufferable agony" while making deliveries safer and speedier. Many of these more sympathetic physicians acknowledged that fear of pain was a dangerous impediment to the birthing process. But not all women were created equal when it came to pain tolerance and sensitivity. That decades-old notion prevailed that the more "civilized" a woman was, the less she could bear the trials of childbirth. Stanton expressed this in 1852 in a letter to Lucretia Mott, after she had given birth easily to her daughter, who weighed twelve pounds. "Am I not almost a savage?" Stanton wrote. "For what refined, delicate, genteel, civilized woman would get so well in so indecently short a time?"

It was racist and classist value judgments like these that compelled Krönig to pioneer *Dämmerschlaf.* He observed that complicated births were widespread in affluent, educated women whose pain tolerance was diminished by fine living and too much thinking. "The modern woman," he explained in a lecture in 1908, "responds to the stimulus of severe pain more rapidly with nervous exhaustion and paralysis of the will to carry labor to a conclusion." Women who carried out "hard mental work" were apparently far more sensitive to pain than those who "earn their living by manual labor." It was among "nervous" women that the use of forceps had increased "to an alarming extent." Even in experienced hands, forceps increased the risk of lacerations, hemorrhages, uterine prolapse, and infections. Injudicious use was tantamount to butchery. Krönig could see no physiological reason for forceps being so overzealously used. He believed the only thing forceps relieved was the mother's pain, which was prolonging labors and leaving them unable to exert enough muscular power to push. For women who were "incapable of enduring the pains . . . to the end," an operative delivery was the only solution.

Krönig remarked that any doctor who observed the "whole course of labor" in a nervous woman of the "better classes" would agree that her pain was *not* advantageous. Obstetricians who could listen to "screams and groans" and still denounce anesthetics were callous or ignorant. Krönig was also concerned about how pain trauma affected women's mental and physical health before and after their babies were born. He believed that pain's memory, and its fearful anticipation, manifested in nervous exhaustion, "numerous body complaints," and "hypochondriacal moods" during pregnancy. This sense of impending doom was heightened by women hearing about their friends' long and painful deliveries. It wasn't the physical sensation of pain that was problematic, he said, but the negative emotions women attached to it.

Boyd was exactly the kind of "civilized" woman Krönig had in mind. She was incredibly nervous about her impending labor. Her sister had suffered terribly for twenty-four hours before her labor properly began, and she was an "invalid" for months afterward. Boyd also believed her "structural defects"—a narrow birth canal—meant she wouldn't escape the forceps. But as soon as she heard about the Frauenklinik, her fears melted away. Boyd was good friends with Mrs. Cecil Stewart, the second American woman to have experienced *Dämmerschlaf.* Meeting Stewart's strong and bonny one-year-old was all the reassurance Boyd needed.

Accompanied by her friend Marguerite Tracy—Stewart's sister—Boyd arrived at the Frauenklinik on a dark midwinter morning. Her "hour had come." The head nurse, who never seemed to sleep, showed her to the confinement room, decorated blue for a boy. There were four "classes" of ward at the Frauenklinik, and the first-class ward was reserved for the most nervous patients. It also happened to be the most expensive. Boyd, a first-class patient, received the highest level of care and the fanciest recovery situation. She went to bed and waited for her labor to progress. By 4:00 p.m. her contractions were stronger and more regular, and her pain was rising. After two hours, the nurse arrived with her hypodermic loaded with "sleep." The pains dragged on, and in time she received her second injection. She fell "dead asleep" almost immediately.

A few hours later she woke up: "I was frightened in a dreamy way, as if I was in a vault, alive, but put away like the dead." She realized she had no pain and worried she had been given the scopolamine too soon. She crossed her hands and wished for sleep. Then the nurse brought her a "brisk and lively" baby boy wrapped in a papoose. "I had wakened from a ten-hour labor believing I had been caught napping and the labor was before me," she wrote. "While my brain was sleeping, my muscles and nerves had been working and I had brought forth the baby . . . by my own efforts." Her birth had been accomplished with "no laceration, no exhaustion," and no dreaded forceps. The next night Boyd had distended pupils, numb fingers, thirst, and sweats from the scopolamine, but otherwise she felt remarkably well. An hour after the birth, she was doing the exercises the nurses recommended to restore her figure. She enjoyed lavish lunches of soup, omelets, boiled beef, cabbage, roast hare, potatoes, carrots, peas, salad, dessert, and beer. Between 10:00 p.m. and 10:00 a.m. her baby was whisked away to the nursery so she could rest. She spent ten days recovering in perfect peace. "The night of my confinement will always be a night dropped out of my life," she wrote.

Unbeknownst to Krönig, Gauss, and the nurses, Boyd was no ordinary patient. She was working undercover for Marguerite Tracy, who was writing an exposé for *McClure's Magazine* with journalist Constance Leupp. They had tried to interview Krönig and Gauss, but the obstetricians were "baffling and obstructive to the last degree." So they based their report on the testimonies of "Freiburg mothers," who, as they put it, "animated" the dry obstetric and gynecological records they had pored over. Boyd embraced her role in bringing the wonders of the "painless child" to American women. If Krönig and Gauss didn't want to divulge their methods to a pair of women reporters, then Boyd would issue a "definite statement" that held as much value as a "laboratory experiment." Before her baby was born, Boyd inhaled all the available medical literature about *Dämmerschlaf*. But her own "confinement" provided insight that no journal could ever "furnish" in "experience or observation."

In June 1914, "Painless Childbirth" appeared in *McClure's*. Tracy and Leupp told the story of the clinical development, practical method, and experience of *Dämmerschlaf*, or, as they christened it, twilight sleep. Photographs of Boyd and Stewart with their "Freiburg babies" graced the pages, along with an image of a naked five-year-old German boy with his arms outstretched, to illustrate how robust *Dämmerschlaf*-born children became. They extolled the safety of twilight sleep, the calm beauty of the clinic, the focused efficiency of the nurses. And even though they found him frustratingly obstinate, they applauded Krönig for bringing scopolamine to obstetrics. "Painless Childbirth" was a call to arms for women to demand that Frauenklinik-level twilight sleep was made available to all women—or at least to those who could afford it. "That all women, 'modern' or 'old-fashioned' would desire that their child-bearing be made painless, if this is possible with safety, it is not open to debate," they wrote.

"Painless Childbirth" was a sensation. Two "laywomen" had exposed a revolutionary birth method that put women first. The following year, Tracy, with Boyd, published *Painless Childbirth*, a book version of the *McClure's* article that included the full testimonies of Boyd, Mrs. Stewart, and Mrs. Francis Carmody, who was the first American to go to Freiburg in response to "the Painless Childbirth propaganda." After reading the article, Carmody immediately phoned her physician, who "heartily endorsed" the Frauenklinik and promised to visit so that he could observe the method. Carmody's husband published a letter in the *Brooklyn Eagle* celebrating his wife's injury- and nerve-derangement-free delivery. He also praised the feast-level meals she consumed three times a day.

News of Freiburg's utopian maternity resort spread like wildfire. Articles about twilight sleep flooded the national and women's press. The *New York Times* credited Tracy and Leupp with revealing a birth method that "lifted . . . [the] primal curse of their sex." In 1913, Krönig and Gauss promoted their work to medical societies across the US. But according to the *Times*, physicians suppressed it because they were reluctant to learn a "delicate and difficult treatment," and even more so to avoid the hordes of expectant mothers who would start asking for it. But now twilight sleep had reached the public, and women were demanding it regardless of physicians' apprehensions. "It is, as far as we know," wrote Tracy and Boyd, "the first time in the history of medical science that the whole body of patients have risen up to dictate to the doctors."

Twilight sleep represented so much more than an innovation in childbirth. Tracy and Boyd promoted "painless childbirth" as a revolution in medicine's perception of female pain. For too long, women's pain, and their emotional relationship to it, had been dismissed and devalued. Male physicians had been the ones to assess it, measure it, and judge how it felt. But the punitive notion that women were biologically condemned to endure pain had no part in the *Dämmerschlaf* narrative. "It was the first time a doctor had ever admitted that I had a bad pain when I had one," Mrs. Stewart wrote. "Just Dr. Gauss's admitting that my pain *was* my pain made me comforted and happy. I felt at last that I had found a place where people realized that pain was pain."

Tracy and Boyd told distressing stories of women driven to extremes of mental illness by their fear of childbirth pain. Pain trauma permeated women's bodies and minds, shredding their nerves and disturbing their systems. But too often physicians dismissed their mental deterioration as "hysterical fear." Gauss believed that most of the nebulous uterine and ovarian symptoms that sent women to their gynecologists were not organic diseases at all but "nervous complaints" caused by the "memories of child-bearing to these organs." Tracy and Boyd agreed: "It is not for nothing that the word hysteria comes from the Greek word for womb," they wrote. "It is this racking of the soul, this distortion of the mind by the nerves which causes imaginary symptoms of uterine diseases." By "blotting out" both the memory and the foreboding of pain, *Dämmerschlaf* would rid women of the disturbances that plagued their bodies and lives, enabling them to love their children—and husbands—free from "morbid brooding." The press embraced twilight sleep as a blessing for marital harmony and birth rates among "civilized" women. "Through twilight sleep a new era has dawned for women and through her for the whole human race," proclaimed the *New York Times*.

When Carmody was awaiting the birth of her baby, she wrote to her women's club, excitedly confirming that everything in the *McClure's*

article was true. Within months, the campaign for twilight sleep became an activist movement, with upper- and middle-class women from
clubs and societies in New York and beyond forming the National Twilight Sleep Association (NTSA). Leading members included Carmody
and suffragist Mary Ware Dennett, the association's vice president.
Several female physicians embraced the cause, including Bertha Van
Hoosen, a Chicago-based obstetrician and gynecologist who objected
to the medical mistreatment of women. At rallies and demonstrations
at women's clubs, theaters, and department stores, NTSA members
evangelized twilight sleep while parading their "Freiburg babies."
During a speech at a New York branch of the department store Gim-
bels, Carmody exclaimed, "If you women want it you will have to fight
for it; for the mass of doctors are opposed to it."

By 1915, handfuls of hospitals and private clinics across the country
were offering scopolamine-morphine. Van Hoosen, who had used
scopolamine as a surgical anesthetic for years, had been overseeing
twilight deliveries at Chicago's Mary Thompson Hospital since June
1914. She analyzed one hundred deliveries and concluded that the drugs
presented no danger to the life or development of the fetus and were of
great benefit to women's bodies and minds. She claimed twilight sleep
improved the life-chances of babies and would fill the country with
"strong, normal" mothers. "It is the greatest boon the Twentieth Century could give to women," she wrote. Despite these glowing endorse-
ments, the practice was massively contentious—not least because demand
was led by "unqualified" women. Several medical journals laughed off
twilight sleep as a craze and a quack scheme. But many physicians raised
genuine concerns about the risks of scopolamine, especially to babies
born with breathing difficulties. Others questioned the unspoken psychological impact of what was happening to women while they were
robbed of conscious control.

In 1915, Hanna Rion, a journalist for women's publications including
Ladies' Home Journal, wrote, "In the old-fashioned days [women] . . . had
no choice but to trust themselves without question in the hands of the
all-wise physician, but that day is past and will return no more. Women
have torn away the bandages of false-modesty, they are no longer

ashamed of their bodies . . ." But Rion's empowering words masked the disturbing dark side of twilight sleep. Women like Boyd and Carmody had experienced the Cadillac of *Dämmerschlaf* care. Their labors were supervised continuously; their scopolamine-morphine doses were belt-and-braces tested. Their aftercare—with its banquet lunches, indulgent "beauty-baths," and uninterrupted sleep—was more like a spa break than a hospital convalescence. But scopolamine, in reality, had absolved them of all control over their bodies. Since their labors happened in private rooms, with only obstetricians and nurses present, no one could testify to what went on behind those padded doors. If the scopolamine worked, there would be no need to know. As Tracy and Boyd admitted, "a description of her perfect Twilight Sleep can never be given subjectively by the patient. She can only report on the imperfect ones."

In 1914, a physician from Illinois bemoaned advocates for flaunting their babies as "evidence" that painless childbirth had "some magical far-reaching influence that changes the physical destiny of the child." He thought women were using their children to suppress criticism of a birth method that wasn't, in fact, painless at all. What they could not speak about was how their bodies had suffered as their minds slept. "The psychic influence on the subconscious mind of the pain of labor felt but not remembered . . . remains for the neurologist to elucidate." The public furor meant many physicians rushed to improvise twilight sleep at their hospitals and clinics. Women were often left alone for hours, restrained to their beds. Often, the scopolamine dose was not enough to abolish the memory of being semiconscious, restrained, and in excruciating pain. While Boyd was in labor, she had Tracy try to listen outside the door, and all she could discern were a few incoherent rambles and the occasional whimper. But as more obstetricians reported on scopolamine births, the brutal truth was beginning to emerge. Van Hoosen designed a sectional bed covered in a canvas screen, which shut out all noise and light. But it also prevented the "patient" from injuring herself when, in the grip of pains, she "throws herself about." She wore a white gown with a "continuous sleeve," basically a straitjacket, that bound her arms behind her back. Her face was shielded with a mask that left only her nostrils and mouth uncovered, and her ears were blocked with cotton wool. Her legs were tied tightly into stirrups, and strips of webbing were wrapped around her open thighs and secured to the end of the bed. Unable to move, see, or hear, she was imprisoned in her scopolamine gloom and entirely at the mercy of her physician.

After World War I broke out in July 1914, twilight sleep became the second most popular subject in the American national press. For the NTSA, campaigning for painless childbirth was a war in itself, a battle for women's right to choose how to give birth, to have their pain taken seriously, and to have their needs placed at center stage. Even though adverse effects were being reported, the NTSA wouldn't be defeated—it was leading a revolution in the medical treatment of women and their bodies. But in August 1915, a terrible tragedy forced the group to lay down its arms. Charlotte Carmody, the movement's most committed campaigner, died after giving birth to her third child under twilight sleep at Long Island College Hospital. She suffered a massive hemorrhage that might not have been caused by scopolamine, but still her death cast a grave shadow. The *New York Times* reported that Carmody's husband didn't blame her doctor or the drugs for his wife's death. The NTSA's mission to have America replicate the *Dämmerschlaf* had failed. But this was by no means entirely down to the NTSA whipping up demand or because obstetricians and physicians felt forced to bend to women's will. The fervor for scopolamine, in fact, had been an essential cog in the fast-turning wheel of obstetric professionalism.

By prioritizing women's birth pain as a symptom that could be cured, twilight sleep transformed childbirth into a pathological process that required operative and narcotic intervention as the norm, not the exception. Scopolamine could be offered only in hospitals and clinics, and twilight births had to be managed by obstetric physicians, most of whom, at the time, were male. For physicians who argued that medical intervention was essential for improving the country's woeful maternal mortality rates, this was a canny way of wresting childbirth from the hands of female midwives. In 1913, Joseph DeLee, the obstetrician who founded the Chicago Lying-In Hospital, issued a rallying cry for childbirth to *always* be medically managed. "Can a function so perilous," he wrote, "that . . . kills thousands of women every year, that leaves at least a quarter of women more or less invalidated . . . that is always attended by severe pain . . . and that kills 3 to 5% of children . . . be called normal?" A few years later DeLee, who became known as the father of modern obstetrics, used the "twilight sleep craze" to justify his "prophylactic forceps operation." For him, the demand for painless births proved that tokophobia—fear of pregnancy—had become endemic. His birth method consisted of sedative scopolamine injections in the early stages, ether in the second stage to relieve pains, an episiotomy—an incision in the perineum and vaginal wall—to allow babies' heads to pass more easily, and, finally, delivery using forceps. Afterward, a woman would have her placenta removed and her episiotomy site tightly stitched. DeLee proposed that these measures should be routine, and he framed their necessity around what *he* thought women wanted: to be left as "anatomically perfect as she was before."

After 1920, DeLee's methods became increasingly popular. "Preventative" intervention was routine in many maternity hospitals. The twilight sleep movement had, in a sense, achieved its ambition to revolutionize childbirth through medical science. But the intention to have women reclaim their bodies from medical control was trampled in the obstetricians' race to transform childbirth into an illness that required drugs, instruments, and brutal procedures. The NTSA died with Carmody, but the spirit of its campaigns continued into the beginnings of one of the most important feminist movements in medicine's history. Demanding twilight sleep was as much about women deciding for themselves how and when they gave birth as it was about being freed from the punishment of pain. In 1915, Mary Ware Dennett, who had led the NTSA, formed the National Birth Control League, the first American organization to campaign to legalize contraception and release women from "the wretchedness of unwilling parenthood."

Dennett had endured three unbearably painful, life-threatening births since 1900. After her first child was born, Dennett was seriously unwell. Her second baby died of starvation at three weeks old. While delivering her third, a little boy, she suffered an internal tear so severe she needed surgery. Dennett was determined to help other women prevent dangerous, unwanted pregnancies. Her own doctor refused to give her advice about birth control, despite advising her not to have any more babies. Since 1873, the Comstock Laws, a set of federal acts prohibiting the trade, circulation, and distribution of "obscene literature and articles of immoral use," especially through the postal service, had been enforced in the United States. Under these laws, promoting information about contraceptives and abortifacients—substances to induce miscarriage—was a federal offense. Dennett was inspired by the activist efforts of Margaret Sanger, the American nurse, sex education pioneer, and birth control activist. In 1914, Sanger was indicted for distributing obscene material through her monthly newspaper, *The Woman Rebel*, which ran for eight issues with the slogan "No Gods, No Masters." The newspaper was a barnstorming call for women—particularly of the working classes—to rise up against the "slavery of motherhood."

The Woman Rebel connected reproductive choice with women's economic emancipation. It radically redefined "a woman's duty" as staring "the whole world in the face with a go-to-hell-look in its eyes," having an "ideal," and speaking and acting "in defiance of convention." Rebel women claimed "the Right to be lazy; the Right to be an unmarried mother; the Right to destroy; the Right to create; the Right to love; the Right to live." The first issue included writing by the anarchist philosopher Emma Goldman, features on notable "rebels" including Mary Wollstonecraft, and advice on picketing for better pay and working conditions in offices, factories, and garment houses. *The Woman Rebel* was also the place to find all the information needed to prevent conception.

Family Limitation contained the same message for women: of taking control of their bodies and rights through informed social disobedience. Pitched as a "nurse's advice to women," Sanger's pamphlet included homespun methods to prevent a missed period. She urged her reader to act immediately if there was the slightest possibility that "male fluid had entered the vagina." She should use laxatives daily and take a few grains of quinine every night to stop the ovum from attaching. For contraception, Sanger recommended condoms, or pessaries and sponges, and douching with Lysol, vinegar, and salt solutions, or freezing cold water. She even provided recipes for pessaries laced with "special ingredients" to "negate the effect of the male seed." Sanger did suggest couples might try "coitus interruptus," but she stressed that this method "requires a man of the strongest will-power." Also, abruptly ending intercourse, Sanger warned, could leave women unsatisfied and nervously tense. Not being able to "complete her desire does her injury."

The Woman Rebel was blasted as "obscene, lewd, lascivious and filthy." Fearing her trial, and a possible prison sentence of five years, Sanger procured a fake passport and sought exile in Britain. In 1915, her estranged husband, William Sanger, was prosecuted for distributing *Family Limitation* after a copy fell into the hands of a detective working for Anthony Comstock, the US postal inspector and anti-vice blowhard for whom the laws were named. William was sentenced to thirty days in prison. Dennett believed William's arrest had intensified progressives' fear of supporting the need for birth control information. But it was crucial that people mobilized now to push the movement forward. And she absolutely shared Sanger's belief that being able to prevent unwanted pregnancies would enable women to enjoy sex.

Marital rape was not a criminal offense in the United States or Britain. Arming women with the knowledge to prevent conception was incredibly significant when their rights over their own bodies were still so limited. When sex "is not desired on the part of the woman and she has no response, it should not take place," Sanger decreed. "This is an act of prostitution and is degrading to the woman's finer sensibilities, all the marriage certificates on earth to the contrary notwithstanding." At the first meeting of the National Birth Control League, one hundred people gathered in the home of Dennett's friend and cofounder Clara Stillman. Dennett spoke passionately about the "precious results" of sex when it wasn't performed for obligatory baby-making. Human beings were not animals; they had no "mating season," no need to produce yearly offspring. Suppressing information about avoiding "the horrors of perpetuating the supply of unwanted babies" was completely detrimental to sexual relations—especially where women were concerned. Only when women were not condemned to needlessly reproduce would they finally enjoy the "physiological, emotional, and spiritual" rewards of sex.

Sanger's mission was to demystify women's bodies from a medical culture guarded by patriarchal moralism and antiquated mythologies. Sex positivity was a crucial part of that mission. In 1915, Dennett wrote her own guide to sex for her fourteen-year-old son. She was dismayed at how moral codes, embarrassment, and lack of knowledge were preventing parents from educating their children about such important matters. *The Sex Side of Life: An Explanation for Young People* detailed the physiological business of sex, conception, and reproduction. Dennett used the proper names for male and female organs and included simple diagrams. She explained that menstruation was not an illness and that wet dreams were completely normal. She also emphasized how important the emotional aspect of sex was and reassured her son that he needn't feel ashamed. Sex, she wrote, "is everything that is highest and best and happiest in human life." But she also warned that sex can "be easily perverted . . . and made the cause of horrible suffering of both mind and body." Dennett was a product of her time. She warned against masturbation and held prostitutes—"bad women," as she called them—responsible for the scourge of venereal diseases. Sex relations belonged between people who loved each other, she said, and love "can't be bought."

Although Dennett blamed and shamed sex workers, she did regard prostitution as more of a social ill than a female vice. If the joys of loving sex were celebrated and encouraged, she wondered, perhaps men wouldn't need to seek such gratification. For Sanger, prostitution was one of the dreadful consequences of economic poverty, which could be relieved if working-class women were allowed to limit their families. "There is no hope that prostitution will cease as long as there is hunger," she wrote in 1913. Sanger, a committed socialist, had worked as a visiting nurse in the overcrowded Lower East Side. In essays published in the magazine *New York Call*, she revealed how Italian and Eastern European families were forced into destitution by multiple pregnancies. Kept in the dark about how to prevent conception, married women sought so-called back-alley abortions. She had attended women left butchered by clumsy curettage, which could cause fatal sepsis. Around a hundred thousand "criminal" abortions were taking place annually in the United States, she claimed, with an estimated six thousand of these resulting in death. Sanger did not support abortion. Birth control, she was certain, would avoid "the wholesale lot of misery, expense, unhappiness and worry" caused by the "economic necessity" that was leaving women with no other choice.

Sanger returned to the United States in October 1915, prepared to face trial. But the following month, her four-year-old daughter died of pneumonia. The charges against her were dropped. The next year, on October 16, Sanger and her sister Ethyl Byrne, who was also a registered nurse, opened the country's first-ever birth control clinic on Amboy Street in Brownsville, Brooklyn. While Dennett's organization was lobbying against the Comstock Laws, Sanger was deliberately flouting them by helping women obtain "safe, harmless information" about how to prevent pregnancies. A promotional flyer, in English, Yiddish, and Italian, urged women who didn't want and couldn't afford large families to come to Amboy Street, where all mothers were welcome. On the day it opened, the clinic welcomed over one hundred women, who, for the registration fee of ten cents, received all the information they needed on reproduction and contraceptives.

An article in the *Brooklyn Eagle* stated that most of the clinic's first visitors had multiple children and struggled to work hard enough to feed them. One explained, "This is the kind of place we have been wanting all the time; I have had seven children, two are dead, and my husband is a sick man." Another said, "It is so much easier to talk to a woman. That is why I never tell my doctor." The clinic saw upward of four hundred women over ten days, until, on October 26, an undercover policewoman visited, leading vice-squad officials to raid the clinic and arrest Sanger and Byrne. After standing trial in January 1917, Sanger was sentenced to thirty days in Queens County Penitentiary, and Byrne, for the same length of time, in the Blackwell Island Workhouse. Upon her release, Sanger told the *Brooklyn Eagle* that the conditions in the jail were horrible, but her sentence made her only more determined to continue her work. Byrne fared much worse. She went on a hunger strike and was force-fed after 185 hours, making her the first political prisoner in the United States to receive the treatment that British suffragists had endured since 1909. The feedings impaired her respiration, lowered her blood pressure, and weakened her pulse. After ten days, Byrne submitted to a meal. She was pardoned on the condition that she promise never to violate the law again. She was so unwell and weak she had to be transported to Sanger's house in an ambulance.

"Margaret Sanger is going back to violate the law all over again," Sanger stated in her *Brooklyn Eagle* interview. In 1917, she founded the *Birth Control Review*, in which she introduced the term "birth control" for the first time. "Shall We Break This Law?" asked the headline. Her answer was yes: the nation's women *had* to break the law to claim their right to voluntary motherhood. Women must rise up against the "merciless machinery" that was destroying their health and vitality. Enforced motherhood was condemning mothers and wives to ill health, invalidism, and death. It was a disease tearing marriages apart and bringing prostitution, child labor, unemployment, and poverty in its wake. And ultimately, this disease would lead to the deterioration of human civilization.

Sanger, undoubtedly, was pioneering. But she held some troubling beliefs. She regarded birth control as a means to stamp out the proliferation of "children born feeble in mind and body" to working-class mothers whose excessive breeding was filling "jails and hospitals, factories and mills, insane asylums and premature graves." In *Family Limitation*, she bemoaned irresponsible childbearing by women with chronic illnesses including the kidney condition Bright's and heart disease, as well as syphilis, consumption, and mental "defects" like insanity, melancholia, and "idiocy." Sanger did want to protect unwell women from difficult pregnancies. But at the same time, she believed birth control would prevent the nation being burdened by "diseased and defective children." While Sanger was exiled in Britain, she met members of the neo-Malthusian movement, including the physician and sexologist Havelock Ellis, who supported "conscious conception" as a way of solving the social and biological "problems" of overpopulation. When Sanger returned to the United States, she began talking about birth control more explicitly as a civilizing force: "The quality of its citizens and not the quantity is the new keynote of civilization," she told the *Brooklyn Eagle* after her clinic opened.

Where twilight sleep encouraged the "better class" of mothers to breed vociferously, birth control was touted as a measure to prevent the "lower classes" from doing the same. Sanger's neo-Malthusian and, later, eugenic sympathies emerged over the years of her activism. But in Britain, these ableist, classist, and racist ideologies underpinned birth control campaigns from the beginning. While in Britain, Sanger met a twenty-three-year-old paleobiologist, suffrage supporter, and women's rights activist named Marie Carmichael Stopes. Stopes was also a committed social Darwinist and a member of the Eugenics Education Society. On July 5, 1915, Sanger gave a talk in London for the socialist organization the Fabian Society. Stopes was in the audience, listening intently to Sanger explain that birth control would give women "the right to own and control her own body" and "do with it what she desires." These words resonated poignantly with Stopes, who was seeking a legal annulment of her marriage to the Canadian botanist Reginald Gates on the basis that it had never been consummated because Gates was impotent. Gates, meanwhile, claimed Stopes was pathologically oversexed and impossible for any man to satisfy.

To prove her case, Stopes had to obtain a certificate of virginity from her physician. He examined her hymen and confirmed that "there has not been penetration by a normal male organ." Who knows exactly what constituted "normal"? Stopes's divorce was finalized in November 1915. Her experience inspired her to write a book educating women about healthy and fulfilling marriages, because, as she put it, she "paid a terrible price for sexual ignorance." By 1917, Stopes had finished *Married Love, or Love in Marriage*, and was searching for a publisher. Most of the larger houses rejected the book outright because its subject—how to enjoy sex in marriage—was too obscene. In 1918, the independent Critic and Guide Company agreed to take it on. And readers were not so shy. *Married Love* went into its sixth printing within two weeks.

Stopes believed marriages were failing because of repressed attitudes toward women's sexuality. Even in "advanced" books of physiology and medicine, the "mysteries of marriage" were concealed by gaps, omissions, and "misstatements of facts." By demystifying the biological, physical, emotional, and spiritual matters of sexual love, she believed she was doing "a service to humanity." For women, her information was a revelation. She explained how desire ebbed and flowed throughout a woman's cycle, and implored husbands to pursue their wives only if desire was mutual and consent affirmative. Empowering women to see themselves as autonomous sexual beings, regardless of what the law of marriage implied, was especially progressive. Some of her stories give an amazing insight into how oblivious many men were of women's wants and needs. One Mrs. G was so frustrated because her husband did nothing except kiss her on the cheek before intercourse. When Mrs. G expressed "a yearning to feel . . . his lips pressed against her bosom," he responded with one solitary peck on the chest.

Stopes thought medicine's promotion of sexual impulses in women as depraved and diseased had instilled such shame in young women that come the marriage night, they were not only completely ignorant about sex but also utterly shocked about what it involved. Stopes knew of women driven to insanity and even suicide by men's forcefulness. *Married Love* was meant to empower women to see sex not as a duty to endure but as a normal, healthy, and enjoyable experience. And like Sanger's, Stopes's sex positivity went hand in hand with her socialist beliefs about family limitation. Contraception wasn't exactly illegal in Britain at the time. Condoms and diaphragms made of sheep guts and vulcanized rubber had been available from specialist shops since the 1800s. But the act of preventing conception, especially among married couples, was morally reprehensible. Stopes abhorred the way that medicine upheld religious dogma prohibiting family limitation, particularly because women were the ones who suffered the consequences. They were forced into poverty by having so many mouths to feed; their bodies and minds were "murdered" by multiple pregnancies; sometimes they were forced to seek "horrible and criminal abortion."

Since 1861, English law upheld the statute in the Offences Against the Persons Act that made procuring, performing, or assisting with an abortion an offense equivalent to murder and rape. Stopes detested how women were criminalized and forced to risk their lives to end pregnancies, but, like Sanger, she didn't advocate abortion. She agreed that educating women about family planning would eradicate the need for abortion and drastically improve women's lives and liberties. In 1921, the year Sanger founded the American Birth Control League—the organization that would become Planned Parenthood—Stopes opened Britain's first Mother's Clinic in Holloway, North London. It was run by midwives and visiting doctors who offered free advice, to married women only, on all aspects of sexual health. The clinic also provided contraceptives, including Stopes's patented diaphragm. On opening day, women queued in the hundreds around the street. In 1925, the clinic moved to central London, and others opened across England. Stopes also appointed midwives to run Mother's Clinics from horse-drawn carriages, to bring services to working-class women who couldn't otherwise access them.

Stopes received hundreds of letters after *Married Love* was published. She was a revolutionary for her advances in contraception and for enabling women to speak openly about their bodies, to articulate feelings and secrets long buried. But vehement eugenicist beliefs permeated her work. In *Married Love*, Stopes avoided mentioning eugenics; but in her 1920 book, *Radiant Motherhood*, she fully embraced her bigoted views. Followers of the eugenicist movement believed that the population could be improved by selective breeding—weeding out hereditary traits deemed detrimental to the future of society. After World War I, across Europe and the United States, scientists and sociologists enmeshed new ideas about the biological bases of emotional, physical, and intellectual traits with strategies for perfecting the human race. Stopes, like Sanger, thought family planning would prevent the generational burden of mental and physical deformities. But unlike Sanger, Stopes perpetuated a blatantly ableist and racist doctrine that was so much more about racial and biological purity than concern for the well-being and living conditions of women and children. She named her diaphragm the "Pro-Race Cap," and later the "Racial Cap" because of her insistence on birth control as a means to achieve "race perfection."

Radiant Motherhood claimed it was "a book for those who are creating the future." Under the guise of women gaining body autonomy and sexual fulfillment, Stopes argued that the state should control *who* produced the country's future. She urged the enforcement of community policies to make "parenthood impossible for those whose mental and physical conditions are such that there is a certainty that their offspring must be physically and mentally tainted." To achieve what she called "the wonderful rejuvenescence and reform of the race," she said that the feeble-minded, mentally deficient, diseased, disabled, half-witted, imbecilic, epileptic, blind, syphilitic, and "half-caste"—the list goes on—should be compulsorily sterilized. Preventative castration for men, vasectomy, was all well and good, but for Stopes, the power and responsibility lay with women.

In 1919, the National Birth Control League in the United States dissolved. Dennett had founded the Voluntary Parenthood League, which continued to lobby for the words "prevention of conception" to be removed from the Comstock Laws. Sanger had distanced herself from Dennett's cause—after all, she had been punished and imprisoned under the Comstock ruling. Dennett disagreed with Sanger's new support for a bill giving doctors and health professionals the legal right to distribute information on birth control. Dennett wanted contraception advice to be available to all women of all social classes. Permitting only doctors to instruct in such matters was tantamount, Dennett believed, to "class legislation." Sanger regarded birth control as a scientific measure, so the backing of the medical community was nonnegotiable. After the war, from 1919, Sanger articulated the need for birth control in terms of what she called "eugenic value." In *Birth Control Review*, she declared that the "unshakable structure of racial betterment" rested with "free, self-determining motherhood." Dennett didn't share Sanger's opinion that birth control was solely a "woman's problem." But as the eugenicist tenor of Sanger's writings became sharper, so did her rhetoric about women's duty to their nation's future. First and foremost, Sanger believed that educating women to limit their families would bring about the "self-development" and "self-reflection" needed to improve "the quality of the race."

Despite her use of terms like "racial regeneration," Sanger did support the provision of birth control to Black communities. In 1929, she worked with the support of W. E. B. Du Bois, the prominent sociologist, civil rights activist, and historian, to open a birth control clinic in Harlem. Du Bois saw birth control as a way for Black women to improve their economic position and to contribute, as he put it, to the intelligence and fitness of "the black race." In June 1932, Sanger published a special issue of *Birth Control Review* on the "Negro Number." It included an essay by Du Bois, alongside others by physicians and health reformers, on the medical challenges faced by low-income Black families—especially those resulting from what Sanger called "high fertility." Sanger, like many of the contributors, believed birth control would improve the high maternal and infant mortality rates and the "poverty and degradation" that disproportionately affected those families and communities. Some writers addressed concerns that birth control could be seen as a sinister eugenic measure to eliminate the "black race." They insisted, instead, that birth control would lead to what physician Walter G. Alexander called "the betterment" of economic, health, and community standards for all "Negro" people, especially Black women.

In the "Negro Number," Sanger couched what she wincingly called "the Negro Problem" in terms of her reformist attitudes toward the economic situations and health challenges of Black women. And she did not withhold her prejudice against the "feeble-minded, the insane, and the syphilitic" having children. In her 1922 book, *The Pivot of Civilization*, Sanger, in a statement on the principles of the American Birth Control League, stated that children should "only begotten under conditions which render possible the heritage of health." Even though she spun these opinions through her concern for women's welfare, her ableism was acute. She supported the sterilization of the "insane and feeble-minded," and anyone with "inheritable or transmissible diseases." Ever the pro-sex firebrand, Sanger insisted the operation was permissible because it wouldn't "deprive the individual of . . . sex expression."

Forced sterilization had been legal in the United States since 1907 in many states. Young women under eighteen, confined to institutions for conditions like epilepsy or for mental illnesses, were among those most often subjected to sterilization, always without consent, and often with no understanding about what was being done to their bodies. The favored method was salpingectomy—to snip, tie, or remove the fallopian tubes. In 1924, seventeen-year-old Carrie Buck was ordered to be sterilized in the Lynchburg Colony for Epileptics and Feebleminded in Virginia. Carrie had become pregnant after being raped by the nephew of her foster parents. She was confined by them immediately after giving birth to her daughter, Vivian, because they claimed she had always been "feeble-minded." Really, they just wanted her out of the way. Compulsory sterilization was made legal in Virginia that year. The colony doctors diagnosed Carrie with a mental age of nine, and her "illegitimate" daughter as "mentally defective." This proved, to them, that Carrie carried hereditary "feeblemindedness and moral delinquency." Carrie's birth mother, Emma, who was held in the same colony on similar charges, was rumored to be a prostitute. Appeals were made against the order to sterilize Carrie on the grounds of "social inadequacy." But in 1927, the Supreme Court, with the testimony of colony superintendent Dr. Bell, ruled that "three generations of imbeciles were enough." Carrie's fallopian tubes were removed against her will. The case of *Buck v. Bell* set a precedent for the legal sterilization of young, impoverished women in more states throughout the 1930s. In 1931, the British Eugenics Society drafted a parliamentary bill proposing the compulsory sterilization of "mental defectives." It was debated in Parliament but never passed. Two years later, the society introduced the Voluntary Sterilization Movement, which encouraged women with incurable illnesses and disabilities to undergo the procedure for the good of the future.

Sanger continued to advocate for sterilization into the early 1930s, principally to limit the suffering of mothers and children. But the language she chose to use was pejorative and dehumanizing. In her speech of 1932, "My Way to Peace," to the New History Society, she proposed that Congress should "keep the doors of immigration closed" to "certain aliens whose condition is known to be detrimental to the stamina of the race, such as feeble-minded, idiots, morons, insane, syphilitic, epileptic, criminal, professional prostitutes, and others . . ." For those who carried "hereditary taints," she recommended segregation and sterilization. And any woman with a venereal disease, chronic heart or kidney condition, or any illness "where the condition of pregnancy disturbs her health" should be placed under the care of "public health nurses to instruct them in practical scientific methods of contraception in order to safeguard their lives." Despite the hard-core tone of these statements, Sanger distanced herself from such beliefs with the rise of the Nazi regime, whose adoption of eugenic programs for the purposes of racial purity disturbed her. Stopes supported Nazi "population science" and even attended a Nazi Party congress on the subject in 1935. Four years later she sent her "Love Poem for Young Lovers" to Hitler, because, bizarrely, she hoped it might be distributed to married couples through German birth control clinics.

It is an anger-inducing reality that the beginnings of reproductive justice were entangled with ideologies about how women—especially Black women, other ethnically diverse women, and vulnerable women—should be controlled and regulated. The birth control movement in America and Britain arose from the impulses and achievements of women's suffrage. Suffragists had always campaigned for women's rights to make decisions about their own bodies, freed from the stranglehold of misogynistic medicine and social inequality. In 1918, the Representation of the People Act enabled women to vote in Britain from the age of thirty in 1918, and from the age of twenty-one in 1928. By 1920, the United States, and most countries in Western Europe, had afforded women the same right. Without the feminist force of decades of struggle against patriarchal superiority, the achievements of Sanger and Stopes would not have been possible. But just as women's suffrage was a divided and divisive movement, particularly when it came to race and class, campaigns for birth control were as complex as they were crusading. Sanger and Stopes absorbed and promoted the era's sociological and medical ambitions to "perfect" the human race, but their ableism and racism can't be excused.

————

Stopes found a "scientific" rationalization for her sinister agenda of optimal motherhood in new theories about "internal secretions." Since the late 1800s, gynecologists and neurologists across Europe explored how female and male traits were determined by mysterious substances, secreted by the reproductive glands—the ovaries and the testes—which were thought to govern characteristics like intelligence, strength, vitality, energy, and even beauty. In 1905, the British biologist Ernest Starling introduced the word "hormone"—from the ancient Greek meaning "setting in motion"—to describe secretin, the digestive substance secreted by the pancreas, which he discovered with physiologist William Bayliss in 1902. "Internal secretions" came to be understood as hormones, molecules that regulate the function of, and communication between, all the organs and tissues of the human body. For Stopes and many others, internal secretions carried an elusive power—particularly when it came to sex and reproduction. Stopes believed that a woman's secretions had "remote" and "undetected" effects on her progeny beyond "material" hereditary factors like looks, eye color, and so on. Women with the best "in-born" secretions, in her opinion, were white and free of diseases of body and mind.

According to Stopes, mental outlook, emotional experiences, and factors like diet, social life, and home environment could powerfully alter secretions and affect the "potentials" of unborn children. And she placed all the responsibility for secretion-optimizing squarely at the ovaries of women. It was up to women to procreate with husbands of "clean and wholesome ancestry." They should eat only simple, nourishing foods, such as butter and oranges, and make sure their "mental state and conditions" were pure and unsullied so that "intellectual and spiritual interest" was transmitted to their babies. To warn readers about how a mother's thoughts could impede a child's potential and result in "racial loss," she told an anecdote about Oscar Wilde—a "genius . . . sullied by terrible sex crimes." Apparently, Wilde's mother had longed for a daughter while she was pregnant. She blamed herself for "molding" his "perverted proclivities" with her own thoughts. Four centuries after the bonkers belief that birth defects were caused by women's depraved dreams and desires, women's minds were still being policed in reproductive propaganda.

The sinister ideologies of eugenics were bolstered by medical ideas emerging from the burgeoning discipline of endocrinology, the study of human hormones. Eugenics had placed women's fertility and maternal "fitness" under its menacing microscope. Like cattle sent to market, women were scrutinized and judged as vessels of the future. But as theories about "female" hormones emerged, a whole new model for achieving idealized states of physiological and psychological womanhood was set in motion. In the years leading up to World War II, in laboratories in Britain, Europe, and the United States, the race was on to define, manipulate, and perfect the chemical essence of femininity.

11

FEMININE RADIANCE

The fact must be borne in mind . . . that the diseases and physical disabilities of women at the present time, though dangerous to health, are not organic," wrote Eliza Burt Gamble, the American scientist and philosopher, in *The Sexes in Science and History: An Inquiry into the Dogma of Woman's Inferiority to Man*. Published in 1916, Gamble's book was a groundbreaking feminist critique of Darwin's evolutionary assessments of male superiority.

Born in 1841, Gamble had been fighting for women's equality since the beginnings of the suffrage movement. She developed rheumatism in her late twenties after her children were born, but she didn't stop agitating against male superiority. Gamble rejected the idea that nervous and hysterical illnesses had anything to do with "structural defects" thought to be innate in the female body. "The diseases peculiar to the female constitution . . . are due to the overstimulation of the animal instincts in her male mate, or the disparity between her stage of development and his," she wrote. Men's brute force and aggressive sexual appetites had shaped the statutes of marriage. With no economic rights or freedoms of her own, "woman became a dependent, a mere appendage." Constant childbearing was both a marital obligation and a "struggle for existence." Men had never endured any "physical process" nearly so "disastrous to life and health." Under these conditions, women had developed "an alarming degree of functional nervousness." Gamble meant nervousness that manifested in the mind, as opposed to "organic" nervousness that arose from the body. But as women's rights to property, occupations, intellectual freedoms, and political participation were increasing, nervousness seemed to be diminishing. For Gamble, this proved that most nervous illnesses were social symptoms. It was pretty difficult to maintain that women were smaller-brained, perpetually sickly weaklings when they had managed, all on their own, to revolutionize their sphere of existence. Besides, women lived just as long as men, if not longer, proving that evolution had in no way "materially injured her constitution."

Amid all the feverish wartime debates about women's reproductive responsibilities, Gamble's arguments against "excessive and useless maternity" were enlightening. Of course, the birth control movement was forged in the same fire. But the doctrine of reproductive choice carried the strong message of a mother's duty—to her country and its future. Gamble didn't believe that childbearing solved any social ills, even when women were in control of it. Women would achieve superiority by cultivating their "higher faculties," not by blindly fulfilling the biological imperative that had oppressed them for too long.

Gamble argued that a woman's intellect, sympathy, and reasoning were far superior to those of her "better endowed and more thoroughly equipped male mate." The differences between men and women had been shaped by social factors, not by evolution. Gamble was arguing against the master of evolutionary theory by exposing how medical knowledge willfully validated female inferiority. But as medicine turned its attentions to "internal secretions," a new precedent was set for defining biological sex differences. And with these theories that femininity was "caused" by mysterious substances came all-new assumptions about women's susceptibility to myriad disturbances and derangements.

The same year Gamble's work was published, William Blair Bell, then Britain's most respected and influential gynecologist, wrote a tome exploring how internal secretions affected "female" health and determined "feminine" characteristics. Emerging endocrinological theories offered a compellingly modern way to redefine medical conceptions of the functions and processes of the female body, and the biological basis of womanhood. Furthering such theories was a surefire way for male gynecologists to position themselves at the vanguard of this expanding discipline. With the war raging and human reproduction foremost in medicine's mind, Blair Bell took it upon himself to reassess "femininity and its causes" in light of the most advanced scientific ideas about the bases of sex difference.

But what exactly *was* a woman anymore? he wondered. Possessing ovaries used to mean a person was female. And the ovaries determined not only female reproductive functions but also all those adorable characteristics that made a human creature a *woman*. The greatest medical masters had decreed it. Back in 1848, the German pathologist, biologist, and social medicine pioneer Rudolf Virchow issued his famous edict about the organ's femininizing power. "A woman is only a woman on account of her generative glands," he declared. "All the peculiarities of her body and mind . . . the gentleness of her voice . . . the depth of feeling, devotion and fidelity, in short, all the qualities that we admire and honor in the true woman, are only a consequence of the ovary." But it was now the twentieth century. Such "sentimental" and "romantic" notions of womanhood no longer cut the medical mustard. Science had marched in to tear aside the "veil overhanging the mystery of sex."

Since the 1890s, European gynecologists and physiologists had been suggesting that it wasn't the ovary itself that determined "femininity" but the substances secreted by it. Endocrinology didn't upend medicine's long-held certainty that women were defined by their biological role in what Blair Bell called "the reproductive economy." Even though the basis of sex was shifting from the organs to their secretions, women were still viewed as humans who possessed the reproductive apparatus labeled "female," and the external characteristics that enticed men to reproduce with them. Blair Bell might have been a scientific powerhouse, but he still believed the healthiest women obeyed their biological destiny and dedicated their lives, and bodies, to bearing and raising children. He was not about to throw the social baby out with the biochemical bathwater. The way he saw it, a biological human female was made into a woman by the secretions that supplied the traits, impulses, and desires of idealized femininity. So how was this different from Virchow's essentialist declaration made more than half a century earlier?

The simple answer is not very much. But by 1916, endocrinology had discovered that female reproductive physiology wasn't supported by ovarian secretions alone. The other endocrine glands—the thyroid; the adrenal or suprarenal glands, which produce adrenaline; and the pituitary, the pea-sized "master" gland at the base of the brain—were all known to play important roles. Virchow located the "causes" of femininity in a single organ; but for Blair Bell, femininity was caused by a complex concert of glandular substances.

Starling and Bayliss introduced the word "hormone" to describe pancreatic secretions in 1905, but the term wasn't widely used until medicine understood more about all the glands of the endocrine system. When Blair Bell wrote his book *The Sex Complex*, secretions held an almost mystical power. These elusive substances were thought to establish sex difference and support reproductive functions, but no one knew exactly *how*. What was known, however, was enough for Blair Bell to elaborate on some choice theories about biochemical femininity. Internal secretions were a sort of magic potion that supplied women with the impetus to make babies and mother them. Femininity was a combination of "special functions"—physiological and psychological—all supported by secretions. So, in answer to his initial question, Blair Bell decided that a woman was a woman because her glands made her feminine: "*femininity itself is dependent on all the internal secretions*."

The discovery of ovarian secretions began two decades earlier in Vienna. Rudolf Chrobak, a gynecologist at the city university's women's hospital, was trying to figure out how to relieve the symptoms of "artificial" menopause in patients who had undergone ovariotomies. Chrobak was a fervent ovariotomist; he reportedly performed 146 since the 1880s, many during hysterectomies. But ovariotomy induced menopause very suddenly, and women who'd had an ovariotomy often suffered far more severely than those going through natural or physiological menopause. Around 1895, Chrobak's enthusiasm soured after women started reporting hot flashes, vertigo, headaches, and other alarming neurological and vascular disturbances. One patient, who was referred to Chrobak in 1895 for an ovariotomy by none other than Sigmund Freud, had to be confined to a sanatorium afterward. Chrobak was determined to help women cope with the aftereffects of ovariotomies. He stopped removing ovaries quite so enthusiastically and looked to advances in treatments for another distressing "women's disease" for inspiration.

Since the early 1890s, physicians in Britain, France, and Germany had been using sheep, cow, calf, and pig thyroid extracts, either injected into the skin or fed, either raw or cooked, to treat myxedema, a chronic disease that affected mostly middle-aged and older women. Myxedema, or hypothyroidism, is known today to be an autoimmune depletion of the thyroid hormone. It is four times more common in women than in men. Before medicine thought to mine the farmyard for supplements, treatments were limited to hot baths, massages to promote "vigorous friction," "good feeding," iron, nitroglycerine, arsenic, and, if the patient was lucky, convalescent vacations in "mild and genial climates." Unsurprisingly, none of these remedies were particularly effective.

For centuries, the workings of the thyroid had been a mystery. But in the mid-nineteenth century, physicians proposed that it regulated the function of the brain and nervous system. One of the earliest clinical papers on myxedema described a ten-year-old girl from an asylum in Lancashire who was barely able to walk or speak. She was diagnosed with cretinism, an old term for deficiencies of growth and learning. When the poor girl died, her autopsy showed she had no thyroid. From then on, absent and deficient thyroids were associated with physical slowness and heaviness, mental ineptitude, dullness, and confusion. For many women with thyroid issues, mental symptoms were so extreme that they were certified insane and sent to asylums.

In July 1891, a fifty-four-year-old "lady" from Dundee, who had lived all her life with her twin sister, was diagnosed with myxedema. For fourteen years she had a swollen face, sluggish digestion, a weak pulse, slow speech, constant pain, and a complete lack of energy. She was plagued by delusions and nightmares and constantly "oppressed by the weight, mental and physical, of her disease." The likeness between her and her sister was so great that it used to be impossible to tell them apart, but her illness had changed her appearance so drastically that it was "difficult to believe they were sisters at all." Her physician, Edinburgh-based physiologist Robert Alex Lundie, began injecting her with a sheep-thyroid extract in November. She improved rapidly; Lundie was reminded "of the fairy tales, where magic potions make the body grow large and small at will." Two years later, she felt lively, strong, and active. She wasn't tortured by confusion, pain, or headaches anymore. She could sew again, when before she couldn't hold her needle. But Lundie was mostly just delighted that her looks had improved. She had lost weight, her face was no longer swollen, her skin was soft and pliant, and her expressions bright and intelligent. And she could resume her household duties. Never mind that she had recovered her mental health, her pulse had regained its pace, and she could walk without a stick. The thyroid extracts had rejuvenated her most pleasant and amenable feminine qualities!

At the time, the thyroid and the ovaries were thought to be in sympathy and work in similar ways. If animal supplements helped patients recover thyroid function, Chrobak wondered, then might the ovaries of cows or pigs have a similar effect? A few years earlier, an eccentric physiologist and neurologist named Charles-Édouard Brown-Séquard, who tried to revive his own secretions with an elixir of dog and guinea pig testes, reported that a Parisian midwife had administered extracts of pig ovaries to herself with good results. In 1895, gynecologists at Berlin's Landau Clinic were considering ovarian therapy for a twenty-three-year-old who'd had her ovaries and fallopian tubes removed to cure pelvic inflammatory disease. After her surgery, she experienced horrendous vasomotor attacks. As often as twelve times a day her head flushed unbearably, she sweated profusely, and she became horribly dizzy. No remedies worked, so her gynecologists procured cow ovaries in the hope that the effects would mirror those of animal thyroids. After the glands had dried out for twelve hours, she was fed a portion—raw. The next day she suffered only five attacks. To make sure the effect wasn't "psychic," she was given a placebo of "scraped meat" (sounds appetizing) on the seventh and eighth days after surgery, and her symptoms got much worse. Chrobak also gave patients extracted tissues of cow ovaries, eaten raw or cooked, or juiced and injected. The Landau Clinic had reported positive effects from ovarian therapy, but Chrobak was frustrated that he hadn't achieved the same miraculous results. So he looked again to thyroid treatments for his next course of action.

In the 1870s, German surgeons who performed thyroidectomies for conditions like exophthalmic goiter, or Graves' disease, in which the thyroid is overactive and enlarged, noticed that patients soon developed "cretinous" symptoms. Experiments carried out to substitute for the absent gland grafted portions of animal thyroid tissues into other parts of the body, and these proved successful. Chrobak decided to test-run similar experiments. In 1896, in a laboratory at the women's hospital, Chrobak's assistant Emil Knauer removed the ovaries from adult rabbits and transplanted grafts of their own ovarian tissue into their abdominal walls. He found that the uteruses of the rabbits who had received the grafts didn't degenerate like they usually did after animals were castrated. Perhaps they were being sustained by some substance from the ovarian tissue being absorbed into the bloodstream?

This innovative suggestion was confirmed three years later by Josef Halban, an Austrian obstetrician and gynecologist who had been conducting similar experiments on newborn guinea pigs since 1897. Halban wanted to find out how the actions of the ovaries affected the female reproductive system. He removed the guinea pigs' ovaries and parts of their uteruses and implanted tissue grafts under their skin at other places in their bodies. He found that the guinea pigs still developed functioning reproductive organs as they grew. "These experiments compel us to assume," Halban wrote, "that a substance is secreted by the ovaries into the circulating blood, which is capable of a specific influence upon the rest of the genital system."

The discovery of ovarian secretions transformed medicine's perception of how the female body worked. By the early 1900s, physiologists in Europe were revealing more about the role of secretions in menstruation and ovulation. The suggestion that the corpus luteum, the gland created in the ovary after an ovum is released, was involved in the ovary's changes during the menstrual cycle and pregnancy was groundbreaking. In 1903, Francis Marshall, a shy and retiring physiologist from the University of Edinburgh who disliked "modern things such as telephones, card indexing systems, typewriters, airplanes and woman students," joined forces with fellow physiologist William Jolly to investigate how ovarian secretions influenced the estrous cycle. Estrus, named after the Latin word for "passionate frenzy," described the period during a female mammal's cycle when she was most fertile and receptive to sex—in other words, when she was "in heat." After castrating dogs, sheep, ferrets, and a monkey and introducing grafts of ovarian tissue extracted from animals in heat, Marshall and Jolly found that estrus was triggered by a secretion from the ovary's follicle cells. This secretion supported, but was separate from, the secretion made by the corpus luteum.

These new ideas about the function of the ovaries were controversial. Some physicians weren't ready to let go of prevailing assumptions that the ovaries were regulated by the nerves. Others thought that messing around with transplants and grafts was dangerous sci-fi nonsense. One American physician thought it was absurd to suggest that "this one little epithelial body contains all the functions known to womanhood." But as endocrinological knowledge progressed into the new century, it was soon understood that the ovary did not work alone. In 1910, Anne Louise McIlroy, the pioneering Irish-born obstetrician and gynecologist, began investigating the cellular basis of ovarian secretions. Two years later, she carried out animal experiments to investigate their role in menstruation, ovulation, pregnancy, and lactation, as well as on female physiology more generally. She concluded that the ovaries acted in close connection with other endocrine glands to maintain the female body's "normal equilibrium." Although the exact nature of this connection remained a mystery, she was certain that the ovaries had "a powerful influence on the body as a whole." For this reason, removing them for "slight pathological affections" and "menstrual derangements" was detrimental to a woman's health, she said. Only if the ovaries were the seat of a life-endangering "pathological lesion" should a physician even consider extirpating them.

In 1898, McIlroy, one of four daughters of a progressive general practitioner from County Antrim, became the first woman to receive a doctor of medicine degree from the University of Glasgow. After graduation she traveled to Berlin and Vienna, honing her skills in gynecological surgery. In the early 1900s, she cared for socially disenfranchised and poorer women at Glasgow's Lock Hospital and Royal Samaritan

Hospital. Her surgical brilliance and research prowess led to her being appointed the first-ever woman gynecological surgeon at the city's Royal Victoria Infirmary, in 1906. When the war broke out in 1914, McIlroy knew her surgical skills would be invaluable on the front line. Women were denied entry to the Royal Army Corps by the British government, and the War Office's response to women physicians who were prepared to serve in a medical capacity was met with customary condescending sexism. Elsie Inglis, a Scottish gynecologist and suffragist, founded the Scottish Women's Hospitals for Foreign Service in 1914, which, through funding from the National Women's Suffrage Societies, was ready to offer two-hundred-bed hospital units, entirely staffed by women, to the war effort. McIlroy would be appointed head of surgery. But the War Office told Inglis to "go home and sit still." Having never allowed antiquated perceptions of their sex to stifle their ambitions, Inglis and McIlroy offered their services to the Allied nations instead. Throughout the war, the Scottish Women's Hospitals enabled around one hundred volunteer women doctors to serve in fourteen countries, including France, Belgium, Greece, Serbia, and Russia.

McIlroy was instrumental in expanding opportunities for women in medicine, and after the war, as England's first-ever female medical professor, she pioneered medical education for women at the London University. She was well-liked and never afraid to speak her mind about medicine's intervention in women's lives. As an obstetrician and gynecologist, she always prioritized women's care—she was a fierce advocate for obstetric anesthesia for all women—and she revolutionized medicine's understanding of toxemias in pregnancy, now known as preeclampsia. But her particular feminism was sometimes contentious. In 1921, she was embroiled in a legal battle with Marie Stopes over comments she had made that Stopes's brand of cervical cap was highly dangerous. McIlroy supported birth control if it was prescribed by doctors, but she feared that its widespread use would make women "slaves" in "sexual matters, for they will remain the instruments of men's uncontrollable desires."

In her endocrinological research, McIlroy questioned the blinkered view of women's bodies as always governed by their reproductive and sexual systems. Far from being the defining factor of femininity, ovarian secretions, to McIlroy, seemed to have a far-reaching effect on women's metabolic health. Although much more research was needed to discern the functions of internal secretions, McIlroy showed that an understanding of women's illnesses and diseases needed to move beyond a fixation with reproduction. Through endocrinological research like hers, women's bodies were emerging anew. The mystifications of the past, which had condemned too many women to dangerous surgical interventions, were being debunked. Blair Bell, to be fair, also agreed that endocrine knowledge was rapidly changing the understanding of women's health. He dedicated many chapters of *The Sex Complex* to the relationship between the female "genital system" and the other endocrine glands. He considered how disorders of the thyroid, thymus, adrenals, pituitary, and pineal glands might affect women's metabolic functions. But ultimately, Blair Bell's interest in using ideas about internal secretions to validate oppressive beliefs about women's bodies, minds, and lives outweighed his concern for women's endocrinological health.

When Blair Bell wrote *The Sex Complex*, women hadn't yet been granted the right to vote. Many were still fighting for our social, civil, and political rights, our freedom to pursue education and professions, and our independence. Blair Bell took a dim view of women's suffrage, believing a woman's place was in the home. Occupations, intellectual activity, political agitation, personal sexual fulfillment, and any other deviation from marriage and motherhood was, in his esteemed opinion, extremely unhealthy for women and society. In light of the ongoing question of women's emancipation, especially during the turbulent war years, Blair Bell thought it especially pressing to "seize upon the evident differentiations" between men and women.

Blair Bell acknowledged that every human being contained elements of both sexes, because each fertilized ovum contained the potential to develop as male or female. And while he admitted that exactly how sex was determined was unknown, he believed it had something to do with the endocrine organs, which controlled the "sexual evolution of the individual." What counted for Blair Bell was how degrees of masculinity and femininity were expressed across an individual's life. And even though he admitted sex was "dimorphic," he didn't think any deviation from what he deemed "normal" was natural or healthy. The internal secretions hadn't yet been isolated. No one knew exactly what they were or how they worked. So Blair Bell devised a diagnostic system for measuring endocrine function based on his ideals of femininity. Inevitably, a woman with perfectly balanced secretions was the very model of a domestic and maternal goddess.

A "normal woman" with the right proportions of femininity wished for nothing more than to find a husband, have a moderate amount of unexciting sex with him, and bear his children. She menstruated regularly, had well-formed breasts, and was wholly feminine in "outlook and aspirations." She obeyed the evolutionary principle of dependence on men and had an "ardent desire to be loved." But an overly feminine woman with excessive secretions sought pleasure and sexual gratification at the expense of maternal instincts. If her ovarian secretions went haywire at puberty, she would become a compulsive masturbator and grow up "sexually insane." Blair Bell recalled a "young lady" who began obsessively recording her sexy thoughts and feelings in a diary. This dangerous practice of journaling soon spiraled out of control. She started dropping lascivious notes in the road so a man might be "induced" to "satisfy her cravings." Her self-respect was "blotted out of her consciousness" by the "overwhelming stimulus . . . flooding her mind."

At the opposite end of Blair Bell's femininity sliding scale were women who desired neither sex nor children. They had deficient secretions and so they lacked the stimulus to reproduce. Their ovaries were shriveled, and they menstruated "feebly." They had flat breasts, coarse skin, heavy bones, and plain features. These kinds of women, he said, could hardly be called "women" at all. Their secretions were of the "masculine type," and all their metabolic functions were directed toward "the necessity of masculinity." These "unnatural individuals" had aggressive and scheming conversational styles. They pursued competitive work, which "normal" women shunned because it was "distinctly injurious to the finer psychological functions connected with [their] biological life." Without a doubt, they did far too much reading and thinking. They might even attempt to emulate the "masterful" male mind. Truly feminine women could never attain "lofty heights of genius," because the normal female mind couldn't stretch that far. But if a woman ever *did* become a genius, she would "no longer be a woman in the true biological sense of the word."

Reproductive endocrinology, over the past twenty years, had shown that secretions were constantly changing throughout the menstrual cycle—during ovulation, pregnancy, and menopause. Blair Bell interpreted this to mean women were metabolically "instable"—as opposed to men, who had evolved "steady and uniform" metabolisms so that they could keep their nerves calm and minds clear while hunting. Women were thought to be more vulnerable to endocrine diseases than men were precisely because their secretions were so changeable. This also meant their "natural" body processes, especially menopause, could be pathologized as metabolic and biochemical disturbances.

For centuries, the demise of a woman's fertility had been regarded as an illness that disturbed the body and deranged the mind. Superstitions about the aging female body, which had haunted women since the witch trials, inflamed perceptions about the destructive consequences of the end of a woman's reproductive life. With their biological and social purpose coming to an end, menopausal women had, historically, been vilified as dangerous or dismissed as useless. Since the mid-nineteenth century, many gynecologists had treated menopause as a pathology. And since they didn't understand what was actually happening during the "change of life," they tended to characterize menopause according to symptoms they observed in older women patients. And they didn't necessarily distinguish between genuine symptoms of menopause and those of other illnesses their patients might have had.

By the end of the century, almost every conceivable physical and mental disturbance affecting older women had come to be associated with the diminishing of their fertility. But as the American physician Andrew Currier pointed out in 1897, menopause was a normal process. Just as they had with menstruation, gynecologists based their pathological opinions on the experiences of the few women who had a "hard time." In its ignorance, medicine had made women fearful of menopause by dramatizing it as "perilous" and "fraught." "Upon this exceptional experience," wrote Currier, "the doctrine of the dangerous and serious character of menopause has been built up." Perceptions of whether women could get through "the change" with ease often depended on what kind of woman she was, how she had lived, and how faithfully she had obeyed her feminine duties. Like menstruation and childbearing, menopause was thought to cause particular trouble for women whose nerves couldn't weather nature's storm. Walter Gallichan, a British writer on female sexual mores and behavior, believed this "normal and natural occurrence" was impossible for "highly civilized" women to cope with. Their "artificial" and "more-or-less abnormal" lifestyles meant the change was "frequently attended by marked aberrations of a mental, moral, and emotional character, and by specific physical disorders."

From the early 1900s, theories about internal secretions radically changed medicine's perception of menopause. Since the change was associated with depleting ovarian secretions, gynecologists framed it as a deficiency disease. By 1910, a woman's average life expectancy was fifty-five. Blair Bell estimated that most began menopause—or the climacteric—between forty-three and forty-eight. Menopause was now a distinct phase in women's lives, and because of the propaganda of the past half century, many absolutely dreaded it. Although Blair Bell did state that menopause was a natural process that didn't have to be debilitating, he also described it as a "critical period" that few women pass "through without some general disturbances." Blair Bell was in the business of medicalizing every process of female biology. It wasn't in his interest to empower women to think of menopause as normal. Since women's health was supported by internal secretions, he believed their diminishment left women vulnerable to myriad distressing symptoms. But it wasn't just women's bodies that were at risk during the "critical period." For Blair Bell, ovarian secretions were the "guiding force of a women's existence." Robbed of the unseen substances that had given her a reason to live, a menopausal woman was superfluous, cast adrift on a sea of mental and physical ruin.

Menopause today is under-researched, misunderstood, and still shrouded in myths and misconceptions. The World Health Organization defines "natural" menopause as "the permanent cessation of menstruation resulting from the loss of ovarian follicular activity." In other words, it means that periods have stopped, and the ovaries are no longer producing eggs. It is a biological process that will be experienced by most people who have ovaries, usually between the ages of forty-five and fifty-five. And yet, maddeningly, medicine still doesn't have enough knowledge and understanding about the varied experiences of menopause to properly support women through it. Derogatory perceptions of aging women and hackneyed stereotypes about menopause making women mad, sad, and even dangerous are woven into the culture of stigmatization and trivialization that still circulates around menopause. Medicine has insisted, over centuries, on metaphors of decline and demise to describe menopause, and its definitions are still haunted by a lexicon of lack and failure. And frustratingly, menopause is usually diagnosed only after menstruation has stopped for more than twelve months. That means the symptoms of perimenopause, which can happen up to ten years before periods end, are frequently misdiagnosed—especially as depression and anxiety. Even for people who are correctly diagnosed, medical ignorance means the diverse physical, psychological, and neurological effects of menopause are often dismissed. Many GPs and clinicians focus on hot flashes, night sweats, and vaginal dryness as the universal markers. But menopause is unique to the person going through it; there is no such thing as a standard experience.

Recently, clinical guidelines around the diagnosis and treatment of menopause symptoms have been improved. Expanding and advancing knowledge about the multifaceted realities of menopause is, of course, crucially important if all people going through it are to be treated with the dignity and care they deserve. But increasing clinical understanding of all the possible psychological and physiological effects shouldn't happen at the expense of respect and appreciation. The current average life expectancy of a woman is eighty-three in the UK and seventy-nine in the US. Menopause marks the beginning of a liberatory, transformative, and empowering stage of womanhood. Myths about the depletion of women's worth that have shrouded menopause for too long should now be consigned to history. Breaking down stigma, shifting perceptions, and allaying anxieties at a medical level needs to go hand in hand with a cultural celebration of what it means to be a woman unbound by reproductive biology.

The sense of fear that is still evoked today by the idea of menopause was built up over centuries. But it was in the early twentieth century, when men like Blair Bell were envisaging "the climacteric" through the lens of new theories about deficient hormonal femininity, that the alarming pathological nature of menopause was ingrained. Blair Bell noted that every woman experienced the change differently. But he also warned women to be prepared for "a long and stormy physiological climacteric." Disturbances to the vasomotor system could cause palpitations, breathlessness, digestive problems, headaches, cold sweats, hyperesthesia (increased sensitivity to pain), and the inevitable hot flashes. If the physiological changes were particularly severe, women might also look forward to a host of "instabilities," including mental lethargy, melancholia, temporary paralysis, hysteric fits, and even full-blown psychopathy. But just as in the nineteenth century, menopausal suffering was considered to be proportionate to how femininely healthy—and socially obedient—a woman was. If she had been overly sexually active, she would suffer far more "violent derangements" than a woman who had limited her passions to the marital bed. Her metabolism would go awry; she would become severely depressed and probably start masturbating furiously.

In the past, the only real treatments were fresh air, moderate exercise, bland diets, loose clothing, no alcohol, and maybe a stay in an asylum. But where nature had shut a door, medical science was opening a window. The discovery of ovarian secretions meant femininity could now be supplemented, restored, and rejuvenated. Since 1899, Ovariin and Oophorin, made from the desiccated ovaries of cows and pigs, had been available in tablet form as treatments for menopausal symptoms and to restore fertility in "sterile" women. The craze for organotherapy in the US, UK, and Europe wasn't limited to ovary and thyroid preparations. Medicine's obsession with the secreting glands led to the development of other organotherapies, made from various animal organs procured from abattoirs and meatpacking plants, for all sorts of women's diseases.

As a treatment for hysteria, neurasthenia (nerve weakness), or ane-mia, a woman might have been offered a pill made of dried-up animal-brain gray matter or red bone marrow. If her periods were heavy or long, or she had uterine fibroids, she might be told to try a dose of mammary gland. Organotherapies, especially ovarian supplements, were wildly popular throughout the early 1900s. But there were serious doubts about whether they delivered any active ingredients. No one really knew what doses would be effective or how long a course should continue. The logistics of procuring the raw materials were complicated, and the ther-apies were costly to produce, which made them prohibitively expensive for patients. As an alternative, many women sought out herbal remedies that promised to relieve the miseries of menopause and restore vitality lost to middle and older age. A hugely popular concoction was Lydia Pinkham's Vegetable Compound, sold in US and UK pharmacies and groceries stores as a cure-all for "female complaints."

The compound was invented by Pinkham herself, an American abo-litionist and women's health activist—think a nineteenth-century ver-sion of today's wellness magnates—in 1875 in her home kitchen. It contained an array of herbs and roots traditionally used to relieve wom-en's troubles, including the flowering plant black cohosh. But the main active ingredient was drinking alcohol. Patented and mass-marketed from 1876, Pinkham's compound was promoted all over ladies' publica-tions and the popular press in advertorials aimed at older housewives. During the late nineteenth century, ads claimed that it could cure all the bizarre illnesses medicine said were endemic: "spinal weakness," "falling and displacements of the womb," "ovarian troubles," and so on. Pinkham even boasted that it could "dissolve" cancerous uterine tumors.

By the early 1900s, the compound's special "adaption" to the "change of life" was its major selling point. Advertorials, like one that appeared in a California newspaper in 1912, used the testimonies of "real" women to promote the compound's "amazing results." "For months I suffered from troubles in consequence of my age and thought I could not live," said Mrs. Emma Bailey. "Pinkham's Vegetable Compound made me well and I want other suffering women to know about it." Mrs. Thorn "was passing through Change of Life and felt very bad. I could not sleep and was very nervous." Pinkham's compound "restored me to perfect health and I would not be without it."

After the war, a medical—and cultural—fascination with human rejuvenation took hold. The glands and secretions not only dictated mental and physical health; they also were thought to govern attributes like energy, intelligence, creativity, morality, and sexuality. Endocrinology had shown that the very essence of humanness could be restored to treat illnesses and diseases. Throughout the 1910s and into the 1920s, endocrinologists carried out glandular experiments to try to "cure" nature's most incurable condition: aging. Since the early 1900s, physiologists and endocrinologists in Europe had been exploring ways to stimulate declining mental and physical prowess in their middle- and older-age patients. Since most of these experiments focused on prized masculine traits like sex drive, intellectual acuity, and bodily vigor, it figures that most of these early therapies were designed for men.

In the 1920s, Harry Benjamin, a German-born endocrinologist and sexologist, started offering rejuvenation procedures in his luxurious clinic on New York's Park Avenue. Benjamin had worked with Eugen Steinach, the Austrian physiologist who developed an operation, similar to a vasectomy, to reignite depleting secretions in older men. The "Steinach rejuvenation operation" became wildly popular, and soon he started exploring ways to stimulate women's generative glands. With his contemporary Guido Holzknecht, leading radiologist at the Vienna General Hospital, Steinach developed a female rejuvenation method using low doses of X-rays directed at the ovaries. Since the invention of X-ray technology and its introduction into medicine in the late 1890s, radiation therapies had been used for gynecological diseases that in the past could be treated only with dangerous surgeries. In the early 1900s, Holzknecht had used X-ray therapy to treat disorders of the uterus and ovaries in older women, and apparently patients reported almost miraculous improvements in their skin elasticity, mental efficiency, and physical energy. Benjamin became the most active advocate of the Steinach operation outside Europe. At first, he performed his procedure only on men. But in 1922, he started providing radiation therapy to a handful of women with severe menopause symptoms, including fatigue, hot flashes, back pain, stiff muscles, and "extreme nervousness." Although his patients claimed they felt much better, Benjamin was cautious about overselling the benefits of the less tried-and-tested Steinach operation for women.

One evening in 1922, the American author Gertrude Atherton came across Benjamin's work in a newspaper article describing how older European women were flocking to have their ovaries irradiated and their youth restored. Atherton was sixty-four and desperate to revive her flagging mental energy. Benjamin thought a course of low-dose X-rays would stimulate "a fresh supply of hormones into the bloodstream." After six weeks Atherton had "the abrupt sensation of a black cloud lifting . . . My brain seemed sparkling with light." She immediately "flung herself" at her desk and "wrote steadily for four hours." Benjamin reported, five months after Atherton received her treatment, that nothing could tire her. Her brain was clear, new ideas "came to her like a flash," and her blood pressure had decreased. In 1923, Atherton brought Benjamin's "reactivization" therapy to the world's attention through her bestselling novel *Black Oxen*. Her main character, a fifty-eight-year-old woman, regained the sexual and mental energy of a twenty-year-old after being "Steinached." Soon, women all over the United States and Europe were imploring Benjamin to release them from "a future menaced with utter fatigue." According to Atherton, Benjamin sometimes waived the considerable fees for his restorative zapping in the most "appealing cases." Within years, female reactivization was combined with diathermy, which delivered heat to the glands and supposedly made them more sensitive to the stimulating effects of X-rays. These procedures caused such a storm that the "rejuvenation of the bodily and sexual powers of men and women" was debated in Congress in 1927. "The question of rejuvenating the fairer sex is of absorbing interest," announced John Kindred, the Democrat representative for New York's Long Island, "To women, youth is even more precious than to men. Yet, for reasons intimately connected with her anatomy, woman's road to the goal of rejuvenation is more laborious than men's."

The Steinach operations, for both men and women, have since been discredited as little more than a powerful placebo, and, especially for those women exposed to X-rays, a potentially harmful one at that. Although there was no proof that the procedure brought about any real biological changes to ovarian secretions, purveyors like Benjamin, and the women he treated, truly believed in the efficacy of the procedure. Many women reported that they did feel genuinely rejuvenated after being Steinached. And although the risks of repeated X-ray therapy was questioned at the time, Benjamin was certain that his meticulously calculated low doses were harmless. But despite the questionable efficacy of female rejuvenation, Benjamin's ambition to enable women to enjoy enhanced vitality after their "dangerous age" was still pioneering. Progressive and caring, Benjamin was the first physician to acknowledge, document, and study gender dysphoria. In the 1900s, he met and became friends with Magnus Hirschfeld, the revolutionary German physician and sexologist who founded the Institut für Sexualwissenschaft (Institute for Sex Research) in Berlin in 1919. Hirschfeld studied, celebrated, and advocated for the experiences and rights of people with diverse gender identities and sexualities. He was also a passionate campaigner for women's rights and defender of reproductive choice and justice. At the time, people who were gay, gender-nonconforming, or trans risked being imprisoned or confined in asylums. Hirschfeld wanted to transform medical and societal perceptions and allow people to live, free from prejudice, according to the gender they identified with. In 1933, the institute was raided by the Nazis as part of the purge on homosexuality, and thousands of books, journals, images, and patient records from the extensive library and archives were burned.

Hirschfeld died in 1935 of a heart attack while living in exile, in Nice, France. Benjamin continued Hirschfeld's work in the 1940s in his clinic in San Francisco, where he treated trans people with hormone therapies. In an era when queerness and gender diversity were demonized and punished by the law and the medical establishment, and people risked being subjected to dehumanizing psychiatric interventions and surgeries to "cure" them, Benjamin pioneered clinical understanding and patient respect. In 1966, he published *The Transsexual Phenomenon*, the first study of its kind, which was instrumental in transforming medicine's treatment of trans people. By 1967, Benjamin had cared for, examined, and corresponded with nearly three hundred people. He urged hospitals and individual physicians to "treat these patients who are still so often cruelly rejected by the medical profession."

Benjamin is one of the most important figures in the history of transgender health and medicine. He deeply understood how cultural concepts of masculinity and femininity affected gender orientation as much as "its biological counterparts, maleness and femaleness." Even before he began researching transsexuality, he respected women's rights to embody and enjoy their femininity in ways that were not dictated by their reproductive biology.

For Benjamin, who fully believed in the healing potential of his procedure, reactivization was a validation and celebration of womanhood that wasn't yoked to childbearing. And his conviction that women's bodies held these transformative rejuvenating forces flew in the face of prevailing medical beliefs that women's endocrine glands were as unstable and defective as their uteruses were once thought to be.

Over the next decade, the seductive mysteries of female secretions were finally revealed. Scientists in laboratories in Germany and the United States raced to isolate the chemical structure of estrus. In 1928, the German pharmaceutical company Schering launched Progynon, the first commercially available estrogen supplement. Progynon pills promised to correct the imbalance in female sex hormones that occurred during menopause and to relieve symptoms like hot flashes, palpitations, and, of course, mood swings. Because it was made from estrogen extracted from the placentas and ovaries of animals, Progynon was expensive and complicated to produce. By 1933, the three properties of the primary female sex hormone estrogen—now known to be estrone, estriol, and estradiol—had been isolated from the urine of pregnant women and also horses. All three were swiftly patented. Since human hormones were easier to obtain, Progynon was made from pregnant women's crystallized urine instead. In the early 1930s, a similar product called Emmenin was launched by Canadian pharmaceutical laboratory Ayerst.

The costs involved in producing medications using active human estrogen were prohibitive, so biochemists started developing synthesized estrogen for medications that could be manufactured more cheaply. In 1941, Wyeth Pharmaceuticals in the United States launched Premarin, so named because it was harvested from pregnant mare urine. Finally, women could be prescribed an inexpensive medication to relieve severe menopause symptoms, where before their doctors might have offered nothing more than a few vaguely reassuring words. Companies such as Wyeth were instrumental in promoting the wonders of Premarin to patients themselves, but they also flagrantly exploited menopausal myths to drum up sales. In early advertising campaigns, Premarin was touted as a relief for husbands burdened by moody, quarrelsome wives. One showed a woman laughing with two men, accompanied by the headline "Help Keep Her That Way." Another, "Husbands Like Premarin Too," showed a couple enjoying a lovely trip in a sailboat above this clanger: "The physician who puts a woman on 'Premarin' . . . usually makes her pleasant to live with once again. It is no easy thing for a man to take the stings and barbs of business life, then to come home to the turmoil of a woman 'going through the change of life.'"

With the discovery of estrogen, many mysteries of female biology emerged into the glimmering light of the future. The essential *stuff* of femininity was tangible and malleable, and now it could be chemically supplemented and enhanced. But despite all the clinical and pharmaceutical advances of the first decades of the twentieth century, old ideas about women's bodies being naturally defective and deficient still pulsed through endocrinological theories. While in the past female nature had been blanketed as "hysterical" and "neurotic," now it was "hormonal." Ingrained beliefs about the far-reaching influence of hormones on women's bodies and minds mean that people with chronic diseases—especially those that cause abdominal pain and affect menstruation—still risk being told that their symptoms are simply the natural consequences of fluctuating female hormones. The persistent myth that women's mental and physical health is at the mercy of their capricious hormones was laid down in the early 1900s, when female secretions were characterized as erratic, mutable forces that needed to be regulated and controlled.

Those early versions of hormone replacement therapies—known as menopause hormonal therapy—were undoubtedly an enormous relief for many women. But the ideology behind the development of drugs such as Premarin was a revision of the centuries-old adage that the healthiest women were the most pleasingly feminine. In the 1950s and 1960s, the effects of estrogen supplementation on women's health—both beneficial and detrimental—would become clear, making hormone replacement therapy a fiercely debated issue in women's medicine. Several physicians in the early 1940s were rightly cautious about the risks of prescribing swiftly marketed, poorly tested synthetic estrogens. But, at the time, many members of the medical community, and women themselves, remained blissfully unaware of the dark realities of the hormone revolution.

12

LIFTING THE CURSE

In 1914, a student at Stanford University was desperately searching for a cure for her period pain. Every month she suffered such awful cramps that all she could do was rest. Her mother had taken her to "every kind of doctor" but "none of them did . . . any good." Then she met Clelia Duel Mosher, Stanford's professor of personal hygiene and women's medical adviser. Mosher asked her to loosen her clothing, lie with her knees flexed, and apply gentle pressure to her abdomen with one hand. She was to breathe in deeply and see how high she could raise her hand by lifting her abdominal muscles, and then observe her hand lowering as she exhaled and her muscles contracted. Mosher asked her to practice this exercise ten times, morning and night, while wearing her nightclothes. She was to make sure her room was well ventilated, and her movements smooth and rhythmical.

At first, the student was skeptical that Mosher's exercises would work. But for the next two weeks she diligently lifted and contracted. The day her period arrived, she anxiously asked her mother to prepare her bed and fill hot-water bottles. "I was so sure that I would have the customary pain that I lay down and waited for it to begin," she recalled. "But it did not begin." She went into the garden to gather greenery for a dance she was attending that evening and promptly fell over a fence. Worried her injury would set off her cramps, she retired to bed. By dinnertime she still felt no pain. She got dressed, went out, and danced the night away. The next day she felt tired and noticed an annoying sense of weight in her pelvis. But she was free of "pain, cramps or any bad effects."

Mosher was born in 1863, in Albany, New York. Her father, Cornelius, was a doctor, and Mosher longed to follow in his footsteps. She attended Albany Female Academy, the oldest girls' day school in the United States, but a bout of tuberculosis when she was a child had weakened her health. She wanted to go to college to study medicine, but her worried father wouldn't allow it. In a converted greenhouse in her family home, she studied botany and horticulture, and soon she was running her own floristry business. By the time she was twenty-five, Mosher had saved enough to pay for her own tuition at Wellesley, a private liberal arts college for women, and one of the "Seven Sisters" founded from the early-mid to late-nineteenth century to offer women an education equal to the male Ivy League. Mosher suffered from ailing health and exhaustion, but she wasn't deterred in her ambitions to become a doctor. By 1900, when she was thirty-seven, she had two master's degrees, a medical degree from Johns Hopkins, and her own private practice in Palo Alto, California. She had achieved what was assumed to be impossible for her; as a woman who had been so unwell, it wasn't expected that she could cope with the rigors of study or the demands of a medical career. Her experiences made her determined to debunk prevailing myths about women's innate physical and mental weakness and fragility.

In the 1890s, while she was completing her master's in physiology, she turned her attentions to menstruation. Like most women of her generation, she would have grown up hearing the message that periods were a shameful illness. Debates around the impact of menstruation on women's mental and physical strength were still highly contentious after Edward Hammond Clarke's provocative stirring of the pot in 1872. Mosher understood that men like Clarke exaggerated a few choice cases of menstrual pathology to argue that all women were terribly impaired by periods. The idea that "the periodical flow of blood from the genital tract" caused "disability and suffering" was so ingrained, Mosher noted, that women whose periods were easy enough often feared they were "abnormal." But she wasn't about to enter into a war of words with physicians who exploited menstrual mythologies to hard-sell female inferiority. Instead, she wanted to show how these narrow-minded but highly influential medical ideas in no way reflected the "normal or even average condition of women." Following in the footsteps of Mary Putnam Jacobi, Mosher looked to menstruating women themselves to prove it.

Mosher began interviewing and examining women like her, college women, about their menstrual experiences. These women were embracing opportunities now open to them in the changing world, and the last thing they or any woman needed was to be impaired by what Mosher called "traditional periodic incapacity." But she knew that simply stating this—as a woman physician—wouldn't be enough to refute ingrained myths that all women were "invalid one week out of four." Armed with hard-won research expertise and advanced scientific knowledge, she devised a methodology to study the physiology of menstruation. Mosher was a solitary person, absorbed in her work and isolated in her research. On her own, in a laboratory at Stanford, she considered reams of findings about women's living conditions, nutrition, sleep patterns, exercise levels, and other activities. She carefully analyzed details of their cycles, flow, pain, and other symptoms, and tabled their blood pressure, respiration, and hemoglobin levels. She also wanted to know how they felt about menstruating; she gave them diaries to record their feelings and sensations and exchanged letters with them regularly. By 1896, Mosher had studied more than 3,350 cycles in over four hundred women. Menstruation had never been explored and examined in such detail or such breadth before. Her "detailed presentation of . . . important facts" proved that menstruation, for the majority of women, was as normal a "periodic" function as sleep, digestion, defecation, and urination. Mosher believed that, unless a woman had an underlying disease, most common period problems were caused not by some inherent female defect but rather by fear and anxiety exacerbated by pervasive medical and cultural myths.

Mosher held the era's restrictive fashions partly responsible for menstrual ill health. She personally shunned buttoned-up, voluminous-skirted outfits in favor of loose, collared shirtdresses—with plenty of pockets—worn with ties and simple brimmed hats. The average skirt width at the time was an incredible thirteen and a half feet. Worn without supports, these hefty garments could cause "pelvic congestion" and enteroptosis—sagging abdominal muscles and intestines. Although corsets had been abandoned by the early twentieth century, the trend for tight girdles and narrow sleeves still impaired posture and joint flexion. Internalized ideas about female physical delicacy also meant that women were not exercising nearly enough. But the most prevalent cause of menstrual incapacity, Mosher believed, was fear. "The terms 'sick time' and 'being unwell' have long been grafted into our ordinary speech . . . The fact upon the mind of constantly anticipated misery can scarcely be measured."

Male gynecologists, the chief peddlers of menstrual misery, had inflated "abnormal" cases and perpetuated the assumption that pain was inevitable. Mosher wanted to normalize, not pathologize. Most women didn't need the opinions of unenlightened physicians who would demand they refrain from moving and thinking. Most healthy women could manage menstruation on their own. Mosher's abdominal crunch regime was designed to gradually strengthen core muscles to help relieve cramps and heavy bleeding. Over the years, she taught her technique—known as Moshering—to hundreds of patients and students, and many women's physicians adopted it in their own practices.

The theory behind Moshering was based on Mosher's master's research into female respiration, which disproved one of medicine's many wildly inaccurate theories. Until 1894, it was believed that women were not anatomically able to inhale and exhale from the abdomen and diaphragm. Several nineteenth-century physiologists also thought women of the "civilized races" had evolved "costal" breathing because of their sedentary lifestyles. Others thought women must be built to respire primarily from their upper chests because the female abdomen was reserved for pregnancy. Surprisingly, physicians didn't twig that being laced into suffocating corsets might have something to do with shallow breathing patterns. By observing one hundred women—fifteen of whom were pregnant—Mosher revealed that women were perfectly capable of diaphragmatic respiration, even into the ninth month of pregnancy. The only impediments were constrictive clothing and medical speculations. At a time when medicine and society still held such a tight grip on women's bodies and minds, Mosher dared to let them breathe.

In 1923, after thirty years of research into two thousand women over more than twelve thousand menstrual cycles, Mosher concluded her study. She published *Woman's Physical Freedom*, a groundbreaking book full of advice to relieve menstrual and menopausal "disabilities." The war had ended, and the world was being reconstructed. It was high time all that nonsense about female weakness, inferiority, and dependence was consigned to history. "Health is the birthright of every woman as well as of every man," she proclaimed, "but until we rid ourselves of some of the hampering traditions . . . the average woman will not attain this birthright." She knew that education and knowledge free of superstition and prejudice were key to improving women's health. And as a feminist physician, she was generating this knowledge by listening to and trusting women. But by 1923, theories about glands and secretions were once again reducing women to inferior biological conditions. What did their subjective feelings matter when hormones could do all the talking for them?

In 1926, the American physiologist Edgar Allen, who contributed to the isolation of estrogen, and the gynecologist J. P. Pratt conducted the first clinical trials of injectable ovarian hormones. Some subjects were going through artificial menopause, and others had amenorrhea—scanty and infrequent bleeding. Finding an effective treatment for women who had undergone gynecological surgeries was undoubtedly important. But Mosher wouldn't have countenanced pumping women full of estrogen simply because their periods were on the light side. She knew of a woman who was instructed by her college physician to abandon her studies for this exact reason. But this was totally unnecessary because she was otherwise perfectly healthy. She went on to bear eight children, all healthy and vigorous.

Allen and Pratt, however, saw amenorrhea as a deficiency disease.

One of their subjects, thirty-one-year-old Miss A.C., had bled lightly and erratically since she was thirteen. After receiving hormone injections for twelve days, she said she menstruated "more than I have ever . . . at one time in my life." Allen and Pratt didn't mention whether she had any other symptoms, fertility problems, or underlying illnesses. Nothing was said about her life, work, or health history. The success of their trial rested solely on whether an idea of "normal" blood flow was restored.

Gynecology's historical obsession with menstruation had made periods the "central idea" of women's lives. And now endocrinology was adding fuel to the fire by parlaying menstruation—and menopause—into new disease categories of deficient and defective hormones. Mosher rejected the notion that ovarian secretions had bearing on strength, intellect, or accomplishments. After her 1920 lecture "Strength of Women," a doctor commented that female secretions must be deficient because women suffered so badly after ovariotomies. Surely female physiological inferiority was indisputable, since women were riddled with hormonal incapacities. To Mosher, this was nonsense. She knew many women who "distinguished themselves during the menopause and afterward" when their ovaries were inactive. Mosher was sixty when *Woman's Physical Freedom* was published. She wasn't about to be trampled by bad science. Before she retired in 1929, her book was reprinted six times across the United States and Europe.

Mosher made the important distinction between "functional" period niggles and the pain and heavy bleeding of gynecological diseases. Throughout the nineteenth century, normal menstruation was frequently pathologized into surgical oblivion, while abnormal menstruation was often dismissed as common or garden-variety women's troubles. But by the 1920s, gynecology had progressed enormously, thanks to advancing biomedical knowledge and treatments. An understanding of diseases that affected menstruation—including uterine fibroids and cancers of the cervix and uterus—was emerging into the scientific light. But even though blood and pain were being taken more seriously as signs of illness and disease, stigma and misbelief still clouded diagnoses.

Since the early 1900s, gynecologists had been trying to fathom the causes of dysmenorrhea, the clinical term for severe menstrual pain. The association of pelvic and uterine pain with hysteria had been waning since the end of the nineteenth century. But gynecologists in the early twentieth century still filtered their assessments of women's gynecological pain through patronizing and punitive assumptions. If a woman's physician couldn't fathom a reason for her dysmenorrhea—like inflammation, muscle spasms, or a more serious underlying condition—she was probably just sensitive and nervous, especially if she was the luxury-living type who cried over the slightest discomfort. For George Ernest Herman, an obstetrician at the London Hospital, dysmenorrhea was a disease unto itself, triggered by "severe spasms of uterine colic" reflecting through the spinal nerves. It was most common in adolescent girls with "highly developed nervous systems" and rare in women over twenty-five. The only "natural" cure was pregnancy, he believed, to quiet the uterus by dilating the cervix. If a sufferer didn't procreate as early as possible, she risked becoming sterile and forever devoid of sexual feeling. He did admit that ovariotomy was the only fail-safe medical solution for dysmenorrhea. But he stressed, "This is a thing seldom to be considered." The procedure was now known to be highly risky and cause horrible aftereffects; but Herman objected because ovariotomy meant losing "the potentialities of marriage and motherhood." If a sufferer was infertile or in pain after having had children, she could "be relieved of menstruation and its sufferings" after the age of thirty-five. But her physician must rule out kidney and intestinal conditions before agreeing to surgery. If he was still certain her pain was menstrual, he had to be completely sure it wasn't "merely a monthly manifestation of psychasthenia"—neurosis characterized by obsessive fears and thought to manifest in physical symptoms—"neurasthenia" (nerve weakness) or, yes, "hysteria."

While dysmenorrhea was seen as a disease of mostly younger women, physicians recognized that when it affected older women, uterine fibroids were probably to blame. The cause of these noncancerous growths of smooth muscle and tissue was still a mystery. Fibroids were thought to be most common in women between the ages of thirty and fifty.

Although smaller fibroids could be harmless, larger fibroids could cause tormenting pain, excessive hemorrhaging, bladder problems, chronic constipation, and pelvic obstruction. The heaviest fibroids were often "the source of much suffering and, occasionally . . . death." But by far the most serious consequence, according to certain gynecologists, was that they "hindered conception" and "prevented convenient coitus."

In the late 1800s, some gynecologists in Britain, America, and Europe turned to electrotherapy to treat fibroids and other complaints such as dysmenorrhea, uterus displacement, menopause symptoms, and neurosis. Electrotherapy was literally a galvanizing force for restoring health to the reproductive organs—and a humane alternative to surgery. Purveyors believed that by placing electrodes on a patient's abdomen and lumbar region, and sometimes inside her body, she would be left "as nature made her, a *woman*, and not a thing." Although some claimed electrotherapy could shrink fibroids, others dismissed it as quackery. By the late nineteenth century, the rise in surgeries for fibroids had eclipsed the electrotherapy craze. A procedure called myomectomy, in which the fibroid was excised through the vagina or abdomen, meant that women would still be able to have children. But if a fibroid was too large, calcified, or septic, women had to submit to a hysterectomy. "Hysterectomy for fibroids is unrivaled . . . for its ability to amend invalid women by the thousands," declared British gynecological surgeon John Bland-Sutton in 1913. "It enables them to lead useful lives, and, if married, to be companions to their husbands."

Bland-Sutton recommended myomectomy only to preserve fertility or for young women eager to marry. But for the middle-aged, it was better to "enter into the pleasures of life" as "wombless women" than crawl into old age beset with fibroids. "Total" hysterectomies, for larger fibroids, involved removing the cervix along with the uterus, and sometimes the ovaries and fallopian tubes. Since the 1870s, this operation had also been performed as a radical treatment for cervical cancer. The "subtotal" hysterectomy, developed in the late 1800s, removed the uterus and part of the cervix, usually through the vagina, and carried fewer risks. But it wasn't an effective treatment for cancer because surgeons weren't able to remove marginal lymph tissue that might become malignant. In the late nineteenth century, seven in every ten women who underwent total hysterectomy died.

By the early 1900s, surgical methods and hygiene had improved, but hysterectomies were still potentially perilous. Bland-Sutton preferred to take the safer vaginal route, but he urged absolute caution because patients could still bleed to death. After surgery, women were in intense pain even if they had been anesthetized (not all were), and many vomited and developed high fevers. Wounds could burst and become infected; internal bleeding and bladder, kidney, and intestinal complications were common. Then there was the ever-present risk that women, said to be emotionally fragile at the best of times, would experience "psychical disturbance" and develop "post-operative insanity." Despite these horrendous dangers and side effects, hysterectomies remained the most popular treatment for fibroids in the early twentieth century.

Over the last century, medicine has come to understand that up to 70 percent of white women and 80 percent of Black women will have uterine fibroids at some point in their lives. Black women are two to three times more likely to be affected earlier in their lives, and to develop fibroids that are larger, multiple, and cause life-limiting, painful symptoms. While fibroids are often small enough to go unnoticed, some women experience extreme pain, heavy bleeding, and pain during sex, which is all too frequently dismissed by doctors. And medicine still has no idea exactly what causes fibroids. Speculation that fibroids might be caused by genetics or increased estrogen has done little to relieve women's suffering, or to ensure they are diagnosed promptly and treated respectfully. Despite there now being different treatment options—pain management and physiotherapy, hormone-modifying drugs (including the Pill), and less invasive laparoscopic surgeries and myomectomies to remove fibroid tissue—many women are told their only options are to deal with the pain or have a hysterectomy.

The myth that a hysterectomy is the only cure for fibroids, laid down more than one hundred years ago, persists to this day. And a hysterectomy still carries enormous risks to a woman's health and quality of life. It can lead to bladder and bowel problems and vaginal prolapse. Removing the uterus places extra strain on the pelvis, causing chronic pain and mobility problems. And it can reduce libido and destroy "sexual sensation." But women are routinely not informed about these serious complications. In the US, it has been suggested that one reason for this insistence on often completely unnecessary surgery is that gynecologists have to perform a minimum of seventy hysterectomies during their residencies. And in the UK, the lack of specialist knowledge, gynecological "culture," and incentives for nonsurgical, pharmaceutical, and therapeutic alternatives are to blame. By failing to address its ignorance and by prioritizing profit, tradition, and convenience over real care for women's bodies and lives, gynecological medicine is still woefully failing women with fibroids.

While Bland-Sutton was extolling hysterectomy's virtues, the innovative surgeon and physician Louisa Martindale was investigating far less invasive options for treating women with fibroids. In 1913, she visited the Freiburg clinic where Krönig and Gauss were revolutionizing gynecological treatments with X-ray therapy. Martindale, Brighton's first female GP, bought her own 200,000-volt machine so that she could treat fibroid disease and breast cancer with "intensive" X-rays. She became one of the first physicians in Britain to pioneer this alternative to traumatizing surgeries. By 1920, she had treated thirty-seven women with "uterine fibromyomata" at Brighton's New Sussex Hospital for Women, which she founded. For middle-age patients whose fibroids were no bigger than a "six-month pregnancy," she considered X-rays "the treatment *deluxe*." Although high doses could cause vomiting and radiation sickness, aftereffects were minimal compared with those from hysterectomies, which took months to recover from. Martindale treated headmistresses and school matrons, an author, a government official, and a businesswoman—all of whom could all ill afford to take time off from their careers. X-ray treatment, she concluded, "improves the health of the patient without interfering with her usual mode of life . . . It does away with the nervous shock of an abdominal operation . . . and most important of all, it is a treatment eminently successful in suitable cases, and is one free from any mortality."

By the early 1920s, X-rays were being used in several British hospitals to treat fibroids and also chronic metritis, inflammation of the uterus caused by a bacterial infection. Plenty of surgeons were still pleading the case for hysterectomy; but for physicians who embraced X-rays, the results spoke for themselves. The treatment was suitable for women who couldn't endure surgeries, like those with anemia, lung and heart disease, and thyroid conditions. X-ray therapy shrunk fibroids, halted bleeding, and brought on a trouble-free menopause with minimal hot flashes. It also offered "glorious possibilities" for treating other devastating diseases. In the 1920s, cancers of the uterus, ovaries, and cervix were the leading causes of death in women. "There is . . . no case in which the Woman Doctor is more needed than in the case of cancer," Martindale wrote in 1922. Owing to their "natural dislike of . . . medical examination" by men, many patients refused to seek treatment until it was too late. If they could consult with a woman doctor, their "terror" would be "allayed," and their lives saved. Women were suffering because of a lack of knowledge, research, and care, and also because the doctor-patient dynamic was rigged against them. She urged women doctors to use their intuition, self-sacrifice, reasoning, and sympathy in the "service of humanity." The advent of X-rays and, later, radiation therapy marked a humane shift in women's medical treatment. Martindale called on "fearless" woman doctors to bravely lead its future.

In 1924, Helen Chambers, the leading cancer expert, gave a lecture to the Medical Women's Federation (MWF), founded in London in 1917 to support women in medicine. Chambers had been researching the effects of radium on blood and tumors at the cancer laboratories of Middlesex Hospital since 1911. During her lecture, "Progress on the Cancer Problem," she suggested that members of the MWF form a committee to explore the treatment of cervical cancer with radium therapy. Martindale joined, along with Anne Louise McIlroy and other esteemed pathologists and gynecologists, including Dr. Elizabeth Hurdon, who observed radium therapy in Europe and used it in her own practice at Johns Hopkins. Over the next four years, the committee traveled between three women's hospitals providing a radiation clinic. They treated over three hundred women and reported fewer recurrences and many full recoveries. But such a chemically hazardous treatment needed a dedicated facility and properly trained staff. In 1928, the committee launched a public appeal to fund a hospital "for the radiological treatment of women suffering from cancer and allied diseases."

Within two years, a property on Fitzjohn's Avenue in North London was converted into a thirty-bed hospital, directed by Hurdon and staffed entirely by women. It was supported by private donations and public organizations, including the Medical Research Council and the British Empire Cancer Campaign, which provided the radium. The treatment was expensive, but beds were reserved for public patients. In 1930, the Marie Curie Hospital, named for the honored physicist and chemist who won the Nobel Prize in Chemistry in 1911 for isolating radium, was opened. For women patients, the option to be treated with radium therapy rather than surgical butchery, by women who understood and respected their bodies, was not only preferable but lifesaving. Women sought help before their diseases became more destructive because they knew they could consult with, and be treated by, a woman. The shame and humiliation that had been instilled in them about their most intimate body parts was allayed. By 1937, nearly one thousand women had been treated for uterine cancer at the hospital. The five-year survival rate for "early operable cases" was 83 percent—the second highest, at the time, of all cancer clinics worldwide. By 1967, when the Marie Curie Hospital was transferred into the Mount Vernon Hospital in Northwest London, it had treated 13,802 cases of cancer, mostly of the cervix, uterus, and breast but also the ovary, vulva, vagina, and rectum. Those incredible women turned the germ of an idea into Britain's first-ever cancer clinic led by women, for women. They revolutionized the care of some of the most devastating diseases of the female body. And they achieved this as feminist activists committed to reforming the medical care and treatment of women, at a time when male surgical prowess was deemed more important than women's health and happiness.

Whether they were debunking antiquated myths or pioneering humane, world-leading treatments, women in medicine made truly radical progress in the early decades of the twentieth century. When physicians like Martindale and Mosher led the charge on women's diseases and body knowledge, they were dedicated not only to improving women's health but also to helping them lead lives free of social oppressions. In Britain in the 1920s, the need to educate women about their bodies and their health became especially urgent. Women were increasingly leaving behind the privacy of home and entering public life. The 1918 Education Act raised the school-leaving age to fourteen, and the Sex Disqualification (Removal) Act of 1919 meant that middle-class women had more opportunities to pursue university education and professions, from medicine, law, and teaching to clerical and administrative work. After the war, many working-class women remained in the labor force. But assumptions that women were physically weak and therefore less productive meant that their wages, even for backbreaking industrial and "sweated" work, were meager. Menstruation was universally acknowledged as an illness that "greatly handicapped (women) in professional and business life." Why treat them well and pay them properly when they're sick for a week of every month?

For the Medical Women's Federation, dismantling punitive falsehoods that threatened women's educational and professional ambitions was a vital cause. Its members spread the word that periods were neither an illness nor a disability through pamphlets distributed to schoolgirls and factory workers, talks at women's clubs, and advertisements in newsletters. The leading members also pursued research projects. In 1915, Dr. Alice Sanderson Clow, a "humane and perceptive" expert on women's physiology who had trained at the London School of Medicine for Women, began her own survey of "normal menstruation" in 2,050 "healthy girls" between the ages of twelve and twenty-two. Most participants were in secondary school; others were enrolled in the teacher training college where Sanderson Clow worked as a medical officer. With dysmenorrhea still high in gynecologists' minds, and negative perceptions of menstruation posing social barriers, Sanderson Clow was determined to prove that periods were not pathological.

At the annual meeting of the British Medical Association in 1924, Sanderson Clow revealed that only 3 percent of the women she interviewed experienced "disabling" period pain. Most discomfort could be relieved with exercise, fresh air, hot baths, and improved hygiene. She firmly disagreed that uterine spasms and mystical causes like "under-developed genital organs" were as common as some male gynecologists claimed. What women needed was accurate, unbiased information. They also urgently needed private lavatories in their schools, factories, and offices so they could wash, change their sanitary towels, and dispose of used ones discreetly. After she read her paper, one male physician confessed that he had been taught that menstruating women were incapable of doing anything. It was absolutely unheard of to suggest one took a *bath*. His mind was blown by a patient who kept up her active regime of cycling during her periods. The panel president revealed that he'd recently been "asked to believe that two-thirds of all women had their pelvic organs misplaced and suffered dysmenorrhea as a result." He was extremely grateful to Sanderson Clow and the MWF for doing all that hard work so that male physicians could "look at the subject . . . with a greater sense of proportion." Amazingly, not all medical men were quite so willing to bow to women's wisdom.

Sanderson Clow held gynecologists' egregious claims about menstrual ill health responsible for the discrimination women faced. Throughout the 1920s, physicians conducted investigations into the pressing question of the "economics of menstruation." In 1928, the British Industrial Fatigue Research Board reported on two years of research into "the effect of the menstrual cycle on working capacity." By measuring women's performances in blind tests, the industrial psychologist Charles Samuel Myers and his assistant concluded that "this physiological phenomenon has, as a rule, no noticeable effect on working capacity among normal healthy women." They also found that menstruation had no bearing on mental acuity. But plenty of gynecologists refused to let go of the idea that menstruation made women mad, sad, and useless. Many believed there was no such thing as a "normal" bleeding woman. By the late 1920s, endocrinological theories about the role of hormones and glands in human psychology had crept insidiously into ideas about women's mental and physical health. No matter what the surveys said, it didn't change the fact that women were at the mercy of their capricious hormones.

In 1928, a thirty-two-year-old mother of two went to Mount Sinai Hospital in New York to see her gynecologist, Robert Frank. For months she had been feeling exceptionally nervous and tense just before her period. Once, when she was eight weeks late, she fitted and flailed as if she were hysteric. Her husband was "considerate and kind," but her illness was tearing her family apart. She had considered taking her own life. Frank couldn't find any evidence of a pelvic condition. She wasn't pregnant or menopausal. Her neurological examination was normal. When her tension was "at its height," as Frank put it, he drew 80 cubic centimeters of her blood. She calmed down immediately, but after a few hours her "hysteria" returned.

What could be transforming this dutiful wife into an insufferable harpy gripped by "suicidal desire"? It must be her bloody hormones. Frank had been studying secretions of sex hormones during the menstrual cycle for a few years. His patient's blood contained twice the amount he would expect to find in a normal premenstrual woman. Obviously, her ovaries needed to be quieted down. Frank administered a course of X-ray treatments, and soon her symptoms subsided. So did her periods. After three years, her estrogen levels were reduced substantially. Her "nervous disturbance"—and the anguish of her poor husband—was mercifully relieved.

In February 1931, Frank addressed the New York Academy of Medicine about the "manifold disturbances" he had observed in fifteen female patients between twenty-four and forty-seven years old. Up to ten days before their periods, all had complained of "indescribable tension." They were restless and irritable and felt like "jumping out of their skin." Their "desire to find relief" drove them to "foolish," "reckless," and "reprehensible actions." When their periods arrived, they usually returned to normal. Frank concluded that an "excessive accumulation of hormone" preceding menstruation was the cause. He had defined "normal" hormone levels after studying the estrous cycle of mice. He named this troubling clinical phenomenon "premenstrual tension" (PMT).

For severe tension, Frank recommended "X-ray toning." The oldest woman in his study underwent "elimination"—a total hysterectomy. In mild cases, or for women who had a few good childbearing years left, he recommended medications to encourage hormonal excretion, laxatives, and heroic amounts of coffee. When he published his findings, he included a helpful chart summing up each patient's main "complaint." F.B., forty-one years old, was an "unbearable shrew"; "husband to be pitied," he remarked of forty-seven-year-old L.H.; A.W., forty-one, was "impossible to live with." In addition to all the "psychoneurosis" these women were inflicting on everyone around them, many had undiagnosed physical symptoms. Seizures, intense pain, fatigue, asthma, heart and lung problems, skin bleeding, and edema in the hands, feet, and face were just some of the conditions he attributed to excessive hormones. By naming PMT as a psychiatric disorder, Frank legitimized the myth of menstrual madness that had haunted women for centuries. But by claiming that so many physical symptoms were also linked to secretions gone wild, he set the stage for many "obscure diseases" to be explained away as hormonal.

Menstruation was the perfect canvas for new ideas about women's changing lives and social roles. As the world faced the devastation of the global depression, "women's work" in stable industries and civil sectors increased. Politically, women's rights had expanded with the passing of the Nineteenth Amendment in the US in 1920 and the Representation of the People Act in the UK in 1928. But socially, a woman's place was still in the home—even when her contribution to the workforce was more valuable than ever. Marriage bars in the US and UK meant that many were forced out of their jobs after they wed. For several female psychologists and psychiatrists, women's emotional relationships to menstruating were expressions of the internal frustrations of being female at a time when gender roles were so conflicted.

While Frank was defining hormonal hysteria, German psychoanalyst Karen Horney was connecting PMT to conflicts between the biological motherhood drive and the psychical rejection of everything it involved—from sex and birth to giving up work and having to care for a child. Helene Deutsch, a colleague of Freud's and one of the first psychoanalysts to specialize in women's health, blamed PMT on the symbolic loss of a pregnancy and the failure of the female imperative to be "a servant of the species." For British psychoanalyst Mary Chadwick, feelings of loneliness, worthlessness, and "extreme unhappiness" were caused by ingrained shame, disgust, and fear about menstruating. Chadwick also claimed period blood triggered "phantasies" about the punishment of women's bodies during the witch trials. These theories wouldn't have been much help to the average woman worried about how her period would affect her ability to work, or the young girl brought up to see her monthlies as a shameful curse. But these psychoanalysts were not calling for ovaries to be yanked out or hormones to be manipulated. Instead, they were revealing how women's menstrual health was affected by an infuriating array of myths, anxieties, and misbeliefs—even though some of their theories are essentialist and reductive by today's standards.

"So much, then, for the background of superstition and mysticism which in previous times so completely befogged the subject of menstruation," wrote American gynecologist Emil Novak in *The Woman Asks the Doctor.* Published in 1935, Novak's book was meant to enlighten readers about the "distinctive biological characteristics" of their bodies. The solution to improving women's health lay with education, especially around body functions "enshrouded in a mantle of mysticism." And there was none quite so mystical as periods. Novak was thrilled that "modern . . . scientific investigation" was "sweeping away the cobwebbery of mystery" that had surrounded women's blood and bodies for centuries. He reassured his readers that there was nothing dirty or defiling about menstrual blood, but he still talked about "soiled" sanitary napkins and the "offensive odor" of menstrual blood. He stressed that periods were "normal" and shouldn't interfere with "life's activities." Even so, exercise, diet, clothing, working hours, and recreation should be strictly controlled if "injurious conditions" were to be "ameliorated." He blamed mothers for coddling their daughters into seeing periods as a "sickness" but in the same breath advised against strenuous studying, since it laid "the foundations for a future life of nervous and perhaps physical invalidism." Novak fancied himself a compassionate progressive, but his book was a patronizing reduction of women's body experiences to a very male and thoroughly medicalized view of "femaleness." He firmly believed that a woman should obey the authority of her gynecologist—the arbiter of knowledge about her "special physiological functions." And a woman who was possessed of a little of this knowledge was a "far more satisfactory patient."

Novak had very particular ideas about menstrual hygiene. In the mid-1930s, a revolutionary tampon with a cardboard applicator, sold under the now-famous brand name Tampax, became available through drugstores, chemists, and mail order. Designed and patented by a GP and osteopath from Colorado named Earle Cleveland Haas, Tampax tampons were the first commercially available form of internal sanitary protection. A US newspaper ad from 1936 welcomed women "To This New Day for Womanhood!" Tampax was pitched to modern, active, energetic women whose lives shouldn't be constrained by bulky pads. Advertisements lauded the tampon's ability to transform periods into a modest celebration of the wondrous possibilities of being a woman. Being able to buy a box of five or ten that could fit in a small purse, for thirty-five cents in the United States, was a watershed moment for menstrual health and hygiene. As well as being wholly more convenient than pads, tampons promised women a discreet and hygienic menstrual experience—a major selling point was that tampons helped keep periods a secret and made them "invisible." But for many medical men, Novak included, the thought that women might risk their decency by submitting to "intravenous manipulation," as he put it, was appalling.

Like many gynecologists and physicians at the time, Novak decided the "internal vaginal tampon" was not suitable for unmarried girls because it would cause pain and injure the hymen. Married women with "loose vaginal canals" would probably find the tampon fell out. Besides the danger of cervical infection Novak associated with "plugging," the idea of women touching their own vaginas was most indecorous. Novak couldn't countenance any woman risking such intimate interference—unless she was a professional dancer. He advised anyone wanting to use tampons to first seek their gynecologist's "diagnosis."

But a huge part of the appeal of Tampax was that women could purchase and use tampons without a doctor's say-so. It enabled women to take control of their bodies and to manage menstruation without medical meddling. After being told for so long that periods were a pathology that impeded women's capacity to think, work, and enjoy their bodies, Tampax promised a kind of freedom. But advertisers were not sleeping on the fact that medical men objected to tampons. Tampax understood that allaying medical anxiety had to be front and center in marketing campaigns. "Your doctor will be able to tell you that Tampax is the most natural and most hygienic method of sanitary protection," explained a 1936 ad. "EVERY DOCTOR should know about Tampax," proclaimed another ad, which also announced that the tampon was "designed by a physician" and was "highly useful to gynecologists." On the one hand, advertising emphasized how tampons freed women to dance, swim, partake in sports, and enjoy "holiday freedom." But on the other, the messaging evoked the attitude of paternalistic protection that surrounded women's bodies in the 1930s. If women wanted fulfilled and productive lives, they better be sure medicine had granted them permission.

In the early years of World War II, as women entered the workforce in huge numbers, tampons were pitched as a means for women to serve their countries unimpaired by their "natural disabilities." One British newspaper ad, from 1942, claimed that without Tampax, it would be impossible for women to partake in the "strenuous struggle for freedom." The underlying message that tampons were beneficial to menstrual health played neatly into new narratives about women's value outside the separate sphere. Serving the war effort was "the task that allows no room for 'off days.'" Users were liberated in their lives and liberated from their body's failings. Tampax was a commercial company; it exploited all kinds of messages to profit from women's bodies. But perhaps the most insidious of all was this idea that tampons transformed women into instruments of labor, whose messy, unpredictable, defective bodies could be regulated to maximize efficiency. Throughout the 1930s, women's bodies, and lives, had been emerging into the spot-light of public health and national progress. Where women were once the private guardians of the home, now they were the public servants of the future. As World War II loomed ominously, women's productive and reproductive bodies would be subject to increasing medical scrutiny, control, and discipline.

13

DUTIFUL AND DISCIPLINED

In 1933, in a small terraced house in County Durham, a thirty-two-year-old woman had just given birth to her seventh child. Like most of the women her age who lived on her street, she was married to a coal miner. The colliery owners provided accommodation for workers and their families, in houses just like hers, in mining towns and pit villages across the north of England. Thankfully, her husband had kept his job in the mine after the recession, but the little housekeeping money had to stretch. She now had nine mouths to feed. Every day at 4:00 a.m., she rose while her family slumbered to weave mats, which she swapped with her neighbors for clothes. Then there was bread to bake, a vegetable garden to tend, and coals to haul from the outhouse. Until 10:00 p.m., sometimes even midnight, she cooked, cleaned, and cared. Her husband was kind, considerate, and devoted to her, but he had to work. She did everything she could to make sure her children were well fed, and healthy.

Her own health, however, had been deteriorating for years. Her shoulders ached from nerve inflammation. Her kidneys were damaged by the Bright's disease she suffered as a child, causing constant headaches, nausea, and digestive troubles. On the advice of the colliery doctor, she had had her teeth pulled to cure her gum disease. Since her last pregnancy, she had recurring cystitis, and her lower-right abdomen throbbed continuously. The doctor had prescribed medicine for "ovarian trouble," and she prayed this would work so that she wouldn't have to go to the hospital for surgery. Who would look after the children? When the local "health visitor," a midwife who attended nursing mothers, babies, and children under five, came to check on her, she was amazed at her "indomitable pluck." Although the woman had been "delicate all her life," she was "extremely careful to preserve . . . whatever strength and health remains for her."

This woman, and many like her, was one of 1,250 participants in a study led by the Women's Health Enquiry Committee (WHEC) into "the incidence and nature of general ill-health among working-class women." Made up of eleven nonpolitical representatives of women's organizations across England and Wales, the committee wanted to reveal the hidden truth about the illnesses, diseases, disabilities, and life circumstances of working-class women across the country. "The woman only comes onto the map of public conscience," declared WHEC member Margery Spring Rice, "when she is performing the bodily function of producing a child." Outside reproduction, women like the thirty-two-year-old from Durham escaped medical "vigilance"; the pain and suffering they bore every day, as they struggled to make ends meet, slipped unnoticed into the cracks of ignorance and inequality.

Throughout the 1920s, women's bodies became the focus of public and governmental attention for the most tragic reason. One in 250 "live births" resulted in a mother's death. In 1932, a committee appointed by the Ministry of Health (MOH) to examine maternal mortality and morbidity published its final report. Of 4,655 maternal deaths studied over four years, an incredible 45.9 percent were avoidable. Many were dying because of inadequate postnatal care, poorly managed labors, and a lack of treatment facilities. But women were also blamed for their own demise. "Negligence of the patient or her friends, in failing to follow the doctor's advice or in ignoring obvious symptoms" was named as a leading cause, especially of fatal embolisms, preeclampsia—or toxemia, as it was known then—and postpartum hemorrhaging.

The WHEC recognized that the MOH report failed to grasp the "complex problems, medical and social," contributing to "damage and disease resulting from childbirth." At the time there were no accurate public records of women's chronic health problems. Health care was fractured and fragmented, especially for people who couldn't access medical benefits under the National Insurance Scheme. Good health was a privilege beyond the reach of so many. Only employed people who made compulsory contributions through their wages were eligible for "free" health services. A husband's benefits did not extend to his wife or children. Unless they were contributing to a private scheme or could afford a private doctor, women had free health care only during pregnancy and for the year they were "nursing mothers." Outside of childbearing, an "incalculable amount" of ill health was unreported, undiagnosed, and untreated.

The MOH report didn't consider the obstacles women faced when seeking medical attention. Nor did it address the impact of long-term illness on maternal health. Instead, it recommended that medical services should be directed toward disciplining girls' bodies to "withstand the stresses and strains inseparable from maternity." Healthy childbearing was the solution to a "healthy race." Women should be taught to obey the "physiological law" of their reproductive destiny from childhood. The WHEC noted that the recent "spate of scientific investigation" at least meant "medical opinion" was "alive to the fact that the function of child-birth . . . is fraught with danger and requires the highest degree of expert study and care." Women's health and welfare was, finally, worthy of "anxious consideration." But while the female body was valued *only* as "the human casket of precious unborn life," the grim realities of women's suffering would remain shadowed.

Beginning in 1933, the WHEC distributed questionnaires through the health visitors so women could describe, in their own words, their experiences of ill health. They also gathered information on housing, sanitation, diet, occupations, housekeeping budgets, daily routines, and leisure activities. In 1939, Spring Rice published the findings in her book *Working-Class Wives*. The most common conditions were anemia, constipation, dental problems, rheumatism, "bad legs," and gynecological ailments including dysmenorrhea, menorrhagia, and uterine prolapse. Around a third had never seen a doctor for their abdominal and pelvic pain, heavy bleeding, or "womb trouble." Many just accepted that such symptoms were women's lot, especially after having children.

Some were frightened of going into a Poor Law hospital; others were unable to because they couldn't leave their children. When women did visit male doctors, they were often told to stop fussing or to go home and rest—which, let's face it, was impossible. One twenty-five-year-old went to her GP about unrelenting menstrual pain only to be told she would "grow out of it." Another couldn't bear discussing her "intimate affairs" with a man. If only she could visit a "woman doctor" she might be relieved of her troubles.

Working-Class Wives presented a wealth of statistics, but it didn't reduce women to anonymous numbers. Instead, it amplified their voices to show how their health difficulties were connected to their economic insecurities. Most of these women shouldered the relentless burden of "sacred responsibility." "The emancipation for which many thousand women have worked in the last hundred years," wrote Spring Rice, "has had little or no effect on the domestic slavery of mind and body of the millions with whom rests the immediate care of a home and family." By shining a light into the "small dark unorganized workshop of the home," Spring Rice wanted to reveal the "stealthy and sinister deterioration" of the housewife's "health and happiness." Many families were forced into desperate poverty by the unemployment crisis. The pressures this placed on mothers and wives, to make do, tend, and provide, meant their "mental and physical well-being" was being "sacrificed." "The constant struggle," explained a housewife from Essex, "has made me feel nervous and irritable and . . . unable to move or even think coherently. This effect of mental strain expressed in physical results seems most curious and I am at a loss to properly explain it to a doctor." Her husband was out of work. Before marriage, she worked as a bookkeeper and typist. She hated to think how her mental state was affecting her children.

The problem of maternal mortality and morbidity would never be solved until health care was freely available during "all the stages of a woman's life," and "for all her ailments." Spring Rice called for maternity clinics to be extended into women's health centers, providing treatment for gynecological disorders, "psychological troubles," and much-needed advice about family planning. Spring Rice believed passionately that women should have the right to control their fertility, especially when their health was at risk. Since 1924, she had been superintendent of the North Kensington Women's Welfare Clinic, which provided birth control. The WHEC reported an average of five pregnancies for each participant. One forty-three-year-old from East London had endured twenty-three pregnancies; nine ended in miscarriage. For years she had suffered anemia, kidney disease, and heart troubles. Although she had been to a hospital, she had never been given any advice about birth control.

The tensions between women's private right to control their bodies and their public duties as mothers of the "race" came to the fore in fierce campaigns around abortion in the mid-1930s. Under the Infant Life (Preservation) Act of 1929, killing a viable fetus was a criminal offense unless the mother's life was at risk. In 1934, 14 percent of "puerperal death" in England and Wales was attributed to "disease and damage" caused by botched operations and poisonous abortifacients. Sanger and Stopes had campaigned for birth control and family planning as the "cure" for illegal and dangerous abortion practices. Now feminist activists were fighting for women to be able to choose to end pregnancies without their lives and liberties being perilously threatened.

In 1934, more than a thousand delegates of the Women's Co-operative Guild congress voted to demand abortion be decriminalized and made as safe and accessible as any other medical procedure. The guild also called for women serving prison sentences for breaking "antiquated laws" to be amnestied. "Children should be born through choice and not because of fear," said Mrs. Day, who moved the resolution. She knew of a woman from Rochdale, a large town in Greater Manchester, serving four years for helping a friend "in dire need." Mrs. Jarvis, seconding the motion, stated that no contraceptive was 100 percent reliable, so women should be able to have an operation performed with "skill and care." Her decision to do this should be hers alone, for "our bodies are our own." Abortion was not legally permitted for psychological reasons unless the woman was certified insane. If she couldn't face raising another child, her economic situation was dire, or her social circumstances were precarious, she had no legal or medical protection.

Abortion rights were a class issue. Women were ending pregnancies regardless of the law. But how much danger this posed depended on their means. Some could afford to pay physicians who performed "therapeutic" abortions under the legal radar. But working-class and poor women had to improvise. If she couldn't afford "female pills" covertly advertised for "menstrual blockages," she might try purgatives such as Beecham's pills and quinine. Many resorted to herbal brews, gin, scalding baths, "indulgence in violent exercise," or, harrowingly, knitting needles, crochet hooks, or scissors. Some inserted pieces of slippery elm bark, a traditional folk abortifacient that expanded when wet, to dilate their cervixes. But it contained bacterial spores that could cause infections and life-threatening sepsis. Even if these unreliable remedies worked, women were often left bleeding, in intense pain, and seriously unwell.

In 1936, a group of socialist feminists including F. W. Stella Browne and the physician and birth control advocate Joan Malleson formed the Abortion Law Reform Association (ALRA). Browne was a radical political writer and lecturer who had been a member of the WSPU. Since the 1920s, she had campaigned for women to embrace their diverse sexual wants and needs. She criticized the ways that women's sexualities were quashed by the "masculine mythology" of social mores and moral ideals. An ardent supporter of birth control, Browne recognized how sex, especially for working-class women, was bound up with fear. It was completely unfair for women to be denied pleasure because of the terror of punishment and potential death, and encouraging avoidance and abstinence was dehumanizing. The year the ALRA formed, the National Council of Women of Great Britain presented a deputation to the MOH urging it to "appoint a representative committee" to investigate abortion and consider what "medical, legal and social" measures might improve the "existing situation." A committee of physicians, politicians, and activists, run by the MOH and the Home Office and chaired by MP and barrister William Norman Birkett, was established. The Birkett Committee began a three-year inquiry into the impact of the country's oppressive laws on the death and disease of women forbidden to choose.

The urgent need for reform became a stark reality in 1938. In the early

evening on April 27, fourteen-year-old Miss H was walking along London's Whitehall when a guardsman from a barracks on Horse Guard's
Parade asked if she wanted to see a horse with a green tail. Once she was
lured into the stable, Miss H was violently raped multiple times by five
guardsmen. She managed to escape and find a policeman, who took her
to Cannon Row police station, where she was examined by a woman
officer. Her internal injuries were horrific. Three perpetrators were identified, and rape committal proceedings began in May. Miss H was pregnant. She saw a gynecologist at St. Thomas' Hospital who refused to
interfere because she had been impregnated by a guardsman and might
be carrying "the future Prime Minister of England." "And anyhow, girls
always lead men on," he wrote in his report.

Miss H's parents took her to see Joan Malleson, who agreed she
should be allowed a "therapeutic abortion." Malleson then wrote to Al-
eck Bourne, a prominent and sympathetic gynecologist at St. Mary's, to
ask if he would "risk a *cause célèbre* and undertake the operation in hospital." The guardsmen had been found guilty and sentenced to penal
servitude—imprisonment with hard labor. Malleson was certain that
public opinion would be "immensely in favor of termination . . . in a case
of this sort." Bourne agreed to perform the procedure for no fee, and told
Malleson that afterward he would turn himself in. On June 14, Bourne
told Chief Inspector Walter Bridger, "I have emptied the uterus and I
want you to arrest me."

Bourne's trial began on July 18 at the Central Criminal Court. He
was charged with "unlawfully procuring the abortion of a girl" under the
Offenses Against the Person Act. Miss H had been subjected to an un-
imaginably traumatic attack. But she was diagnosed as "normal" and
"healthy." The injuries she sustained would not have made childbirth
difficult, the court heard. Bourne had to convince the jury that he had
upheld his duty to preserve Miss H's health. He argued that the "circumstances of the conception" implanted "seeds of terror" in her mind. Even
though the pregnancy wouldn't *technically* endanger her life, it would
doubtless condemn her to a life of incurable "nervous, psychoneurotic . . .
and secondary physical illnesses."

The judge, Mr. Justice Macnaghten, reminded the jury that "the desire of a woman to be relieved of her pregnancy is no justification for performing the operation." But he asked them to think carefully about the extraordinary facts of the case. Miss H was a child. Parliament had recently raised the age of consent from an alarming twelve to sixteen. Her pelvic bones were not fully developed. It was not only illegal but medically "undesirable" for her to bear a child. Common sense must prevail when considering the mental anguish that a girl of such "tender years" would suffer by being forced to "carry in her body" the consequences of this terrible rape. The jury still had to determine whether Bourne had caused "the death of the child" in "good faith" for the "purpose of preserving the life of the mother." The jury adjourned for forty minutes. Bourne was found not guilty.

Bourne's acquittal was an important step on the long road toward reproductive justice. But it was a tentative one. Responses to the case revealed how abortion in the eyes of the law and the medical profession was still by no means a woman's right. When the Birkett Committee published *The Abortion Report* in 1939, it recommended that therapeutic abortion was legally justified if a doctor was acting to avert "serious ill-health" rather than only to prevent death. It also acknowledged there was "widespread sympathy" for permitting abortion for victims of "unlawful" sexual conduct—rape and incest. But first, the sexual conduct in question had to be decreed unlawful. If a girl or woman felt supported enough to report her assault, judgments about her social status, morality, and sexuality clouded whether she was believed. "Abortion cannot be justified merely on the strength of an allegation that pregnancy is due to rape," the report stated. Even if she was underage, the Birkett Committee didn't think she was automatically entitled to a termination. Such permission would be a "direct temptation to loose conduct among young girls." The despicable views of Miss H's gynecologist—that young girls led men on, gave consent despite their protestations, and understood "quite well" what they were doing—were depressingly pervasive.

Before the introduction of "Rape Shield" protection laws from the late 1970s in the US, details of a woman's sexuality and sexual history could be used as evidence during trials to discredit her accusation of rape, assault, and abuse. It wasn't until 1999 that laws restricting the use of complainants' sexual history as evidence were formalized in the UK. Today, a woman's credibility can still be impacted by perceptions of her character, actions, behavior, clothing, and appearance. Victims are often humiliated and belittled by judgments under cross-examination. Imagine how unbearable it would have been to seek justice for sexual violence when the law was influenced by such cruel and prejudiced attitudes. Justice Macnaghten described Miss H as "an ordinary decent girl, brought up in an ordinary decent way." At the beginning of the trial, the attorney general confirmed she had been a virgin. Her respectable parents didn't have a clue about how to procure an abortionist. If Miss H had been of "the prostitute class" and endured a similar ordeal, Bourne almost certainly wouldn't have performed the procedure. Shockingly, he would have refused point-blank if Miss H were "feeble-minded," since "she would not have suffered mental distress in the pregnancy." Besides, the "quality" of a child born to a mentally unwell woman, or one who had to earn a living through sex work, "was no concern of his."

The Birkett report ultimately left the interpretation of the law to the discretion of doctors. Therapeutic abortion was a medical procedure, warranted only when a physician "diagnosed" the mental or physical destruction a pregnancy might cause. The committee didn't recommend the law be changed, only "clarified." Cautious doctors were not obligated to agree to an abortion unless they believed a woman's life was indisputably in danger. But if they did, they at least had some legal protection. Most criminal convictions for abortion at the time were issued not against medical doctors but against "laywomen" abortionists.

In Macnaghten's opinion, there was a massive distinction between the benevolent actions of a respected physician and the people who "did it for money." The judge had recently overseen a case in which a "woman without any medical skill" traveled to London to procure "the miscarriage of a pregnant girl." Her fee was 2 pounds and 5 shillings—just shy of £114, or about $155, in today's money. Seconds after she administered her instrument, "the victim of her malpractice was dead on the floor." Unlike this "predatory harpy," Bourne was a "highly skilled" surgeon who agreed to perform an abortion "without fee or reward" because of his commitment to "the alleviation of human suffering." Demonizing "unqualified" women while lionizing professional men was a tale as old as medical history. And neither the legal nor medical establishment of 1930s Britain was about to admit how important the care and services of laywomen were for those whose bodies were not their own.

While there were certainly abuses, not all abortion providers were the grasping, anatomically illiterate butchers the report painted them to be. Many women performed abortions to save lives, not squander them. And not all professional doctors were quite so charitable as Bourne was. The Birkett Committee reported that between 2 and 3 guineas, equivalent to about £127 to £190 today—approximately $172 to $257—was the average fee for a doctor or a layperson. Some high-end gynecologists charged upward of 100 guineas, comparable to well over £5,000 today. Women would always find a way to procure abortions, the committee agreed. And they rarely did so for "selfish" reasons. Married women ended pregnancies because of poverty, unemployment, and health problems. Some single women couldn't face the stigma and hardships of being an unwed mother. The report didn't recommend any solutions to the social and economic difficulties behind rising abortion rates. Nor did it hold the law in any way accountable for maternal injury, illness, and death. It was more convenient to blame "unskilled" abortionists. And sadly, it was more important to uphold moral righteousness than to protect society's most vulnerable women.

Thankfully, this wasn't the view of all the committee members. Dorothy Thurtle, the Labor Party politician and women's rights activist, believed the fundamental reason that working-class women sought "non-medical abortionists" had been overlooked. In her minority report, she explained that "a high degree of fertility" impelled many to defy the law. And until this problem was "considered courageously and honestly little advance will be made." Thurtle was vice president of the Workers' Birth Control Group (WBCG), an association of members of the Labor Party and affiliated groups, which lobbied the MOH to "recognize birth control as an essential part of Public Health work." Since 1927, Thurtle had campaigned for scientific contraceptive advice to be freely available to all working people through local health authorities and maternity centers. The majority of the committee remained ambivalent about the need for "reliable . . . harmless and simple to use" contraceptives for all—not just the middle class and well-to-do who attended birth control clinics, or private doctors who "give information to those who can pay for it." Some committee members cautiously agreed that accessible "birth control advice" might "alleviate the difficulty" of illegal abortion. But detractors, especially those involved with religious organizations, feared the unrestricted "spread of contraception" would "intensify the evil."

The objections heard by Birkett from pro-life doctors were ludicrous. Dr. Mary Caldwell of the Union of Catholic Mothers claimed diaphragms caused mental illness, cancer, and womb enlargement. A Welsh gynecologist claimed that he knew a woman who developed "acute eroticism" after receiving a pack of condoms in the post. These notions were not taken seriously, but the committee still upheld conservative attitudes about who should be allowed contraception. Only married women whose health would be impaired by pregnancy should be allowed birth control through public health authorities. Once again, a woman's feelings, life circumstances, and right to decide didn't come into it. Contraception was a medical matter, and it was up to a medical professional to "diagnose" its need.

For Thurtle, the "refusal to extend . . . facilities to those who desire to space their families" was a "counsel of despair." The WBCG also recognized that "excessive child-bearing" damaged women's bodies and minds in far more insidious ways than the medical establishment acknowledged. But even for a progressive organization like the WBCG, contraception was a public necessity rather than an individual right. This sense that women should control their bodies to relieve the country's medical and economic burdens permeated the interwar control movement. Back in 1930, the WBCG joined with other campaign and voluntary groups to form the National Birth Control Council (NBCC). Across twenty clinics, the council provided information to "married people" so they could "space or limit their families and thus mitigate the evils of ill health and poverty." Yet again, only those who obeyed their socially ordained duties were deemed worthy of birth control.

Since the end of the nineteenth century, the birth rate in Britain had been gradually decreasing, in line with the "demographic transition" that happened across Western Europe and the United States. The reasons for this transition are complicated, but many sociologists and historians have linked fertility decline to the expansion of women's rights, education, and employment opportunities. And the culture around reproduction had also shifted from quantity to quality. As women gained more knowledge about their bodies and their fertility, they were better equipped to limit the size of their families. But by 1939, in Britain the birth rate had shrunk, worryingly, below replacement levels. Anti-feminists could now argue that reproductive choice was not only religiously and morally abhorrent but nationally destructive. The NBCC changed its name to the Family Planning Association to shift its purpose from fertility limitation to life-quality improvement. But the world was hovering on the brink of history's most devastating war. Progress toward reproductive autonomy was about to be subsumed by the elevation of women from subservient wives and mothers to heroic home-front defenders.

In the spring of 1941, the Ministry of Labor called on women between the ages of eighteen and sixty to register for voluntary service. That December, the National Service (No. 2) Act conscripted women, for the first time in British history, to serve in the war. At first, single women and widows between the ages of twenty and thirty were called up. They could enter the industrial workforce in engineering, transport, or munitions, or join the auxiliary departments of the Air Force and the Royal Navy, as clerks, mechanics, codebreakers, or operation planners. Many became nurses or hospital support staff, teachers or cooks. Thousands volunteered for the Women's Land Army, which cultivated soil, grew crops, worked in dairies, and managed forests. By 1943, 90 percent of single women and 80 percent of married women were employed, many in roles previously barred to them on the basis of sex. Their contribution to auxiliary services freed up men for military duty, and their labor was vital for ensuring that agricultural and industrial production flourished.

The war expanded the lives of many women. Miraculously, the idea that women were too physiologically and mentally fragile to carry out "men's work" faded away. But while women were filling the boots of the male labor force, they were also "conscripted" to keep the home fires burning. Initially, women with children under the age of fourteen didn't have to enter service. But from 1941, more nurseries were opened to enable women to work, though women still had to fulfill their social purpose and "natural" destiny as housewives and mothers. Feminine domestic labor was rebranded from invisible drudgery to a publicly valued part of the war effort. As the minister of food Lord Woolton explained in a radio broadcast to "the housewives of Britain" in 1940: "We have a job to do . . . No uniforms, no parades, no drills, but a job wanting a lot of thinking and a lot of knowledge, too. We are the army that guards the Kitchen Front."

With birth rates in free fall, women were also expected to step nobly up to the procreation plate. The government intervened with welfare provisions to encourage women to produce and nurture citizens of the future. Postnatal care had been improved in response to the epidemic of maternal mortality and morbidity. Public hospitals made space for more maternity beds. In 1940, the Ministry of Food (MOF), which controlled rationing and food distribution, started providing free milk to pregnant women, nursing mothers, and children under the age of five. From 1941, food welfare schemes were introduced so that everyone receiving free milk was also entitled to supplements of cod-liver oil, orange juice, and vitamin A and D tablets. "The raw material of the race is too valuable to put at risk" the MOF declared in 1943.

It was tremendously important that mothers and babies were provided for during the scarce-and-stricken war years. But at the same time, maternity was becoming ever more medically controlled and socially supervised. Women, after all, possessed the "raw material" of reproduction—and that material had to be regulated and disciplined to give the next generation the best chance of growing fit and strong. A 1941 ad for the MOF's welfare food scheme, headed "Welcome Little Stranger," told pregnant women that "the very best welcome you can give your baby is a beautiful body, a contented disposition and a healthy, happy mother." Although this idea of maternal-health perfection permeated the pronatalist agenda, overtly eugenic discourse around reproduction had—publicly at least—quieted down since the late 1930s. The fascist program of racial hygiene and national purity, enforced by the Nazis, brought the chilling consequences of eugenic theories into a horrifying reality.

In 1933, the Nazi Party passed a law legalizing the eugenic sterilization of *lebensunwertes Leben*, "lives unworthy of life." Women and men with chronic diseases and disabilities—epilepsy, manic depression and mental "deficiency," schizophrenia, Huntington's chorea, hereditary blindness, deafness, and congenital "physical deformities"—were to be sentenced to *Hitlerschnitt*, Hitler's cut. Any women thought to possess some deficiency that was detrimental to the future of the Third Reich were subjected to tubal litigation—the tying of the fallopian tubes—and later, to the destruction of the ovaries using X-rays. Many women forced to abort their babies were also sterilized without their consent. The law permitted the use of force on any person who didn't submit.

Sterilization criteria became a measure of social and racial cleansing. Anyone deemed deviant or degenerate, including women of ethnic minorities, those who were unmarried or poor, had many children, relied on welfare, or engaged in sex work were targeted. During the Holocaust, Jewish and Roma women held in Auschwitz and Ravensbrück were the victims of sickening mass-sterilization experiments conducted by research gynecologist Carl Clauberg. He injected the ovaries of hundreds of women, mostly mothers, with formaldehyde—which caused unbelievable pain, inflammation, internal bleeding, and very often death. He was trying to perfect a way to sterilize up to one thousand women a day in the nations the Nazis planned to conquer. From Block 10 of Auschwitz, where Jewish people were held for medical experiments, physician Horst Schumann selected young women to endure prolonged doses of X-rays to their ovaries. Many died from radiation exposure.

The Nazi eugenics program was the logical conclusion of regarding women as nothing more than reproductive material. These unthinkable atrocities were only part of the suffering meted out to women for the purposes of biological research. But abuses of this kind were not contained to the Nazi regime. The 1933 law was heavily inspired by the compulsory sterilization law modeled for the United States in 1922 by Harry H. Laughlin, superintendent of the Eugenics Record Office, the epicenter of eugenic propaganda. Couched as a means of promoting "the health of the individual" and the "welfare of society," Laughlin's law was a racist and ableist plan to weed out "undesirable" traits that didn't fit his vision of a strong, white America. Since 1927, when seventeen-year-old Carrie Buck lost her appeal against her compulsory sterilization order at the Lynchburg Colony in Virginia, twenty-seven states had passed laws permitting eugenic sterilization in mental institutions. Any "defective" person afflicted with "hereditary forms of insanity"—namely "idiocy, imbecility, feeble-mindedness or epilepsy"—could be forced to undergo a salpingectomy or a vasectomy.

Vulnerable and disenfranchised women were the targets of these procedures. Sexual "looseness" and promiscuity were interpreted as symptoms of a chillingly broad category of feeblemindedness. This meant young women who had suffered sexual violence risked having their fertility stolen because they were seen as "manifestly unfit" to become mothers. California, which had the highest rates of compulsory sterilization in the United States, performed the majority of procedures on young women "diagnosed" as "dependent, delinquent," and mentally deficient. At the Sonoma State Home, they were often forcibly admitted just to be sterilized and promptly "released" because they could no longer propagate welfare-draining offspring. After the Depression, eugenic lawmakers framed sterilization as a solution for the country's economic burdens. But in reality, these despicable practices were designed to rid America of people who, in the white supremacists' opinion, were not deserving of life.

From the 1930s, racist beliefs about biological and social inferiority legitimized the mass sterilization of Black and other ethnically diverse women. Poverty, the eugenicists insisted, was a disease spread by populations who were incapable of controlling their sexuality and childbearing. To "cure" this disease for the benefit of whites, thousands of Black, Indigenous, and Latinx women were cruelly robbed of their bodily autonomy. The most rampant reproductive racism in California was forced on Mexican women branded as "hyperfertile" and "criminally inclined." In 1936, at the Pacific Colony state hospital in Spadra, now Pomona, a sixteen-year-old Mexican girl was sterilized because she was a "mentally deficient . . . sex delinquent" with "truant and disciplinary problems." She'd had a child when she was only fourteen. Her IQ, according to the Pacific Colony psychiatrist, was "high moron level."

In the Southern states, poverty scapegoating and racial hatred fueled crusades to steal the reproductive rights of thousands of Black women in the name of social improvement. Five thousand of the eight thousand "mentally deficient" people sterilized in state institutions in North Carolina in the 1930s and 1940s were Black, and 85 percent were women. Beginning in the 1930s, the Mississippi state government swerved the limits of eugenic laws by allowing surgeons and gynecologists to perform "therapeutic" salpingectomies and hysterectomies without patients' consent or knowledge, after childbirth or during procedures like appendectomies. This operation, known as the "Mississippi appendectomy," was practiced for decades.

Dehumanizing misbeliefs about Black women's bodies and minds had justified inconceivable sexual and reproductive abuses against them for centuries. Under the guise of post-Depression public health measures, Black women were once again being denied the right to control their own bodies. From the late 1930s, eugenic ideas underpinned many interventions into Black women's reproductive rights. At one end stood the racist eugenicists, those appalling apologists for medical violence, who demonized Black mothering, sexual behavior, and susceptibility to illnesses and diseases. On the other end were the reformists who saw birth control as a way for Black women to take charge of their fertility and reduce health problems associated with "excessive" childbearing.

For years, Margaret Sanger had been championing family planning and contraception for women and communities whose lives and health were impacted by economic insecurity. In 1930, her Birth Control Clinical Research Bureau joined forces with the National Urban League, the civil rights organization advocating for the rights of Black communities affected by racial discrimination, to open another birth control clinic in Harlem, home to thousands of Black people and families who had

migrated from the Southern states since World War I. Sanger was well
aware that the legacy of medical exploitation, eugenic ideologies, and
racist segregation made Black people suspicious of white-led interventions into their bodies and lives. To help secure people's trust and "determine the best methods . . . for educating the public concerning the
aims and purposes of Birth Control," Sanger appointed an advisory
council of fifteen Black social and medical leaders to help run the Harlem clinic. One council member was May Edward Chinn, the first
Black woman to graduate Bellevue Hospital Medical College and, at
the time, the only Black female physician in Harlem. During her internship at Harlem Hospital in the late 1920s, Chinn went on emergency calls with local ambulance services, tending the sick and injured
in overcrowded apartment houses. Segregation rules meant private hospitals in New York refused to treat Black patients and barred Black
physicians from practicing, so Chinn set up her own practice after her
internship. By the time she was appointed to the clinic council, she was
an established community physician. She often treated patients in their
homes, turning kitchens and bedrooms into makeshift operating theaters where she and a surgeon performed essential procedures under the
low glow of battery-operated lamps.

With the expertise and on-the-ground knowledge of respected figures like Chinn and Mabel Staupers, the Harlem-based nurse who
revolutionized the profession by breaking down barriers of racist discrimination, the Harlem Clinic provided family planning advice, contraceptives, and gynecological care to thousands of women. But it wasn't
until 1933, when the clinic employed Black nurses, physicians, and social workers, that women felt comfortable and supported enough to
attend in larger numbers. But the huge tensions that existed around the
"aims and purposes" of birth control had not gone away. Sanger, like
many eugenically minded reformers, still saw reproductive discipline as
a route to "racial betterment." For Black communities, leaders, and
health professionals, birth control was one way to begin to overcome
"the unequal economic and political relations between Blacks and
whites." Sanger genuinely believed that education around family planning and contraception would improve the living conditions and health

of Black women. But she also promoted the idea that societal ills would be solved by regulating and controlling Black women's reproductive freedom.

Sanger, in so many ways, was a revolutionary. In 1933, she helped bring about a revision of the Comstock Laws' blanket ban on contraceptive distribution. She arranged for a package of pessaries to be imported to Hannah Stone, medical director of the Research Bureau, knowing it would be confiscated by US Customs. When *United States v. One Package of Japanese Pessaries* went to court in 1936, the judge ruled that the contraceptive had been obtained for medical rather than obscene purposes. Physicians were then permitted to supply birth control to patients for health preservation only. For decades, Sanger had seen how a lack of access to contraceptives was diminishing the health of women, especially those suffering from poverty and deprivation. But she wrongly believed that Black women were ignorant about family planning and needed the guidance of a white-led organization like hers to "recognize the need" for limiting their families. In 1936, after funding cuts led to it being taken over by the New York Committee of Mothers' Health Centers, the Harlem Clinic closed its doors. But Sanger's ambitions to bring about "racial betterment" with birth control didn't waver. The following year, she started devising plans to bring clinics, services, and outreach to impoverished communities in South.

In 1937, the National Emergency Council was appointed by President Roosevelt to examine the "economic conditions of the south." "The low-income belt of the South is a belt of sickness, misery, and unnecessary death," the council reported. The especially high rates of disease and ill health among Black communities, the report stated, "was not due to physical differences between the races" but "greater poverty and lower living conditions." At the time, Sanger was the honorary board chair of the Birth Control Federation of America (BCFA). She felt it was the organization's duty to help women "improve their immediate situation" by bringing services to areas where access to birth control was restricted and segregated. Sanger knew birth control would not alleviate the "special social and economic pressure" Black women faced. But she did believe it could help tackle the "attendant loss of life, health and happiness that spring from these conditions." Her experience with the Harlem Clinic had taught her how important it was to gain the trust of communities first. So in 1938 she devised a plan to have Black physicians and nurses run local clinics, while Black ministers, trained by the BCFA, would advocate for the new services and allay people's fears. In a letter to Clarence Gamble (of the Procter and Gamble dynasty), a board member of BCFA, Sanger wrote, "We do not want word to go out that we want to exterminate the Negro population, and the minister is the man who can straighten out that idea if it ever occurs to their more rebellious members." Gamble replied, "Let's appear to let the colored run it."

The "Negro Project," as it was known, was controversial and contentious from the very beginning. The BCFA formed the Division of Negro Service in 1939 and invited prominent Black educators, politicians, and physicians to sit on an advisory council and publicly endorse birth control. One was Dorothy Boulding Ferebee, an obstetrician, a civil rights activist, and "one of the outstanding Negro women physicians in the country." But as had been the case with the Harlem Clinic, the Negro Project was ultimately controlled by white organizers. Rather than following Sanger's engagement and outreach idea, the BCFA wanted to integrate birth control into existing health facilities supported by Roosevelt's New Deal. The BCFA appointed a white male, Robert Seibels, chair of a committee on maternal welfare within the South Carolina Medical Association, to set up demonstration clinics in rural Berkeley County and Nashville, Tennessee. The BCFA employed Black nurses to work in clinics and educate women about the new services. But to actually get ahold of contraceptives, women had to visit white doctors. Sanger disagreed with the BCFA's insistence that the project was delivered by white-male outsiders. Seibels dismissed her as a "dried up female fanatic." The clinics were not well attended because women, understandably, were reluctant to consult with white doctors about such intimate matters. The Negro Project funding folded in 1942.

Sanger's intentions—to educate and empower—were realized far more effectively by activists who actually understood the health concerns and life experiences of Black women. Contrary to Sanger's infantilizing opinions, Black women had been practicing birth control, of their own volition, for decades. Community leaders and health activists had been organizing services for segregated communities across the country since the early 1930s. In 1941, Ferebee became chair of the Committee of Family Planning within the National Council of Negro Women, the organization founded in 1935 by Mary McLeod Bethune to support Black women's civil, political, and economic rights. Since 1935, Ferebee directed the "Cotton Field Clinic," which brought medical care to plantation workers in Mississippi. She endorsed birth control as a means to improve health and welfare, and she also stressed the importance of grassroots education and community support. She proposed a "well-rounded, well-planned public relations program," led by Black physicians, nurses, ministers, and teachers in "personal, daily contact with the masses of the Negro."

The obstacles imposed upon Black women's access to and use of birth control couldn't be overcome by outsider programs of persuasion and coercion, especially if they were white-led and smacked of "race suicide." "The existing medical and social problems of the Negro," Ferebee declared, "are . . . problems of the nation." If "family planning" was "vital to the . . . welfare of the mothers and babies of this country," it was even more so for women paying the price for systemic injustice with their bodies and their lives. As Ferebee insisted, birth control was an essential part of preventative health care and a human right.

When Sanger first started campaigning in the early 1900s, she framed voluntary motherhood as a way for women to reclaim their bodies and lives from medical and social control. But for her, birth control for Black women was a vehicle to drive social improvement rather than an individual, autonomous right. The prewar birth control movements in Britain and America centered on the idea that women's bodies needed to be disciplined to relieve the conditions of poverty and deprivation associated with overpopulation. This responsibility was imposed not on white middle-class mothers but on Black women and other ethnically diverse women, marginalized and disenfranchised women, the working class, the vulnerable, and the poor. As the influential American activist and philosopher Angela Davis wrote, "What was demanded as a 'right' for the privileged came to be interpreted as a 'duty' for the poor."

The United States entered the war in 1941. Amid anxieties about declining birth rates, the BCFA changed its name to the Planned Parenthood Federation of America. As in Britain, the organization's emphasis shifted toward the importance of family planning in securing the healthiest, happiest citizens of the future. Promotional material encouraged married couples to "have as many children as their health and economic circumstances justify." But oppressive ideologies about what *kind* of women were fit to bear the "children of tomorrow" still lurked beneath wartime pronatalist agendas. As women's bodies and lives remained under the glaring spotlight of public health, medical and social tensions continued to rise between their private rights and their public duties.

14

CONTROL AND PUNISH

In 1941, a twenty-five-year-old woman from Cleveland, Ohio, was engaged to be married. But before she and her fiancé could be granted a marriage license, she had to prove she was not infected with syphilis. So she went to a clinic to have the Wassermann test, a blood test for syphilis antibodies named after the German bacteriologist who developed it in 1906. She was certain the test would be negative. She was saving herself for marriage, and she didn't have any suspicious symptoms or health worries. But the test was positive. She "denied any sexual exposure," but her physicians didn't listen. The Wassermann test was supposed to be watertight biological proof. Her fiancé called off the engagement.

For nine months, from April 1942, she received over forty injections of medications, including neoarsphenamine, an arsenic derivative used to treat syphilis since the 1920s. When a physician performed an internal examination, he confirmed she was a virgin. The "introitus"—the opening to her vagina—would only "admit one finger." Four subsequent syphilis tests came back negative. But the physicians would not let that initial positive go. She had more blood tests and a painful lumbar puncture to draw spinal fluid. All these tests were normal. But a sample of "special blood," sent to another hospital in Cleveland, turned out to be positive. Between August 1943 and December 1944, she received seventy more injections. When this treatment ended, her tests came back negative. At long last she was declared free of an infection that she never even had. The tragic truth about the disease that *was* lurking in her body, the disease hidden behind the false-positive syphilis diagnosis, wouldn't be revealed for years.

Ohio was one of thirty-three states that enforced premarital screening legislation since 1938 as part of a nationwide campaign to curb the rise of syphilis. When it first emerged in the late fifteenth century, this devastating disease had been shrouded in mystery, prejudice, and fear. From the sixteenth century, syphilis was known to be transmitted through sexual intercourse, and it remained one of the most widespread infectious diseases. But its association with moral degeneracy and sinful behaviors meant it had sunk into the margins of medicine. Sufferers were marked by disfiguring sores that ravaged facial features. If it was left untreated, disease-causing bacteria could invade the bones, heart, liver, and nervous system, causing blindness, brain damage, and an excruciating death. European nations blamed syphilis epidemics on invading armies. In England it was called the "French disease"; in France, the Spanish disease; in Russia, the Polish disease; and so on. By the nineteenth century, its spread was generally blamed on female sex workers—remember the violations of the Contagious Diseases Act?—because it was epidemic among the military in times of war. Sex workers were framed as deviant hosts, transmitting their sin to innocent, courageous soldiers.

Syphilis was a sinister enemy to health and decency, thwarting treatment at every turn. And because so little was known about where it came from or how to cure it, certain communities and populations were scapegoated as the disease's vectors. Into the twentieth century, as high rates of syphilis mortality and morbidity among Black communities in the South were acknowledged, medical authorities perpetuated racist misbeliefs about "sexual impetuosity" to explain it away. It's hardly surprising that no concerted effort to eradicate syphilis had been made when it was associated with, and blamed on, people medicine had historically marginalized, demonized, and ignored.

But in the early 1930s, as the United States faced the impact of unemployment and poverty on the nation's health, syphilis was brought out of the shadows. Surveys conducted by the Public Health Services suggested that one in ten Americans had the disease, with around half a million new infections contracted every year. Since no screening programs existed, many sufferers had no idea they had it until the disease took its most destructive hold. Another study suggested that 18 percent of all deaths from heart disease, the leading cause of death in the United States next to cancer, were actually caused by complications from syphilis. Undiagnosed and untreated syphilis was not only a waste of life; it was a waste of money. Thomas Parran, the physician and public health expert who launched the "war against syphilis," estimated that the annual cost to US taxpayers for treating syphilis patients in medical facilities was around $15 million. For all those confined to institutions for insanity, paralysis, and blindness, the cost was reportedly between $40 and $50 million every year. The country could no longer afford to let this "unmentionable moral scourge . . . rot the very foundations of physical and mental wellbeing." Parran was appointed US surgeon general in 1936. He made it his mission to bring the true costs of syphilis to public attention and unite medical professionals, state governments, and citizens in a mass effort to rid America, once and for all, of this "great plague."

Parran was determined to wrestle syphilis from the moral closet and treat it like any other public health threat—with medical research, public education, prevention, and cure. But this didn't mean the syphilis slate was suddenly wiped clean of social and biological prejudices. Women were not the only targets of syphilis trace-and-control programs. Men were also required to have Wassermann premarital tests in many states. But women's bodies were the main sites of discipline and control in attempts to flatten the VD curve. A huge number of new cases every year were attributed to "children born afflicted . . . innocent victims of the transmission from parent to child." One of the purposes of screening was to prevent unwitting carriers from passing the disease to their "progeny." If a woman, like the twenty-five-year-old from Ohio, was identified as a carrier, her marriage license was withheld until she had undergone a noxious arsenic and mercury treatment and was declared "cured."

Years before premarital laws were enforced, many hospitals and clinics demanded that pregnant women be tested for syphilis. Prenatal screening, enshrined in the legislation of many states from 1938, is now a routine part of preventative health care for pregnant women across the US, and in the UK under the NHS. A blood test for sexually transmitted infections including syphilis, hepatitis B, and HIV is usually performed at the first prenatal medical appointment. Of course, it is important that any underlying infections that might be transmitted from mother to fetus are identified and treated as early as possible. But the responsibility for ensuring the health of an unborn baby still lies with mothers, not with fathers. At present, the US Centers for Disease Control (CDC) recommends regular STD screening for pregnant women, sexually active women who are under twenty-five or engage in so-called high-risk behaviors, and gay and bisexual men. But for heterosexual men, at present, STD screening is entirely voluntary. Women are still expected to shoulder the responsibility of sexual health. The availability and acceptability of routine testing means women, importantly, have independent control over their own bodies. But today's preventative health care is yesterday's regime of control and punishment.

In the late 1930s and early 1940s, amid fears about declining birth rates, motherhood and childbearing were promoted as patriotic duties. But economic pressures and the impending war made many women reluctant to bring more children into the world. In the early war years, federal funding for maternity services and health insurance provisions for working women was increased. Prenatal care, hospital births, and postnatal care were now accessible for those who wouldn't otherwise have been able to afford it. The idea that medicine was there to protect and defend the health and well-being of mothers and babies was an essential aspect of the pronatalist culture sweeping America. And if the country was to be replenished with the fittest citizens, then women's bodies—the vessels of the future—had to be as regulated, disciplined, and *clean* as possible.

In 1941, the American Committee on Maternal Welfare promoted the Mother's Charter, a bill of rights for potential mothers everywhere. Headed "The Defense of Mothers Is the Defense of Nations," the charter proclaimed that every woman fulfilling her "obligation" of "creating and sustaining new life" was "entitled to health and protection for herself and humanity." It was also her responsibility to uphold the "inherent right" of her baby "to be born without inherited or transmitted diseases." "Premarital and preconceptional . . . examination" was a mother's duty and a wife's privilege. Submitting to state-controlled medical supervision was surely a small price to pay for eternal marital health and happiness. A poster promoting "full medical examination for VD before marriage" depicted a bride leaning beatifically against her groom underneath the headline "Happiness Ahead—for the Healthy but Not for the Diseased." Once again, the preservation and success of the idealized social units of marriage and family lived and died with women—with the control of their bodies, with the surveillance of their biology.

If syphilis screening was intended to protect mothers and wives, it meant something completely different when women who deviated from marriage, motherhood, and monogamy were targeted. Anxieties about the threat VD posed to the military led to fierce propaganda campaigns warning soldiers off "good-time girls," "pickups," and "streetwalkers." Posters featuring femme fatales with cigarettes clasped between bright-red lips, headlined "She May Be a Bag of Trouble" and "Booby Trap," spelled out in no uncertain terms that "A Minute with Venus" was not worth "A Year of Mercury." "Loose" women were depicted as seductive vamps hunting for prey to unload their penis-destroying diseases upon. Men were the victims; women the perpetrators. The "promiscuous" woman as vector of infection was a well-trodden cultural trope, and during the "war against syphilis," it was thoroughly exploited. If syphilis was the scourge of decent masculinity and family harmony, then women who languished outside the lines of socially prescribed femininity were targets for blame and shame.

In 1941, the US Office of Community War Services formed the Social Protection Division to "safeguard" the armed forces and civilian population against the "hazards . . . of venereal diseases." The division focused on stamping out not only prostitution but "sex delinquency." Health officials had the power to confine any promiscuous woman, regardless of whether she was soliciting sex or not, and force her to be tested at one of the new quarantine hospitals or rapid detection centers.

If she didn't submit, a court order would force her to. Women who tested positive were detained and given intravenous high-dose anti-syphilitics like Salvarsan, an arsenic-derived "magic bullet" developed in the early 1900s. Detention was meant to last until the cure was affected, but it could be indefinite. These measures were spun as "community activities directed toward the protection of women from sexual exploitation and the social rehabilitation of prostitutes and other sexually delinquent women." The ethical violation of forcing women to endure a nonconsensual medical procedure didn't come into it. The preservation of public health and morality, in the feverish 1940s, was sacrosanct.

Long-held social mythologies about women, their bodies, and their susceptibility to illnesses crystallized in these wartime health campaigns. Medical discourse reflected and validated the age-old belief that the healthiest women were the most socially obedient. Margery Spring Rice's shrewd observation that women "only come into the public conscience" when performing "the public duty" of motherhood rang especially true in early 1940s America. The female body, in the eyes of medicine and society, was reproductive above all else. And early in the war, women's reproductive bodies were machines that could be tuned to best perform their vital functions. Federal funding for medical research, stimulated by Roosevelt's post-Depression New Deal programs, meant new discoveries about etiology and epidemiology—the how and why of diseases—were emerging in laboratories and clinics. But just because science was demystifying some of history's more baffling chronic diseases, it didn't mean that oppressive social mythologies about women's bodies, minds, and lives suddenly disappeared. The perception that women's primary purpose was to reproduce was very much upheld in the age of clinical advancement. And in the late 1930s, amid fears about declining birth rates, women's duty to replenish the stricken population wasn't contained to social health crusades. The pronatalist agenda permeated new understandings about one of the most mystifying and misdiagnosed "diseases of women"—endometriosis.

The symptoms of endometriosis, including agonizing pelvic and abdominal pain and heavy menstrual bleeding, had been documented since the beginnings of medical time. But myths about women's blood and pain had always prevailed over serious attention and thought. Beneath wandering and suffocating wombs, ovaritis, pelvic insanity, menstrual madness, and straight-up hysteria, endometriosis lurked—unseen and misunderstood. Endo began to be recognized and studied as a distinct disease in the late 1800s. But it wasn't until the 1920s that its biological causes were considered.

In the early 1920s, John Sampson, a gynecologist at Albany Hospital, peered through his microscope at biopsies of endometrial tissue growing as cysts on and surrounding his patients' ovaries. Sampson coined the term "endometriosis" in 1927, in a paper based on 293 cases studied over five years. He theorized that menstrual blood, containing sloughed-off bits of endometrial tissue, sometimes flowed back through the fallopian tubes and implanted onto the surface of the ovaries and the peritoneum (the membrane lining the abdomen), where it grew and spread. Sampson's "retrograde menstruation" hypothesis stuck around for decades. But it didn't explain what caused the pathology in the first place. Endometriosis remained, as it does to this day, "a riddle of etiology" for perplexed gynecologists.

After Sampson named the disease, a renowned Boston gynecologist named Joe Vincent Meigs had "worked and puzzled about" endometriosis. Meigs had specialized in gynecological surgery and research since he received his doctor of medicine degree from Harvard in 1919. After residencies at Massachusetts General and the Free Hospital for Women in the town of Brookline, which, since 1875, was dedicated to caring for poor women, Meigs became clinical professor of gynecology at Harvard Medical School. At the forefront of knowledge about gynecological disorders and diseases, Meigs turned his attentions to endo precisely because it remained such a riddle. It was absolutely in his professional interests to advance his standing as a clinician, and his reputation as an arbiter of knowledge, by unraveling this most enigmatic disease. In an editorial published in 1938, Meigs explained that endometriosis diagnoses were becoming more frequent among private patients. And those patients, as opposed to women of lower income who were treated in public hospitals, happened to be more well-off types who were prioritizing their education and careers. The increase of endo, Meigs surmised, "might be due to delayed marriages and to lack of early and frequent child-bearing."

All those years of working and puzzling led Meigs to conclude that endo was a "physiologic response to persistent . . . menstruation." Unless interrupted by the "normal" state of pregnancy, menstrual hormones were constantly stimulated—which encouraged endometrial tissue to grow outside the uterus. Since endo caused a "definite lowering of fertility," young women with the slightest "stigma" were urged, as they had been for centuries, "to marry and bear children early." Meigs admitted that the "economic difficulties of the day" were not exactly encouraging. But unless they wanted to become "abnormal," they should procreate as soon and often as possible, "even though their finances are limited." "Normal girls" over twenty-three who hadn't had babies were playing endo roulette. "The monkey mates as soon as she becomes of age and has offspring until she can no longer have any or until she dies," he mused. "Menstruation in this animal must be rare." It must be wrong, Meigs wagered, for female human animals with basically the same physiology to "put off child-bearing until 14 to 20 years of menstrual life have passed."

In April 1941, Meigs gave a presentation on endo to the American Surgical Association in which he compared four hundred gynecological operations at his private practice with four hundred similar cases at Massachusetts General. Endo, he announced, was markedly more frequent in "well-to-do" women than in poorer patients "of that social status that marries early and has children frequently." By "well-to-do," he meant white, educated, and middle to upper class. He urged private doctors to recommend "early marriage" and suggested wealthier fathers give their eighteen-year-old daughters their inheritance, so they were financially free to procreate vigorously. Meigs laced his literature with these kinds of inferences throughout the 1940s. As the understanding of endometriosis began to expand, and more gynecologists published clinical studies, Meigs kept on banging his eugenic, paternalistic, patriarchal drum.

In September 1941, Atlanta-based gynecologist Walter Holmes

reported on eighty private patients diagnosed with endo since 1930. Holmes didn't use endo as a stick to bash single and child-free women with. Instead, he focused on the disease's "devastating effects," diagnostic challenges, and possible treatments. Meigs's report from earlier that year mentioned "pain" only twice—once to acknowledge dysmenorrhea as a symptom and once in a list of signs of infertility. Holmes, meanwhile, noted all the different sites and severities of his patients' pain. He confirmed that pain wasn't associated with only menstruation; 25 percent were in pain almost constantly. And their pain wasn't only pelvic and abdominal; it radiated to their backs, groins, hips, thighs, kidneys, and stomachs. They also suffered many debilitating symptoms, including constipation and bladder problems, fevers, digestive disorders, headaches, dyspareunia (pain during intercourse), and nervousness. Most hemorrhaged profusely during their periods, and many bled throughout their cycles. But for some, periods seemed normal. Since the symptoms and signs of endo were so diverse, Holmes stressed how important a "carefully taken history" was. Only by talking to women, and listening, would the disease be properly understood.

Since the end of the 1930s, gynecologists and pathologists realized that endometriosis could creep and spread beyond the ovaries and abdomen. Endometrial tissue had been found in the round ligaments of the uterus, the bowels, colon, rectum, cervix, bladder, lymph nodes, and lungs. Women didn't yet go for routine gynecological checkups or Pap smears. Diagnostic imaging techniques like transvaginal ultrasounds were tomorrow's world. Sufferers were often only diagnosed after treatment for another gynecological or pelvic condition, like uterine fibroids. By the time many found out they had endo, it had become "invasive and destructive." The only real treatments were aggressive, mutilating surgeries or irradiation therapy. Sixteen of Holmes's patients, all between ages thirty and sixty-two, had undergone ovariotomies; while thirty-eight, between ages thirty and fifty, had undergone hysterectomies. Although many were relieved of their endo symptoms, they suffered the vasomotor disturbances of artificial menopause. Over two-thirds of the women who endured radical surgeries experienced "extreme nervous symptoms" afterward. Younger endo sufferers faced a difficult choice:

forgo having children or endure excruciating pain and many other symptoms. Holmes noted that endo caused fertility problems, but he didn't once suggest the pregnancy cure: "Patients . . . deserve a frank discussion of their condition with explanation of the cause of their . . . discomfort and other . . . symptoms." Kudos to Holmes for treating his patients as human beings and not as reproductive machines.

Holmes understood how important it was for gynecologists to appreciate that endo was not a one-size-fits-all disease. Today, endo remains one of the most frequently misdiagnosed, misunderstood, and medically stigmatized chronic diseases affecting women. Across the world, 10 percent of women of reproductive age live with it. Women today wait an average of seven and a half years from first reporting their symptoms to receive a correct diagnosis. There is still no cure. And as Holmes astutely observed, the "factors of prevention" remain "unknown." It's staggering, and shocking, to realize that the diagnostic and pathological mysteries that still impede the care of people with endo have been well known since at least the 1920s. Endo is as much of an etiologic riddle today as it was in 1941. What has been reinforced over time, and is now firmly entrenched, is the sexist perception that endo is a "career woman's disease." This disease has been the subject of intense clinical and biomedical speculations for decades. But one ignorant misbelief has held fast: endometriosis is a punishment for women who dare to deviate from the biological imperatives and social duties marked "female."

After Holmes's paper, Meigs trotted out his nonsense that endo was a "physiologic response to an abnormally uninterrupted menstrual career." Women who put off having children had only themselves to blame. Young women should stop fussing about their careers and get on with obeying "nature's rules." Previous generations of mothers and grandmothers who obeyed the laws of nature weren't riddled with it, were they? Meigs was seemingly oblivious to the fact that endometriosis wasn't diagnostically confirmed until the late 1920s. He didn't acknowledge that its symptoms had been documented for centuries. Holmes, by focusing on the diverse symptomology of endo, showed how much about the disease went unnoticed when gynecologists viewed it only through the lens of reproduction. And, as in Britain in the late 1930s,

American researchers were only beginning to uncover the realities of female ill health—realities eclipsed by medicine's almost exclusive focus on women as child-bearers.

Back in 1935, two leading American epidemiologists initiated the National Health Survey. Six hundred unemployed workers were recruited across nineteen states to gather data on illnesses and impairments suffered by household members. When the project closed in 1941, researchers had interviewed 737,000 households, making the survey the largest investigation into ill health conducted in the United States. The results showed that the Depression had taken a significant toll on the health of Americans. Among communities whose access to medical services, care, and treatment was diminished, the situation was devastating. By illuminating the hidden social and economic costs of illness, especially chronic illness, the survey showed that poor and working-class people urgently needed publicly funded health care and insurance benefits. It also revealed how little was known about illness, disease, and injury in certain demographics—including women who could not afford private medical care.

David E. Hailman, a statistician from the Public Health Services, analyzed data on "the prevalence of disabling illness" among "female workers and housewives." Women endured more chronic and communicable diseases than men. Mortality rates were higher for men, but women experienced far more "sickness." When Hailman published his findings in 1941, he showed that this remained true even when female-specific puerperal and genital causes were taken out of the equation. Housewives—women whose "main duty" was caring for the family and home—suffered disproportionately with cardiovascular, kidney, and liver diseases; rheumatic conditions; nervous and mental illnesses; cancer and tumors; and undiagnosed chronic conditions. Women also experienced more "disabling" communicable diseases, syphilis included. But since syphilis often went unreported, Hailman wasn't able to give separate figures of its prevalence. Hailman's report wasn't a qualitative investigation like *Working-Class Wives* was. But through uninflected facts and stats, his findings reflected something very similar to those of the Women's Health Inquiry Committee. Outside reproduction and sexual health, virtually no attention was being paid to women's illnesses and diseases.

Evidently, being overlooked and ignored when they weren't doing their sacred duties had distorted understanding of women's bodies and minds in troubling ways. So little was known in the late 1930s about the causes and courses of the chronic diseases Hailman described. As the country faced up to its public health challenges, federal funding began to be poured into biomedical research. During the war years, the need to advance scientific understanding of communicable and chronic diseases became even more pressing. The Committee on Medical Research, formed in 1941, coordinated the nation's efforts to prevent, diagnose, treat, and cure. Medical science teetered on the brink of a scientific revolution. For women whose illnesses and diseases had been shrouded in assumptions, misbeliefs, doubts, and prejudices, the advances of World War II promised sweeping changes. But just because objective science was about to transform and expand medical knowledge, it was no lightning rod for change—especially where social and cultural attitudes toward women were concerned.

PART THREE

1945–PRESENT

15

PUBLIC HEALTH, PRIVATE PAIN

September 1945 marked the end of World War II. As Britain and the United States tried to come to terms with their devastating losses, their governments focused on preserving and protecting human life. When the Labour Party won the 1945 UK general election in a landslide victory, Prime Minister Clement Atlee appointed Aneurin Bevan as health minister. For Bevan, the provision of health care and medical services for all the country's citizens, regardless of wealth, was at the top of the agenda for postwar welfare reform. In July 1948, Bevan inaugurated the National Health Service at Davyhulme's Park Hospital, Manchester. For the first time, all health care, medical treatment, and medicines would be free at point of use from "the cradle to the grave." "Everyone—rich or poor, man, woman or child—can use it or any part of it," announced a leaflet sent to every household. "But it is not a 'charity.' You are all paying for it, mainly as tax-payers, and it will relieve your money worries in times of illness."

Park Hospital (now Trafford General) was one of 2,751 of Britain's 3,000 hospitals—previously run by local authorities, charities, or the church—taken into public ownership and funded by national insurance taxation. As nurses formed a guard of honor, Bevan entered Park Hospital on the morning of July 5, holding the keys ceremonially presented by Lancashire County Council. The first patient he met was thirteen-year-old Sylvia Diggory, who was being treated for acute nephritis (inflammation of the kidneys). She had been moved from the children's ward after an outbreak of measles to a veranda near the main entrance. A photograph of Sylvia talking with Bevan, as a ward sister and nurse look on proudly, marked the beginnings of the most important achievement for British people in history. Sylvia became the first hospital patient treated by the NHS. Her care would have cost £17, equivalent to about $23; her father earned only £5—just under $7—a week. "Bevan asked me if I understood the significance of the occasion," she explained later. "[He] told me it was a milestone in history—the most civilized step any country had ever taken, and a day I would remember for the rest of my life."

An information film, broadcast on BBC television, showed a young mother perusing her NHS leaflet. Wearing a floral dress, trench coat, and natty hat she visits her GP, who sits at his office desk wearing a suit and tie, to have her family's application forms signed. Another, instructing viewers to "choose your doctor now," showed a woman talking with her similarly besuited physician while balancing her young son on her knee. In the wake of the war, housewives were morale-boosting backbones, rebuilding the country child by child, meal by meal, task by task. Domesticity had been respun as an invaluable national duty. The NHS promotional campaign capitalized on this image of the socially responsible, modern housewife. Taking charge of her family's health, by making sure her husband and children were all NHS patients, was just one of her valiant duties.

As well as emphasizing how valuable women were to the welfare of the family—and the country—these campaigns also reinforced gender divisions in barefaced ways. Women played a privileged role as caregivers, but men remained the experts and the authorities. When the NHS was launched, the majority of hospital doctors and general practitioners were white, male, upper-middle class, and privately educated. Social and welfare reform didn't mean that traditional medical beliefs underwent a progressive overhaul. Undeniably, the NHS was an enormous benefit for women, especially those who had been the victims of healthcare inequality. Women such as those surveyed by the Women's Health Equality Committee, who were forced to neglect their illnesses, diseases, and injuries because of economic insecurity and lack of health insurance, could now receive comprehensive GP care, hospital treatments, dental procedures, surgeries, and prescription medications. "It was such a relief, particularly to women with young children who could not afford to call the doctor out," recalled Mary Dowlding, who began work as a receptionist at a GP surgery in Kent the day the NHS was launched. But the NHS also inherited the legacy that women were child-bearers, first and foremost, so their health-care needs pivoted around their reproductive functions.

The pronatalist belief that reproduction and motherhood were women's primary duties was still prevalent in the late 1940s. In 1947, the baby boom in Britain peaked at just over one million births—a dramatic increase from 1941, when only 695,000 babies were born. At the very beginnings of the NHS, women could consult their doctors about all their health concerns, but the clinical and biomedical understanding of many chronic diseases was still in its infancy. The most significant immediate changes in women's health care occurred around maternity and childbirth. Under the NHS, GPs became the first port of call for pregnant women. Where before they might have engaged a private obstetrician or a midwife, now GPs were providing the kind of structured clinical postnatal care that continues today. At their local doctors' surgery, women received their diagnosis of pregnancy; they were given Wassermann tests for syphilis and blood-group workups; they were offered advice on pregnancy symptoms such as nausea and vomiting and educated about what was happening in their bodies at each stage of their pregnancy. While the reform of maternity care contributed to massive improvements in maternal and infant health, it also shifted the culture of childbirth from home to hospital. With the care of childbirth being handed to NHS GPs and hospital authorities, the specialist care and intimate knowledge of midwives was subsumed by new regulations. And women—still very much the vessels of the future—were more subject to medical scrutiny, supervision, and surveillance than ever before.

In the United States, postwar debates about the need for universal health care were championed by President Harry Truman. After Roosevelt's death in April 1945, Truman—his former vice president—was sworn into office. In an address to Congress in November 1945, Truman

discussed his proposals for including "health security" in his Economic
Bill of Rights. Through a payroll-tax funding system, similar to the one
adopted in Britain to support the NHS, Truman wanted every person
in America to be given the "right to adequate medical care and the
opportunity to achieve and enjoy good health." Before and during
the war, maternity-reform initiatives, such as the Emergency Maternity
and Infant Care program, led to hospital birth rates increasing by 78.8
percent. Expanded access to insurance coverage under the Blue Cross
scheme meant more working-class women could now access clinical
care during pregnancy, birth, and the postnatal period. Truman, in his
address, stated, "Public health and maternal and child health programs
already have made important contributions to national health. But large
needs remain. Great areas of our country are still without these services." But as the 1935 National Health Survey had shown, a huge
amount of untreated illness and disease, unrelated to reproduction, was
impacting women who faced economic insecurity. Beyond maternity
and child health, women, especially young women, were suffering from
"widespread physical and mental incapacity." Universal health care, and
with it an increase of doctors and hospitals, medical education and research, would make, for the first time in American history, "good health
equally available to all citizens."

Sadly, Truman's social-reformist vision floundered amid fierce criticism and suspicion. Fearing that such a socialist move was part of a
Communist plot, the Republican-controlled Congress rejected Truman's proposal in 1946. But increased federal funding did mean hospitals were expanding, and clinical research was flourishing. Alongside all
the new medications, vaccines, treatments, and diagnostic methods that
emerged during the war years, clinical discoveries were also exposing
some inconvenient truths about medicine's past failings, especially related to serious chronic diseases in women.

In 1946, the woman from Ohio who tested positive for syphilis during her premarital screening in 1941 fell ill with a wracking cough. An
X-ray showed she had chronic bronchitis. Her hemoglobin levels were
low, and a course of iron tablets made no difference. Her doctors decided to repeat the Wassermann test, which was positive. By 1948, she

was constantly weak and feverish. Presuming she still had syphilis, her doctors prescribed penicillin, which had become widely available in the early 1940s after it was produced to treat Allied troops fighting in Europe. But this treatment made her even sicker. In 1949, she was admitted to the Cleveland Clinic. Her blood count and pressure were through the floor. She stayed in the hospital for just over a month. Her progress, according to her notes, was "stormy." She was discharged on June 15. But her doctors hadn't noticed that her pericardium, the lining around her heart, was filling with fluid. She died at home on July 15.

"Case 3," as she was identified in the clinical report, was one of hundreds of women who developed mysterious symptoms after testing positive for syphilis. As it turned out, the Wassermann test was not an "infallible scientific method" for confirming syphilis. In fact, false-positive reactions were common, often in women with underlying, undiagnosed chronic diseases. But since the shape-shifting syphilis antibody showed up in a patient's blood years before her symptoms appeared, she would be automatically diagnosed with and treated for syphilis while her chronic disease lay latent in her body. The fallibility of the Wassermann test was well known by then. But one of the most destructive diseases hidden beneath its false-positive bias was only just beginning to be understood.

Case 3 died from complications of systemic lupus erythematosus (SLE). SLE, usually just called lupus, had appeared in medical writings since the ninth century, when it described scaly, livid skin rashes resembling wolf bites. "Lupus" is the Latin word for wolf, and a prescient metaphor for what the disease turned out to be: an autoimmune condition caused when a person's own antibodies viciously attack their own cells, organs, and tissues. Since the mid-late nineteenth century, when lupus was identified as a systemic disease that could damage the body beyond the skin, medicine understood that it was overwhelmingly more common in young and middle-aged women than in men. But until the 1940s, the etiology of lupus remained a mystery. Physicians had been toying with the idea that the immune system could produce an internal toxic reaction, a sort of allergy to the self, from the early 1900s. But this confounded medical logic. Immune cells were supposed to protect against disease, not cause it. But in 1948, immunologists at the Mayo Clinic found an autoimmune cell in the bone marrow of a woman with systemic lupus. They named it the LE cell. For those who believed autoimmunity was plausible, there was now a way to explain many symptoms that had been misdiagnosed in women, often with disturbing results. When the LE cell was discovered, immunologists and rheumatologists recognized that systemic lupus affected women disproportionately; what they didn't understand was why. Today, 90 percent of people living with lupus across the world are women between the ages of fifteen and forty-four. And although medicine speculates that female sex hormones and immunological differences might be to blame, the exact reasons remain a mystery.

Just before she died, Case 3 received a blood test that showed she had the LE cell. Her lupus had gone untreated for years while her vulnerable body was pumped full of mercury, arsenic, and penicillin. The stigma of being diagnosed with syphilis left her severely depressed. After her fiancé left her, she became a recluse. Her tragic history was revealed in a study conducted at the Cleveland Clinic of five patients, all women, who developed SLE symptoms after Wassermann false positives. Other clinics hastily followed up with patients who might have suffered the same fate. In 1948, supported by a grant from the National Institutes of Health (NIH), two chronic disease specialists from Johns Hopkins began a study of 148 patients wrongly diagnosed with syphilis since the late 1930s: 104 were women; 9 had verified SLE, and 36 were strongly suspected of having it.

When the specialists Joseph Earle Moore and W. Beale Lutz published their report in 1954, they included "life tables" of a sample of patients with suspected SLE to show how their diseases had manifested since their Wassermann tests. A twenty-two-year-old was misdiagnosed with syphilis during a routine pregnancy screening in July 1949. Two months later, she suffered "depressive psychosis" and underwent electroshock therapy. In November, when she was five and a half months pregnant, she had a "therapeutic abortion." By the time her blood revealed the LE cell, she'd had another abortion and endured years of

arthritis in her fingers and hands. Thankfully, her lupus went into remission after her diagnosis in 1954.

The following year, Moore and two other chronic disease specialists,
named Laurence E. Shulman and James T. Scott, published another
report that included the "major clinical manifestations" of lupus. It was
clear that lupus was a diverse disease that expressed in many different
ways in the bodies and minds of their false-positive patients. As well as
creeping into the joints, skin, eyes, heart, kidneys, lungs, and blood vessels, lupus evidently had serious effects on mental health. A cluster of
women had been placed under psychiatric care after being "diagnosed"
with syphilis. One, aged thirty-one when her SLE was confirmed, had
been seriously unwell since her early teens with constant migraines and
painful swelling in her legs. Rather than admit they were baffled, her
doctors decided she was "maladjusted" and sent her to a psychoanalyst.

Over the next year her physical symptoms continued, and she became severely depressed. A physician suggested she might have SLE,
but her psychiatrist was having none of it. He refused to refer her for
laboratory tests and instead diagnosed her with schizophrenia and
treated her with electroshock therapy. When her mental health didn't
recover, they tried to "cure" her by inducing an insulin coma. This painful and humiliating "therapy," introduced into psychiatric treatment in
the late 1920s, was supposed to promote mental clarity in patients with
schizophrenia. Failing to see any improvement, her psychiatrist admitted her to a psychiatric hospital where surgeons cut away part of the
frontal cortex of her brain in a brutal procedure called topectomy. After
being locked up for two years, she was finally admitted for biological
tests, which showed she had the LE cell. She was treated with steroids,
and her disease went into remission. She was declared "OK" by another
psychiatrist, although she still suffered some "emotional instability."

It is unbearable to imagine how much these women suffered because
of misdiagnoses and clinical ignorance. Moore, Shulman, and Scott
showed that lupus was not a rare condition and that its varied symptoms
made it very hard to diagnose. They also revealed that lupus could manifest psychologically and neurologically, making undiagnosed women

vulnerable to "perhaps unnecessary psychiatric treatment." What an understatement. And even though the LE test could confirm the disease, women still had to grapple with doctors' assessments of their "bizarre" and "puzzling" symptoms before the possibility of lupus was even entertained. It was far easier to blame a woman's unnamed pain on maladjustment, emotional instability, psychosis, or hypochondriasis than to admit to not knowing the cause.

It's no wonder women's mental health deteriorated after shameful syphilis diagnoses followed by years of doubt, dismissal, and pain. Pain is the most enduring symptom of lupus. In the absence of a clinical sign that could be observed and interpreted by a doctor, a woman's pain was presumed to exist only in her head. In the 1950s, pain was not a clinical sign. Pain felt by a woman with undiagnosed lupus was nothing more than a subjective sensation. Pain couldn't be visualized on an X-ray; pain didn't sediment in a test tube. But the age-old question of what to *do* with women's pain, now that diagnoses could be made by biomedical evidence rather than speculations and assumptions, was raising its rather inconvenient head.

The discovery of autoimmunity collided with another radical movement in medical thinking: the study of the relationship between emotional experiences and chronic diseases. Back in 1935, Helen Flanders Dunbar, the American psychologist, published *Emotions and Bodily Changes*, a pioneering book in the history of modern psychosomatic medicine. The term "psychosomatic," from the ancient Greek words for mind and body, described any illness that manifested in physical symptoms thought to originate from psychological causes. It emerged from clinical research, such as Dunbar's, into the ways that certain unexplained diseases were influenced by troubling life experiences. Unlike hysteria, psychosomatic illness was not a social construction to pathologize unruly and undesirable aspects of femininity. It didn't imply that a sufferer's symptoms were feigned or fictitious. But while Dunbar's work was innovative, it set the stage for psychological diagnoses to be made instead of physiological ones when it came to elusive chronic diseases. And many of those diseases had substantial—and vastly misunderstood—emotional effects on sufferers.

It wasn't until after World War II that the impact of trauma on health really came to the fore. In 1950, Franz Alexander, the Hungarian American psychoanalyst, described the "Holy Seven," a group of diseases he believed were psychological. Three affected mostly women and, it would turn out, were autoimmune: thyrotoxicosis, excess production of the thyroid hormone that causes Graves' disease; rheumatoid arthritis; and ulcerative colitis, a gastrointestinal disease that causes inflammation in the colon. So even before the biomedical origin of these diseases was discovered, their symptoms—pain, digestive issues, nervous exhaustion, etc.—had a psychosomatic reputation. By associating those diseases with emotional rather than organic causes, female sufferers were vulnerable to not only dismissal and doubt but to barbaric, pointless psychiatric interventions. These included the topectomy—which the unnamed lupus patient endured in 1951—and the lobotomy, in which surgeons drilled into the brain and severed connections in the prefrontal cortex.

In 1935, the Portuguese Nobel Prize–winning neurologist António Egas Moniz reported success after performing twenty lobotomies for mental illnesses including depression and melancholia. Shortly after, his peers, American neurologists Walter Freeman and James Watts, joined forces to deliver "psychosurgeries," sometimes twenty-five times a day, to relieve mental pain. The lobotomy craze took hold in clinics, asylums, and hospitals across the US, the UK, and Europe throughout the 1940s and into the 1950s. An estimated forty thousand to fifty thousand occurred in the US, and around seventeen thousand in the UK. The most common justifications for prefrontal lobotomy were emotional tension, depression, obsessive compulsions, anxiety, hypochondriasis, and psychosis. "Schizophrenic states" including "excitement" and "restiveness" were also, the neurologists claimed, "strikingly modified" after the procedure. Undue concern with one's own "feelings, sensations, and reactions" were symptoms in every one of these conditions. Women who dared express their mental and emotional pain—pain that doctors couldn't explain—made ideal lobotomy candidates.

By 1942, 75 percent of the patients Freeman and Watts had lobotomized were women. At the time, more men than women were confined to US psychiatric institutions. But the symptoms the lobotomists claimed to cure with their brutal, inhumane procedures were inordinately feminized. In 1947, they reported on twenty cases performed since 1936; sixteen were women, and eleven of those housewives. Like the ovariotomy and the clitoridectomy, lobotomies were endorsed as a way of keeping unwell women out of asylums, which, at the time, were woefully overcrowded. In an era when a mentally healthy woman was a serene wife and mother, any behavior or emotion that disrupted domestic harmony could be interpreted as a justification for a lobotomy. Almost all the housewives were described as suffering from depression. And the success of the lobotomy was measured according to how obligingly they resumed their household duties. For physicians faced with "agitated," "anxious," or "obsessive" women, the lobotomy was a quick-fix solution for "bringing the patient back to earth and the enjoyments thereof." In a surgery lasting roughly an hour, the neurologists promised to prevent "years of invalidism" by cutting off the "emotional component" of mental disorders. "Easier than curing a toothache," newspaper articles gleefully claimed. According to Freeman and Watts, the lobotomy was a success if the patient reverted to an almost childlike state. She might laugh and swear and have temper tantrums, but what a small price to pay for a life free from imaginary illnesses and burdensome thoughts. One patient's husband described his lobotomized wife as "full of don't-give-a-damness." The lobotomy had stolen her ability to make meaning of what mattered.

Despite Freeman's and Watts's claims to success, the lobotomy was often fatal. And if a patient did survive the procedure, it could completely rob her of any quality of life. Several of the housewives died either immediately after the operation, or a few years after. Some took their own lives. One, age forty-eight, was still "indolent" and "sarcastic" after her second prefrontal lobotomy, so she was confined to an institution for eighteen months. Another, unable to be relieved of her "emotional tension," was left to "deteriorate" in a psychiatric hospital, where she endured electroshock treatment.

Freeman and Watts continued to endorse the transformative effects of psychosurgery even though many members of the medical establishment were rightly cautious and disapproving. For families trying in vain to find treatment for their wayward wives and difficult daughters, the lobotomy—despite all the controversy—was an appealing last resort. In 1941, Rosemary Kennedy, sister of John F. Kennedy, was lobotomized by Freeman and Watts at George Washington University Hospital. She was twenty-three years old. Born starved of oxygen, Rosemary had suffered all her life with learning difficulties, seizures, mood swings, and intense anxiety. Before her father, Joe Kennedy, took her to see the neurologists, Rosemary's behavior had been "erratic"—she was confined to a convent, and the nuns reported that she had been sneaking out to bars at night and consorting with men. Rather than risk the family's reputation, Joe Kennedy insisted on the surgery—regardless of the objections of her sister Kathleen. Rosemary remained awake while Freeman drilled two small holes through her skull, before severing her prefrontal cortex. Afterward she was unable to walk or talk. She was sequestered away to a psychiatric facility, out of sight and out of mind. Over the years, she regained a little of her motion and fragments of her speech. In 2005, Rosemary died, at the age of eighty-five, in a hospital in Wisconsin. Her lobotomy was kept secret until 1987.

Later in the 1940s and early 1950s, surgeons and neurologists across the United States resorted to lobotomies to treat the "intractable" pain of chronic diseases, from cancers and kidney disorders to neuralgia and multiple sclerosis. The object wasn't to take a patient's pain away but to literally sever her emotional connection to it. Freeman and Watts heartily recommended lobotomy to physicians as an alternative to narcotic pain relief, for they fully believed that chronic pain in organic diseases was mostly in the mind. "In many cases the attitude of the patient," they proclaimed, "is more disabling than the disease itself; the fear of pain, greater than the pain." Since women were already assumed to exaggerate their pain with their excessive emotions, female chronic illness sufferers were especially vulnerable to being referred for psychosurgery when the extent of their pain exceeded their physicians' patience.

At the University of Oklahoma School of Medicine between 1950 and 1954, three women aged twenty-eight, thirty-two, and forty-three, identified only as "housewives," underwent prefrontal lobotomies as "cures" for ulcerative colitis. The neurosurgeons concluded that their ill-nesses were exacerbated by psychological distress. The forty-three-year-old was so depressed that she tried, twice, to take her own life. The twenty-eight-year-old, "an obsessive-compulsive individual with . . . severe chronic anxiety," suffered particularly badly with her colitis during "serious conflicts with her domineering mother." And the thirty-two-year-old, "an overly meticulous individual," was "excessively" concerned about "inconsequential situations in everyday life." The surgeons de-clared each patient effectively cured. But there is no mention of how the procedure affected their lives or how it made them feel. Their stories are lost to the surgeons' bravado.

"We are sufficiently encouraged by these results to continue to carry out the procedure," the neurosurgeons concluded. They saw no reason why lobotomy shouldn't be encouraged for all hopeless cases of colitis. Before its autoimmune cause was discovered, ulcerative colitis—like many other gastrointestinal diseases throughout history—bore the stigma of being "all in the mind," partly because the stomach, since an-cient times, has been associated with negative emotions. Today, medi-cine understands the more complex interactions between brain and body that can adversely affect conditions like irritable bowel syndrome. But chronic diseases like colitis and Crohn's remain difficult to identify and treat; and patients—especially women—are often misdiagnosed with anxiety. In the 1950s, the lobotomy was championed as another of those revolutionary cures that didn't just treat the symptoms of a disease but ripped it out right at the roots. In reality, the lobotomy was medically sanctioned silencing, to stop women from voicing how, and where, and why it hurt.

16

MOTHERS' LITTLE HELPERS

S top Emotional Suffering in Chronic Disease," blared an advert by Wallace Laboratories in 1959, for its wonder drug, Miltown. Available since 1955 as a cure-all for anxiety, depression, nerves, and fatigue, Miltown—a trade name for meprobamate, the first widely distributed minor tranquilizer—became the most popular medication prescribed by US doctors after just one year on the market. The earliest ads show exactly whom Wallace imagined the happy-pill popper to be: a housewife struggling with the demands of running her home, raising her children, and keeping a smile on her husband's face. Promotions for this "miracle cure for anxiety" appeared in magazines such has *Cosmopolitan* and *Ladies' Home Journal*. Scores of editorials promised that Miltown would alleviate domesticity-disturbing tensions. And women needn't worry—the tranquilizer was endorsed by doctors as a harmless, non-habit-forming way to gain "a renewed ability to enjoy life." Leading health writers employed by public relations companies penned articles claiming Miltown helped "frigid women who abhorred marital relations" to "respond more readily to their husbands' advances." It goes without saying that most marital difficulties were blamed on some dysfunction of a woman's body or mind. And women's magazines were complicit in convincing readers that unsatisfying sex wasn't their man's problem.

In "Tell Me, Doctor," a column in *Ladies' Home Journal* in the 1950s, gynecologist Henry Barnard Safford offered frank advice to married couples on problems they were too frightened to share with their physicians. Whether the question was on sex, conception, infertility, gynecological cancers, or abortion, Safford was on hand with his white-coat expertise. In one story from 1956, a couple hasn't had "satisfactory . . . relations" in three months of marriage. The man goes into Safford's office and complains that every attempt "has ended disastrously . . . Both of us want a family . . . But what is a man to do, Doctor, when even at the beginning . . . she has a real spasm—and I mean an actual convulsion?" Safford proceeds to talk to the man's wife alone. "It is clear you are suffering from dyspareunia," he tells her, using the clinical term for pain during intercourse. "This condition is commonly accompanied by *vaginismus.*"

Vaginismus, where the muscles of the vagina tighten and spasm involuntarily, makes any kind of penetration—sexual, inserting a tampon, a Pap smear—exceedingly painful, if not impossible. And the pain is not contained to the vagina; it can extend to the pelvis and radiate through the muscles of the back and legs. The association of penetrative sex with pain can be intensely traumatic; one of the main causes today is thought to be emotional trauma from past sexual abuse and violence, internalized shame around sex and intimacy, or a difficult childbirth experience. But the condition has many possible physical causes too, including gynecological illnesses and diseases, pelvic injuries, and even certain medications. Today, up to one in ten people with vaginas in the UK, and as many as 20 percent in the US, experience pain during sex. But since sexual dysfunction is not prioritized as a medical concern unless you happen to be a heterosexual, cisgender man, vaginismus is frequently misdiagnosed as anxiety. Combinations of psychological counseling and physical therapy—like pelvic-floor strengthening and training with dilators—can be really effective treatments. But until medicine creates a culture where the impact of sex on women's minds, bodies, health, and lives is properly researched and respected, vaginismus sufferers risk being dismissed out of hand before their condition can be properly diagnosed and effectively treated.

The silence and shame around sexual dysfunction in women that persists today means many people with vaginismus avoid seeking medical help at all. But when they do, they are frequently told to go home and relax, use lubricants, and loosen up with a few drinks. These attitudes that women's sexual pain and trauma could be overcome if they stopped being so neurotic have hardly progressed since the 1950s. When Safford's column ran, vaginismus was thought to be entirely psychosomatic. When diagnosing the causes of the couple's sexual difficulties, he placed the blame squarely with the wife. And rather than attempt to understand anything of her intimate relationship with her body and sexuality, he informed her she was scared of pregnancy, terrified by intercourse, and harboring a female inferiority complex. "Oh, but I don't feel that way, Doctor," she replied. But Safford insisted he knew better. If she wanted to save her marriage, she must conquer the "problems" in her "mind." And in the 1950s, women were told they could achieve this simply by popping a pill.

Blaming marital conflicts on female biology and psychology wasn't a new idea. For decades, the severity of premenstrual tensions and menopausal disturbances had been measured according to husbands' distress. What *was* new was manipulating women into medicating themselves to keep their men happy. Miltown advertising created an image of a white, middle-class, modern housewife who couldn't afford to let her unruly body and mind disrupt her hard-won domestic bliss—or her femininity. And much like the women featured in Safford's column, Miltown users took charge of their health by bowing to the paternalistic authority of male doctors. When Safford's book *Tell Me, Doctor* was published in 1955, the cover featured a half-dressed blonde bombshell pouting while the doctor brandishes his stethoscope. "If I Had Only Known!" gasps the back cover, above a woman cast in shadow, cross-legged on the floor, biting her nails. Truly feminine women, according to *Tell Me, Doctor*, didn't shy away from revealing private details of their bodies and sexualities. Rather than languish in ignorance, they submitted willingly—and nakedly—to medical expertise. Women who did as they were told were informed, enlightened, and bountifully healthy. A visit to a doctor, and his prescription pad, was promoted, weirdly enough, as an empowered act.

Like Premarin, the estrogen supplement rushed to market in the

1940s, Miltown was designed to smooth over and quiet down women's burdensome feelings and troublesome symptoms. In the medical press, the drug was touted as a remedy for chronic pain, asthma, arthritis, rheumatic illnesses, gastrointestinal conditions, and multiple sclerosis. The idea that a patient's emotional life could exacerbate and even cause many of these illnesses had gained enormous traction since the end of the war. Miltown capitalized on the idea that women's psychological woes—anxiety in particular—were symptoms of nothing more than life-role dissatisfaction. In a 1960 medical advert for Meprospan (another brand of meprobamate), a woman sits at her physician's desk, gazing down at her clasped hands. She is a "tense, nervous patient," tormented by "recurring states of anxiety which have no organic etiology." One 400-milligram capsule, taken at breakfast, leaves her calm enough to go grocery shopping. Another sees her through the preparation of her family's evening meal. And since she has "enjoyed sustained tranquilization all day," she remains "relaxed, alert, and attentive . . . and able to listen" at the PTA meeting. Then she can sleep, "undisturbed by nervousness or tension."

By 1955, chronic pain, asthma, and gastrointestinal disorders were lodged in the psychosomatic imagination. But an organic pathology, autoimmunity, had been identified for two diseases of unknown etiology, lupus—a "rheumatic disease"—and rheumatoid arthritis. The rise in hospital medicine, clinical specialisms, and funded research meant that sufferers of these diseases, long suspected to affect mostly women, could be properly diagnosed and treated. But both lupus and rheumatoid arthritis often began with exactly the kinds of symptoms meprobamate claimed to cure—fatigue, insomnia, nerve weakness, anxiety, depression, cognitive confusion, and muscle weakness. The link between the immune system and multiple sclerosis (MS), the most common neurological disease in America at the time, had been known about since the 1940s. But women sufferers were frequently misdiagnosed with "hysteria" at neurology clinics well into the 1950s.

Today, MS is known to be three to four times more common in women than in men. The disease was first documented by Jean-Martin Charcot—who brought female hysteria to clinical and public attention in the late nineteenth century—in 1868. To this day, MS, like most diseases associated with autoimmunity, is incurable, and its exact cause remains a mystery. And despite being known to be more prevalent in women since the 1940s, the reasons for this gender disparity are still not properly understood. Medicine assumed, for most of the late nineteenth and early twentieth centuries, that MS predominantly affected men. Of course, this was a misapprehension caused by medicine's insistence that men's neurological and motor symptoms were deserving of diagnostic attention, while women, with their delicate female nerves, must be manifesting such symptoms in their minds. Gender bias still affects diagnoses of MS. The disease begins with nonspecific symptoms that relapse and flare, including pain, fatigue, and muscle weakness, and it can be incredibly difficult, and long-winded, for sufferers to be correctly diagnosed. Women with MS are particularly vulnerable to having their "unexplained" pain and neurological symptoms misdiagnosed as somatization disorder, a mental illness manifesting in physical symptoms for which no cause can be found. In the 1950s, if a woman went to her doctor complaining of crashing exhaustion, aching muscles, a fogged mind, and trembling hands, a tranquilizer was the perfect foil. Why bother puzzling out the cause of her cryptic symptoms when a pill might just shut her up?

Meprobamate was introduced to Britain in 1956. It quickly overtook barbiturates as the most popular medication for women with anxiety, insomnia, weak nerves, and unexplained pain. But statistics showed barbiturates were being overprescribed by the NHS—with deadly consequences. Between 1954 and 1956, barbiturate overdoses caused the accidental death, or suicide, of 217 women in England and Wales. Alarmed medical editorials warned of the dangerous side effects and habit-forming realities of this "placebo . . . to assuage doctors' anxieties." Meprobamate, the manufacturers claimed, was less toxic and in no way addictive. But it was extortionately expensive. In the House of Commons in November 1956, ministers argued that the NHS was being unduly stretched by prescription demands for this "American encroachment" for "hypochondriacs and neurotics." But far more alarming were the physical and mental costs. Meprobamate caused many side effects, including blurred vision, drowsiness, and nausea, and, as it turned out, it was definitely habit-forming. But despite the evident dangers, tranquilizer use skyrocketed. And the majority of users were women. One psychiatric physician questioned whether the tranquilizer trend reflected a genuine rise in mental ill health. If this were the case, then meprobamate offered doctors an all-too-easy fix. Instead of being worked through in therapy, root causes were simply "obscured in a thick cloud of chemically induced tranquility." But the psychiatrist also pointed out that drug companies were claiming that almost every mood and feeling, from tiredness and irritability to apprehension and excitement, were "syndromes" that only their pills could cure. Women, the main consumers of these drugs, were not stupid. They were not blindly gulping pills because a magazine advert told them to, nor were they so easily convinced that their every emotion was pathological. Women were facing a very real crisis of identity, of selfhood, now that society expected them to feather the nest for war-torn husbands and repopulate the human race.

Many women—at least the white, middle-class ones who embodied the era's ideals of domestic femininity—had experienced the new responsibilities and relative freedoms of the war years. Their opportunities had expanded with political emancipation, education opportunities, and employment rights. But their mental and physical health was crumbling under the pressures of motherhood and homemaking. Companies peddling meprobamate were cunningly adept at pathologizing the paradox of postwar femininity. Educated housewives had more disposable income, life chances, and "labor-saving devices" than their mothers dreamed of. Yet they were overworked, overwhelmed, and beset with functional disorders. "Is anxiety and tension fast becoming the occupational disease of the homemaker?" one Miltown medical ad asked. And if so, what could be the cause? Was it unrealistic to "grant that she is socially, politically, and culturally equal while continuing to demand domestic and biological subservience?" Yes. Was it unfair to expect her to "shoulder the guilt burden of this child-centered age without unraveling around the emotional edges"? Again, hard yes. But Wallace was in the business of making a profit, not redressing gender inequality. "Whatever the cause," the ad declared, "it helps to add Miltown to her treatment—to help her relax both emotional *and* muscular tensions. It's no substitute for a week in Bermuda, or for emotional readjustment. But it will often make the latter easier for her, as well as for the physician."

The new cultural stereotype of the anxiously unwell housewife fueled the production of benzodiazepines, such as Valium, Librium, and Serax, introduced to Britain and the US in the early 1960s. Benzos were not thought to induce dependence. Ads cribbed the latest ideas about the relationship between domestic strains and mental ill health, and they were stunningly gendered. One ad, by Wyeth, featured a woman slumped behind prison bars of mop and broom handles. "You Can't Set Her Free, But You Can Make Her Feel Less Anxious," the headline exclaimed. Serax could relieve all the tension and irritability arising from her "sense of inadequacy and isolation." In a few pills' time, she could cope perfectly with her "day-to-day problems." Drowsiness, dizziness, fainting, rashes, nausea, lethargy, edema, slurred speech, and altered libido were just a few of the small-print side effects.

Benzo advertising constructed a very specific female patient—ravaged by imaginary illnesses, emotional excesses, and unease about her place in society—who could be "cured" with sleep and silencing. As with those women labeled "hysterical" in the nineteenth century, she was being coerced into submitting to a potentially harmful cure for a problem invented by medical men. The PR companies behind tranquilizer campaigns knew that modern housewives were in the grip of a mental health crisis. Ads paid lip service to their struggles—but they also gaslit women into thinking the problem lay with their inability to adjust to their "natural" role. Medicine, for centuries, had cleaved to the idea that embracing domestic motherhood—and its attributes of docility, submissiveness, and self-sacrifice—was the healthiest state for a woman's body and mind. Yearning for a life beyond the broom-and-mop prison had always been considered dangerously pathological. Like all those unnecessary gynecological surgeries and punishing treatment regimens imposed on unwell housewives throughout history, tranquilizers were promoted as a surefire way to make frustrated women submit peacefully and pleasantly to their socially ordained duties.

One woman was about to explode the medical and cultural myth that femininity equaled health, happiness, and harmony. In 1957, the psychologist, writer, and activist Betty Friedan began researching the education experiences, subsequent choices and roles, and general life satisfaction of women who graduated Smith College, her alma mater, in the 1940s. She had set out to disprove the very nineteenth-century notion that higher education "fitted us ill for our role as women." But her study "raised more questions than it answered." Many felt conflicted about their rights as women and their roles as wives and mothers. For too long, women had been told they could "desire no greater destiny than to glory in their own femininity." For centuries, but particularly since World War II, "feminine fulfillment" had become the "cherished and self-perpetuating core of American culture." But women were cracking under the pressure.

Psychologists, physicians, and drug companies claimed the problems lay with women's inability to accept and embrace their feminine roles. Modern domestic femininity was a privilege, the experts said. "From the beginning of time, the female cycle has defined and confined woman's role," stated a 1960 *Newsweek* article. "Though no group of women has ever pushed these natural restrictions as far as the American wife, it seems she still cannot accept them with good grace." Women who wanted more, who *needed* more, felt guilty, ashamed, despondent, restless. Their mental and physical health was ravaged by the sense that they should be content with their husbands, homes, and children. In her 1963 book *The Feminine Mystique*, Friedan called this "the problem with no name."

"If I am right, the problem that has no name stirring in the minds of so many American women today is not a matter of loss of femininity or too much education, or the demands of domesticity," Friedan wrote. "It is far more important than anyone recognizes. It is the key to these other new and old problems which have been torturing women . . . and puzzling their doctors . . . for years." When women confessed to their doctors that they were always on the brink of crying, or got so angry it scared them, they were diagnosed with "housewife's syndrome." If their skin broke out in hives and rashes, it was called "housewife's blight." The numbing tiredness that "took so many women to the doctors in the

1950s" was labeled "housewife's fatigue." Many suffered in silence or turned to tranquilizers to blot out the "strange, dissatisfied voice . . . within them." It felt less painful this way.

Friedan called for women to vocalize the problem, to speak with their stirring voices: "It may well be the key to our future as a nation and a culture." *The Feminine Mystique* was an instant bestseller and tremendously influential. It raised consciousness about gender inequalities and energized the 1960s women's rights movement. In 1966, Friedan became one of the founders of the National Organization for Women (NOW). She served as NOW's first president and authored its inaugural statement of purpose. In the wake of the landmark Civil Rights Act of 1964, which outlawed racial segregation and employment and education discrimination based on race and sex, NOW was committed to achieving "true equality for all women in America" as part of "the world-wide revolution of human rights." "We believe the time has come to move beyond the abstract argument . . . about the status and special nature of women which has raged . . . in recent years," Friedan wrote. "NOW is dedicated to the proposition that women, first and foremost, are human beings, who, like all other people in our society, must have the chance to develop their fullest human potential."

Friedan, in her NOW statement, addressed how Black women faced the harshest social and economic injustices, especially in the workplace where they were "the victims of the double discrimination of race and sex." But in *The Feminine Mystique*, she did not embrace an inclusive view of womanhood. The "problem" was middle-class, heterosexual, and white. She was speaking to, and about, privileged domestic femininity; and in doing so, she erased the voices and experiences of ethnically diverse women, working-class women, child-free women, and "women without men." Friedan called for the women *she* was addressing to answer the voice that cried out for "something more than my husband and my children and my house." But she ignored the fact that Black and other ethnically diverse women would be expected to labor inside the homes of those who followed Friedan's clarion call out into the world of work, of thought, of action.

In 1988, bell hooks, the American social and feminist activist, writer, and professor, called out Friedan's myopic vision in her pathbreaking essay about the limitations of white feminism, "Black Women: Shaping Feminist Theory." Writing about the way discourse such as Friedan's shaped the white-supremacist tenets of the mainstream feminist movement, hooks explained: "Much feminist theory emerges from privileged women who live at the center, whose perspectives on reality rarely include knowledge and awareness of the lives of women and men who live on the margin." While hooks did see *The Feminine Mystique* as a "useful discussion" of the impact of sexism on a "select group of women," crucially she revealed how its influence set the precedent for a generation of feminist activism that assumed Black women "did not exist."

Medical attitudes toward mental ill health had routinely ignored the diversity of women's lives and experiences. Theories about female neuroses frequently assumed the sufferer was white and affluent, while the plight of working-class women and Black, Asian, and other ethnically diverse women was scarcely, if ever, thought about seriously. Since the nineteenth century, physicians had claimed that nervous weakness was a disorder unique to "civilized" women, whose delicate constitutions couldn't cope with high-paced industrialized life. Friedan was right to challenge the notion that women were mentally unwell because their fragile nerves couldn't handle the demands of modern living. But through her narrow vision of femininity, she reinforced medicine's historic racist assumption that neuroses and emotional disturbances exclusively afflicted white, privileged women.

Three years after *The Feminine Mystique* was published, American gynecologist Robert Wilson published a "revolutionary little book" that turned out to be almost as sensational. *Feminine Forever* claimed "a new biological destiny" was possible for "every human female." Women had suffered enough, he said, because of "male indifference to anything exclusively female." In the "male-oriented culture," anti-feminist beliefs still dictated that women were inferior, irrational creatures whose sexuality—outside reproduction—was a Very Big Problem. Medicine upheld a "lack of basic sympathy" for women. But Wilson was not tearing down the clinical curtains and demanding doctors redress their biases. Instead, he wanted women—white, middle-class, married, and domestic—to take charge of their own health and happiness by not allowing their bodies to become dried-up husks when they hit forty. Menopause, Wilson believed, was not only curable but "completely preventable": "Every woman alive has the option of remaining feminine forever."

For Wilson, the end of a woman's fertile years signaled the demise of all her desirable and valuable attributes. She was no longer a woman at all, not when all the psychological and physiological factors that determined her attractiveness to men were deteriorating. Her bones weakened and her vagina became "stiff and unyielding." Her whole body was "mutilated" by symptoms so "obscure and bizarre" that her physician was "hopelessly puzzled." As well as suffering hot flashes, night sweats, insomnia, and bladder problems, the menopausal "unwoman" was nervous, irritable, amnesiac, melancholic, probably alcoholic, and definitely always weeping. But now, Wilson claimed, she could escape "the horror of this living decay." With the help of synthetic estrogen, menopausal husks could become true women again: beautiful, vibrant, agreeable, sexually willing, and not remotely hysterical or hunchbacked.

By the 1960s, the belief that women were governed by female hormones elicited by the ovaries, and men by male ones from the testes, had been overturned. The hormonal basis of sex difference wasn't nearly so clear-cut. Since the late 1930s, endocrinologists and biochemists had accepted that female and male bodies produced both female and male sex hormones. Women's bodies were far more hormonally complex than previously imagined, and ovaries were not the definitive source of "femaleness." But where male bodies were seen as hormonally stable, female bodies were subject to constant fluctuations. Estrogen, with its reputation as the primary female sex hormone and the agent of femininity, could be enhanced to make women's bodies more regulated and medically manageable. "Estrogen therapy doesn't *change* a woman," Wilson wrote; "On the contrary, it keeps her from changing." Wilson's propositions were hardly new. Menopause had been framed as a deficiency disease since the early 1900s, and menopausal estrogen therapy had been available for just shy of twenty-five years. But Wilson wasn't recommending that women took supplements like Premarin only during "the change." He was urging them to adopt the "hormone cure" from their mid-thirties to prevent menopause from happening altogether.

Every physical, emotional, sexual, or social ill a woman suffered, Wilson claimed, was caused by her depleting or deranged femininity. And since it was scientifically accepted that hormones influenced most body functions and many mental traits, it was easy for Wilson to claim that estrogen therapy delivered astounding transformative effects. Amid the explosive arguments about how traditional femininity was making women mentally and physically unwell, Wilson valiantly stepped in to defend it. Just like tranquilizers, estrogen therapy was a way to trap women within the traditional domestic sphere, or at least make them conform to it willingly. For estrogen was the chemical drip-feed of the most socially acceptable feminine attitudes and behaviors. "Women rich in estrogen tend to have . . . the ability to think out problems effectively, resistance to mental and physical fatigue, and emotional self-control," Wilson wrote. "In a family situation, estrogen makes women adaptable, even-tempered, and generally easy to live with."

The action of estrogen was known to have a carcinogenic effect by the late 1930s. Debates had ensued about the cancer risks of both natural and synthetic estrogen. Wilson knew that advocating long-term preventative estrogen was controversial; and women themselves were obviously cautious. With his pseudofeminist hat on, he argued that prejudices about older women's sexuality were fanning the fires of medical apprehension. By invoking the "bogeys" of breast and uterine cancer, detractors were trying to stop older women from enjoying emotionally harmonious and sexually fulfilled lives. Now that women's average lifespan was seventy-five years, medical purists and moralists had no right to withhold the "freedoms" of lifelong femininity. Why should women tolerate the depravations of "castration" when they could reach their "full personal potential"? Estrogen-enhanced women were masters "of their own destiny." Feminist activists, at that very moment, were busting the myth of feminine fulfillment wide open, so Wilson's appropriation of the language of women's liberation was a pretty shrewd marketing tactic. And marketing it was.

Wilson's research foundation received substantial donations from pharmaceutical companies, including Wyeth-Ayerst, the manufacturer of Premarin. But this wasn't disclosed to his readers; journalists reported on Wilson's "sponsorships" in the late 1960s, but the facts weren't confirmed until 2002, when Wilson's own son revealed that Wyeth-Ayerst "had paid all the expenses of writing 'Feminine Forever.'" Wilson's book, it turned out, was little more than an advertorial; he was essentially being paid to sugarcoat synthetic estrogen as totally natural, absolutely not carcinogenic, and entirely beneficial. Sure, he remarked, a study conducted in France in 1939 showed that estrogenic substances had a cancer-producing effect on mice. But women are not mice, Wilson helpfully reminded. He even went so far as to claim that estrogen therapy, "far from causing cancer, tends to prevent it." In 1966, the Food and Drug Administration (FDA) investigated Wilson for his wild and baseless claims that estrogen therapy cured menopause and prevented aging, and found that he was misleading the public about the uses of the drugs he touted. But *Feminine Forever* wasn't pulled from the shelves, even in drugstores, where it could still be sold as long as it wasn't displayed alongside any prescription medications. Within seven months, *Feminine Forever* sold more than one hundred thousand copies. Premarin prescriptions skyrocketed. But, as was the case with tranquilizers, women were not flocking to estrogen therapy because of some persuasive medical man. Therapies like Premarin offered relief from symptoms that many women suffered through with next to no support from their doctors. Women had every right to be sexual, mentally vibrant, and energized beyond their reproductive years. Many feminists embraced estrogen therapy as a liberation. But the realities of estrogen therapy had not only been downplayed but officially suppressed. Women were regaining control of their bodies, but they were also being deliberately misled about synthetic estrogen's effects.

Estrogen's potential to liberate women from social and sexual constraints had been unleashed in 1960, when the FDA approved Enovid, the first hormonal birth control pill, as a contraceptive. British women were granted the same permission in 1961, when Health Minister Enoch Powell announced that the drug's UK counterpart, Enavid, would be available from doctors. This little pill, made of synthetic estrogen and progesterone, was world-changing. For the first time, women could reliably take charge of their own fertility. Being able to choose when and if they had children freed women to expand their education opportunities, pursue careers, and wrest control of their lives—and sexualities—from reproduction. They could marry later or not at all, enjoy sex with men without the pressures of becoming pregnant, and release themselves from the fears and risks of ending a pregnancy that was unwanted. But women in the early days of the pill faced a battle for their right to take it.

At first, Enovid and Enavid were cautiously prescribed for menopause symptoms and menstruation disorders, including endometriosis; pregnancy prevention was listed as a side effect. Wilson even claimed that no women taking Enovid "beyond her child-bearing years" would "ever experience the menopause"—and the FDA took him to task over it. Birth control clinics could provide the pill, but at a cost. Most physicians in the UK and US prescribed the pill only to married women when their pregnancy would be harmful. The British government left decisions to the discretion of doctors, many of whom were wary about doling out medication that was not for a disease. And many also shared the opinion of the Church, that the pill would invalidate the sanctity of marriage and was tantamount to abortion. Historical fears that women's sexual freedom would lead to the destruction of moral and societal values pervaded medical, religious, and governmental attitudes toward the pill from its very inception. For now, women's right to reproductive and sexual autonomy remained controlled by medicine and, by extension, the oppressive hands of church and state.

From the 1930s, Margaret Sanger had been dreaming of the perfect contraceptive—a cheap, harmless, foolproof biological method that masses of women anywhere in the world could use. A pill swallowed every day was the ideal alternative to tricky diaphragms, foams, and powders, which Sanger, in typical eugenicist fashion, thought far too complicated for "intellectually retarded" women and "slum-dwellers" to use successfully. This pill, she imagined, would prevent women from resorting to sterilization; it would liberate sex from reproduction; and best of all, women's husbands and partners wouldn't even have to know about it. In the early 1950s, Sanger secured a grant from her friend, the biological scientist and women's rights campaigner Katharine Dexter McCormick, to fund pharmaceutical research into hormonal contraceptives. Sanger gave the grant to Gregory Pincus, an endocrinologist and experimental biologist working in a lab in Massachusetts, so he could begin developing a pill using progestin, a newly synthesized form of progesterone, the "female" steroid hormone secreted by the corpus luteum after ovulation. By 1954, Pincus was confident the ingredients were in place for an effective pill. He recruited gynecologist John Rock to conduct a small clinical study to see if it induced "pseudopregnancy" in his infertile patients. Rock and Pincus had to go under the radar because researching and distributing contraception devices and information was still a criminal offense in Massachusetts. But the FDA would approve the pill only if a large-scale clinical trial on human women was conducted. Pincus and Rock had to find a legal way around the obstacles while still satisfying the FDA. "We need a cage of ovulating females to experiment with," McCormick wrote to Sanger.

The first trial of Enovid was conducted in 1956 on the island of Puerto Rico, the US unincorporated territory, which already had a network of birth control clinics. It was also one of the most densely populated and poverty-stricken areas of the world. Women living in new housing projects in "slum-clearance areas" made, for Pincus and his team, ideal guinea pigs. They had a genuine need for reliable and safe contraception; many had large families and had to resort to sterilization. Many were also unable to read and write, so if they could use the pill effectively, then it was simple enough for any woman to follow the regimen. Participants were told, by hospital social workers and clinic nurses, that they were being invited to try out a new free "medicine that would keep them from having children they couldn't afford." As long as they were forty or under, married, living with their husbands, and had had at least two children, they were eligible. "We all jumped on it quickly and didn't look back," remembered Delia Mestre, one of the participants, fifty years later.

But Mestre and hundreds of others were not told that they were test subjects. They were not able to give informed consent, and they were not made aware of possible side effects. Their bodies would reveal what those side effects really were. By 1958, 830 women living in projects in the suburbs of San Juan, including Río Piedras and Humacao, a farming region on the island's east coast, had tried the pill. Edris Rice-Wray, director of the Puerto Rico Family Planning Association, was in charge of the study. In her first report on the Río Piedras trial of 221 women in 1957, Rice-Wray revealed that 17 percent of participants suffered symptoms including nausea, dizziness, gastrointestinal problems, bleeding, vomiting, and headaches. It "causes too many side-effects to be accepted generally," she concluded. But Pincus and his team dismissed these complaints as the "emotional super-activity of Puerto Rican woman." They were interested only in whether Enovid prevented conception. Seventeen women got pregnant during the trial, but according to the researchers, this was due to the pill not being correctly taken: "We have had not one single pregnancy that could be attributed to method failure." Many women stopped taking the pill altogether because it was making them so sick. The lowest "rates of withdrawal," Pincus remarked, were in one of the Humacao projects, where a social worker "had the women under her control in almost every sense psychologically."

The women of Puerto Rico were regarded as submissive enough to be coerced into continuously taking an unchartered drug. "Why didn't anyone let us make decisions for ourselves?" asked Mestre. When synthetic estrogen—mestranol—was added to the potent progestin mix in 1957, Enovid contained up to three times as much estrogen and at least ten times the amount of progestin as today's combined birth control pills. By 1961, the year after the FDA licensed Enovid as a contraceptive, reports from Britain, Los Angeles, and New Jersey of women suffering pulmonary embolisms and thrombosis emerged in the medical press. By 1963, 272 cases of thrombosis and thirty deaths among users of the pill were reported. But the FDA still approved Enovid for long-term use. In 1964, Searle—the company producing Enovid—was forced to add a disclaimer into the pill packet leaflets stating that thrombophlebitis and pulmonary embolism were an "occasional occurrence," but "a cause and effect relationship had not been demonstrated." Three women in the Puerto Rico trial died suddenly of heart failure and pulmonary embolisms. Their deaths were not properly reported in the trial findings, nor were they investigated. No autopsies were ever conducted.

The Puerto Rico trials ended in 1964. For seven years, Pincus and his team had been fine-tuning Enovid by experimenting on women denied the truth about what they were submitting to. But the abuse and control of Puerto Rican women's bodies and fertility, by medicine and the state, didn't begin or end with the pill. Pincus's interest in the pill wasn't a social one; he wasn't driven to create it because he embraced women's liberation in life and sex. He was an advocate for scientific interventions into population control. Racist fears of overpopulation among Latinx communities had motivated interventions into Puerto Rican women's reproductive choice and freedom since the late 1930s, when contraception was legalized, and laws passed permitting eugenic sterilization. Sterilization, endorsed and supported by the US government, was voraciously promoted to women as the best method of family limitation. By 1970, around a third of the women in Puerto Rico had been sterilized, many without their express knowledge or consent. *La operación*, as it was known, took place in hospitals after women gave birth, in family planning centers funded by the US government, and in birth control clinics for women workers set up in factories owned by American corporations. The pill trials, motivated by eugenic ideologies of population control and race perfection, were part of the historic and ongoing exploitation of Latinx women. And during those years of pill trials, the health and trust of women in Puerto Rico were abused in the race to market and sell this modern, reliable, liberatory contraception to women everywhere.

In 1967, the NHS Family Planning Act was passed in the UK. Contraceptive advice and devices were now available through local health authorities for all women over the age of sixteen, regardless of socioeconomic or marital status. The act also made abortion, for the first time in history, legal for up to twenty-four weeks of pregnancy. For most of the 1960s, in all US states, it was illegal to prescribe the pill to unmarried women under the "age of majority"—twenty-one—without parental consent. By 1969, when many states permitted oral contraceptives for "mature minors," at least 6.5 million American women, and more than

13 million worldwide, were taking an oral contraceptive. The invention of the pill was nothing short of a revolution for women, for their bodies and their lives. But it was also an experiment mired in ethical violation and information suppression. The more women who took the pill, the more health risks came glaringly to light.

The link between thrombosis and elevated hormone doses could no longer be called "speculative." In medical literature and clinical studies, television programs, newspaper features, and magazine articles in the UK and US, the dangers of one of history's most game-changing drugs were becoming frighteningly clear. Physicians often dismissed women's concerns when they reported nausea, leg pains, swelling, and mood swings; others feared the threat of cancer or the long-term risks of artificial hormones. But women were beginning to speak out, in letters to magazines and responses to surveys, about their fears that the pill was having untold effects on their bodies and minds. "Medical specialists at first tended to discount such unscientific comments, attributing them to the vagaries of women," reported the *New York Times* in 1969. "But now doctors are listening intently."

The American journalist, author, and activist Barbara Seaman, a vocal reporter on women's health issues, knew exactly how vital it was for women to be given clear, unbiased information. In 1959, her beloved aunt Sally died of endometrial cancer just before her fiftieth birthday. Sally's doctor strongly suspected her death was caused by years of taking Premarin for menopause symptoms. Ten years later, Seaman published her first book, *The Doctors' Case Against the Pill*, which revealed the truth about how the pill had been forced to market, the risks of synthetic hormones, and the catalog of side effects suppressed by the FDA. She also inspired a generation of women to demand to know why they had been deliberately misled about a drug they were so readily prescribed.

Seaman's findings inspired a series of congressional hearings led by US senator Gaylord Nelson, which ran from January to March 1970. The Senate committee was all white and all male, an egregious omission considering that the pill was taken only by women. At the time, around nine million women in the US alone had taken some form of contraceptive pill. Hugh Davis, an obstetrics and gynecology professor, told the

committee, "Never in history have so many individuals taken such potent drugs with so little information about the actual and potential
hazards . . . We are in fact embarking on a massive endocrinologic experiment with millions of healthy women." An influential male doctor's
insight was important, but it was no compensation for the complete lack
of female voices among the experts invited to testify. On January 23, the
first day of the hearings, Alice Wolfson, a feminist political activist, was
seated in the audience with fellow members of the DC Women's Liberation. Before the hearings began, they handed out leaflets asking the most
urgent questions: "Why are drug companies deliberately withholding
available information on side effects?" "Why is our government's solution
to world hunger to control population rather than redistribute resources?"
And why, they demanded to know, was there no pill for men?

These very good questions are still being debated today. The possibility of a male pill has been considered, researched, and trialed for almost
as long as the female pill has existed. In 2000, a team of scientists from
the University of Edinburgh reported that they had developed and were
trialing a male pill reported to be 100 percent effective. But aside from
a lack of funding, and the fact that hormonally suppressing male fertility is complicated, the major obstacles in the way of a male pill are
cultural conditioning and gender biases. Male libido, for example, is
valued and protected as an important part of their overall health. "Interference" with "sexual desire, feelings and behavior" was one of the
major concerns raised in a 1980 World Health Organization study into
the "acceptability" of the male pill. And ultimately, throughout history,
reproductive responsibility has been thrust upon women. From the beginning, the pill was couched as a way for women to take control of
their own bodies and their fertility. But this also means the costs—
physical and mental—remain women's burdens. And in a medical culture that dismisses and trivializes women's mental and physical health
concerns, it is far easier and more convenient to make women continue
to carry those burdens.

DC Women's Liberation offered men at the hearings the opportunity to share the load, if only symbolically, by taking one of the pills
they had attached to their leaflets. "Let's see how you feel about these

questions when you have one of those pills circulating in your body!" one protester exclaimed. After a male doctor declared that "estrogen is to cancer what fertilizer is to wheat," the protesters shouted, "Why are you using women as guinea pigs? Why are you letting the drug companies murder us for profit and convenience?" Members of the audience broke out in riotous applause, but Senator Nelson commanded them to keep quiet and sit still. They would not keep quiet. "We don't think the hearings are more important than our lives!" Nelson ordered the women to leave. They refused, so he demanded everyone leave. The hearings were reconvened under police guard and closed to the public.

On March 7, three days after the Senate hearings ended, DC Women's Liberation held their own pill hearings in a local church. Speakers included a contraceptive research clinician, a psychologist investigating the impact of the pill on sex drive, a social worker involved with the Puerto Rico trials, a "welfare mother" testifying "about the coercive use of the pill," and Barbara Seaman. All were welcome to come hear "previously suppressed information" and learn the "sexist-racist-imperialist reasons behind that suppression." In their opening statement, they explained, "It is not our mission to have all women of the pill discard it . . . Our mission . . . is to rise up, as women, and demand our human rights. We will no longer let doctors treat us as objects to be manipulated at will . . . We will no longer tolerate intimidation by white-coated gods, antiseptically directing our lives."

Today—nearly twenty-five years after researchers and activists forced this first wave of legislative change and pharmaceutical transparency—the effects of oral contraceptives are still not fully understood. Myths and mystification have circulated around the pill for decades, and in many ways, people taking it are still experimental subjects. Since its side effects are so individual and variable, there has been a dearth of information about how the pill affects physical and mental health. There is evidence that the pill can cause thrombosis—as was made clear in the 1960s—increase blood pressure, and heighten the risk of breast and endometrial cancer in certain people. But the more subjective side effects, especially those linked to mood, sex drive, and emotional well-being, remain frustratingly unclear. Links between pill hormones and depression, anxiety, suicidal ideation, and psychosis have recently been explored in major clinical and research studies. A small study conducted at the Albert Einstein College of Medicine, in New York, in 2019 showed that pill hormones might actually be shrinking the hypothalamus, the part of the brain that regulates mood, libido, and sleep cycles. For the many who report debilitating psychological and mental side effects but are dismissed by doctors and GPs who prioritize insistence on the pill's safety over patient experiences, these new studies are a vindication. But until medicine acknowledges, unambiguously, the evident connections between mental ill health and hormonal contraceptives, we will remain in the dark about the impact of the pill on our minds and lives.

DC Women's Liberation members were demanding, as women still are today, that their voices be heard. Wolfson and her comrades had all been on the pill; they had all been to their doctors with problems; they had all been told to carry on taking it. And they courageously took on the patronizing authority of the male medical establishment to force real change. In the wake of the hearings, the FDA announced that pill packages would be required to include an insert detailing all possible side effects and also contraindications—any symptoms, existing conditions, or disease histories that might make taking certain medications harmful. Many medical professionals balked at having their expertise undermined by some leaflet. Pharmaceutical companies objected to what they thought to be scaremongering tactics that would put women off taking the pill. But women across the United States paid close attention to the proceedings on Capitol Hill. They, too, had been fobbed off by doctors when they reported strange pains, creeping depression, and sickness in their stomachs. Use of the pill dropped by 18 percent, and women started demanding answers from their gynecologists. By the mid-1970s, the estrogen in combined pills had been reduced to about a third of what was in the original Enovid. Progestin levels were decreased by as much as 85 percent. It wasn't until 1977, after the FDA agreed that comprehensive information about the hormone levels of estrogen therapies must be included in every package, that manufacturers had to follow suit. Legislative change was slow, but the tides of grassroots change had already turned. Thanks to those fearless researchers, journalists, rebels, and dissenters, women everywhere were empowered, many for the first time in their lives, to question the blind authority of medicine. The women's health movement was born. Over the next decades, health feminists would come together, all over the US and the UK, to collaborate and campaign, advocate and organize. At community, grassroots, and national levels, women would courageously and creatively begin to challenge, dismantle, and rewrite centuries of medical oppression, suppression, and mystification.

17

OUR BODIES, OUR SELVES

"It is important to understand that mystification is the primary process here," explained *Women and Their Bodies*, a course book written and researched by a group of women from Boston in 1970. "It is mystification that makes us postpone going to the doctor for 'that little pain' since he's such a 'busy man.' It is mystification that prevents us from demanding a precise explanation of what is the matter and how exactly he is going to treat it. It is mystification that causes us to become passive objects who submit to his control and supposed expertise."

The authors first met on Sunday, May 11, 1969, at the New England Regional Female Liberation Conference. During "Women and Their Bodies," a workshop organized by health activist Nancy Hawley, they talked openly about their experiences with doctors. They shared "their frustrations at how little they knew about how their bodies worked." The women decided to form the Doctor's Group so that they could continue, together, to understand and unravel medicine's hold over their bodies and minds.

By 1970, women's lives were more regulated by medicine than ever before. Social progress had intertwined with cultural attitudes to such an extent that many aspects of women's freedoms and rights were controlled by medical gatekeepers. Sexual liberation was afforded by the pill. Estrogen therapy maintained "feminine" health after menopause. To be relieved of pain during labor meant submitting to medically supervised births. The Doctor's Group and all the other women at the heart of the feminist health movement were not rejecting these advances—far from it. But they were pushing back against the culture of mystification that prevailed in male-dominated medicine. So much knowledge about their own bodies was withheld behind that veneer of paternalistic professionalism. Women's health and lives depended on breaking down barriers of secrecy and evasion. And as milestones like the pill trials had shown, real change happened when women listened to other women, created their own knowledge, and bravely put their heads above the parapet.

"We discovered there were no 'good' doctors and we had to learn for ourselves," explained the Doctor's Group. They read medical books and clinical journals, met with health professionals, and distributed questionnaires to friends and peers. Every week, they shared what they had learned about topics including "patient as victim," sexuality, anatomy, birth control, pregnancy, postpartum care, and abortion. "For the first time, we were doing research and writing papers that were about us and for us. We were excited and our excitement was powerful. We wanted to share . . . the material we were learning with our sisters."

In 1970, they compiled their papers into a 193-page book to share with their sisters in Boston and "across the country." Printed by the radical publisher New England Free Press and costing seventy-five cents, *Women and Their Bodies* was a health-feminism manifesto and an anatomy guidance manual for women, by women. In 1971, *Women and Their Bodies* was renamed *Our Bodies, Ourselves*, and its price reduced to thirty cents. That year it sold over 230,000 copies. It tackled issues that had been taboo for too long, like VD, abortion, orgasms, masturbation, and the diversity of sexuality. It spoke plainly about the injustices of the US health-care system, drug company profits, and gender imbalances across the medical establishment. It also encouraged women to touch, explore, and learn to love their bodies, and to realize how "chauvinistic" medical and social attitudes alienated "woman from her body." "What are our bodies?" asked the authors of "Anatomy and Physiology," one of the chapters of *Our Bodies, Ourselves*. "First, they *are* us. We do not inhabit them—we *are* them (as well as mind)."

The women's health movement energized hundreds of groups,

communities, networks, and organizations across the US. Health feminism was not one unified voice fighting for the same issues and concerns. The movement was as diverse and complex as the women involved. Some formed pressure groups to advocate for women's voices in the health-care system, or to lobby the FDA and the American Medical Association against unethical practices and information suppression. In 1975, Alice Wolfson, with Barbara Seaman, health activist Belita Cowan, and Mary Howell, the first woman dean of Harvard Medical School, formed the National Women's Health Network (NWHN) to do just that. Others fought back by affording women the right to make decisions about their bodies. The Jane Collective, founded by Heather Booth in Chicago in 1969, was an underground support network that helped women procure abortions. Abortion was illegal in the majority of the United States, forcing many women to take life-threatening measures. Flyers around the city asked "Pregnant? Worried? Call Jane." After learning how to safely perform surgical procedures including dilation and curettage, members of Jane carried out the abortions themselves in rented apartments across the city.

Women involved with chapters of NOW, like feminist lawyer Carol Downer, also took women's prohibited rights into their own hands by learning and sharing abortion methods and vaginal self-examination techniques. While observing a woman having an IUD fitted at an illegal abortion clinic in LA in 1971, Downer felt "awestruck" at seeing a cervix for the first time. At a clandestine meeting of the newly formed LA Abortion Task Force at the Everywoman's Bookstore in Venice, California, Downer lay on a desk, inserted one of the plastic speculums she had swiped from the clinic, and showed the women how to examine their own cervixes. The Pap smear, named for one of its early inventors, pathologist George Papanicolaou, had been used by gynecologists to detect cancerous cervical cells since the late 1940s. May Edward Chinn, the only Black female physician in Harlem in the 1930s, was also instrumental in the development of the Pap smear. Chinn met Papanicolaou while she was completing her master's degree in public health at Columbia in 1933. During her years caring for marginalized communities in Harlem, she witnessed the misery of untreated cancer, especially among women. She became determined to contribute to research into its early detection and diagnosis, and during the late 1940s and 1950s, she continued to work with Papanicolaou on cytopathology—the study of cells and tissue fragments—as a method of detecting and diagnosing precancerous cervical cells. Chinn's name, sadly, was not attached to the smear test that today saves the lives of thousands of women. But her contributions to the discipline of cytopathology mean she deserves full recognition as one of the most important figures in the history of early cancer detection for women.

It wasn't until the 1960s that Pap smears were introduced into preventative medicine campaigns and women were encouraged to have them as part of their routine gynecological exams. Despite setbacks and controversies, the Pap smear enabled early detection of a devastating disease that, historically, was often diagnosed only when it was too late. But as health feminists revealed, many women couldn't bear being so intimately scrutinized. *Our Bodies, Ourselves* reported that only 12 percent of the "women in this country who ought to have Pap smears" were getting them. Vaginal and pelvic examinations reinforced feelings of "vulnerability and helplessness," objectification and embarrassment, especially when they were performed by male gynecologists—which they usually were.

In September 1972, Downer gave an address at a meeting of the American Psychological Association about how sex discrimination was impacting women's experiences as patients and their health. With her friend and collaborator Lorraine Rothman, Downer had helped create an early abortion device called Del-Em, a less invasive and far less traumatic alternative to dilation and curettage (D&C), the abortion method in which the contents of the uterus are removed surgically. Consisting of a plastic cannula, a syringe, and a glass jar, the Del-Em enabled women to remove their own uterine tissues in a process known as "menstrual extraction." After starting a self-help clinic in LA in 1971, Downer and Rothman traveled the US demonstrating the Del-Em and self-examination. As Downer explained to the American Psychological Association, the self-help movement was "met with outstanding success." In groups of six, women met over six weeks to share information about birth control, sexual health, and cancer. All the participants were given a speculum and shown how to use it. "We are enthusiastic about how much we have learned, and how much more comfortable we feel about our own bodies," said Downer. By touching and seeing themselves, women were creating their own "direct knowledge." Armed with that knowledge, women would no longer be shamed into silence and passive acceptance. They could question their doctors' decisions, think carefully about the medications they were prescribed, and begin to overcome the inhibitions that stopped them from seeking preventative care. "The day of the all-wise male gynecologist is over," announced Downer.

Self-help was a hugely important part of "a giant upsurge of interest in women's health care." Whether they were campaigning for reproductive justice, the end of male medical supremacy, drug-company transparency, safe contraceptives, or natural childbirth, health feminists were united in their fight to reclaim medical knowledge with their own hands. "At this point in our history," wrote Barbara Ehrenreich and Deirdre English in 1973, in their influential text on the historical disempowerment of women in medicine, *Witches, Midwives, and Nurses,* "every effort to take hold of and share medical knowledge is a critical part of our struggle." Women had never been "passive bystanders" in medicine. The medical sexism being exposed on Capitol Hill, in advocacy groups, books, pamphlets, and on bookstore tables, galvanized women to reveal the forces behind "deep-rooted, institutional sexism." "Our enemy is not just 'men' or their individual male chauvinism: it is the whole class system which enabled male, upper-class healers to win out and which forced us into subservience," Ehrenreich and English wrote.

Preventing women from legally and safely ending unwanted pregnancies symbolized, *Our Bodies, Ourselves* stated, "the oppression of women in America and the lies that support it." For health activists fighting against abortion laws, the first step was legislative repeal. But women were calling not just for a change in the law but for a complete shift in medical and cultural attitudes toward women's right to choose. In the mid-1960s, one in six pregnancy-related deaths in the United States was caused by unsafe abortions. Systemic sexism, which valued women's reproductive duties over their human rights, was too often a death sentence. In 1959, the American Law Institute drafted a proposal to make abortion legal if the pregnancy occurred after rape or incest, or if it would endanger the woman or her baby's health. Several states, including Mississippi, Colorado, California, and North Carolina, reformed abortion laws based on the institute's model in the late 1960s.

In 1970, Hawaii enshrined women's right to choose, independent of medical decisions. New York passed a law allowing abortions up to twenty-four weeks. After years of campaigning, consciousness-raising, and legal and medical debate, the US Supreme Court finally made the landmark decision to protect women's constitutional liberty to end pregnancies, at least in the first trimester, in January 1973. *Roe v. Wade* recognized abortion decisions as part of the Fourteenth Amendment, which protected citizens' right to privacy. In the second and third trimesters, state governments could still intervene depending on the health of the mother or the fetus. Three months later, *Ms.* magazine published a crime-scene photograph of Geraldine "Gerri" Santoro, who died, aged twenty-eight, in a Connecticut motel room after her lover, Clyde Dixon, tried to induce abortion with a catheter and a textbook. Dixon fled when Santoro began hemorrhaging, leaving her alone to die. *Ms.* printed the photograph of Santoro in the center of the full-page headlined "NEVER AGAIN." *Roe v. Wade* was an unprecedented leap forward, but abortion remained, as it does today, at the center of intense political, cultural, and religious ideological battles. The feminist health movement energized women, lawmakers, politicians, and the medical community to courageously defend our body autonomy, biological freedom, and life choices. But those rights are precarious and vulnerable. Appointing Supreme Court justices who would overturn *Roe v. Wade* was one of the campaign promises made by the forty-fifth US president in 2016. With the sad death in September 2020 of Ruth Bader Ginsburg, the strongest defender of abortion rights and women's autonomy on the Supreme Court, the haunting possibility that *Roe* could be overturned has edged closer to becoming a reality. The fight to call our bodies our own continues.

In 1972, the authors of *Our Bodies, Ourselves* incorporated as the Boston Women's Health Collective and negotiated a publishing contract with Simon & Schuster. The book was translated into many languages after its first commercial distribution in 1973. Its powerful message of self-help, reproductive and sexual freedom, and medical demystification was incredibly inspiring for British feminists. Unlike in the US, UK citizens had access to universal health care. Treatments, medicines, diagnoses, and preventative health care were freely available through the NHS. And since 1968, when the Abortion Act came into effect in England, Wales, and Scotland, women have been allowed to request legal abortions from NHS providers for up to twenty-three weeks and six days of pregnancy. Women in Northern Ireland were withheld this right until October 2019, when abortions, carried out by a "registered medical professional," were finally decriminalized. And following the landmark referendum result in the Republic of Ireland on May 26, 2018, abortion, at up to twelve weeks' gestation, was legalized for the first time. But the abortion acts in the UK and Ireland are still regulated by criminal law. Abortion is legal as long as two registered practitioners have determined, "in good faith," that the pregnancy has not exceeded its twenty-fourth week, or that its continuation would result in mental or physical harm to the mother or baby. Abortion may be a legal right, but it is one that is afforded to us only through an interpretation of the law by the regulation of medical authority. In 1974, the UK government appointed a committee, chaired by Justice Elizabeth Lane, to investigate the Abortion Act. In its report, the Lane Committee rejected "abortion on request." Women, they decided, couldn't cope with the "burden of making their own decisions." It was "in the interests of the patient as an individual" to leave the decision to doctors. The committee also recommended limiting abortions up to twelve weeks and upholding physicians' power to make diagnoses of pregnancy. Limitations remained at twenty-four weeks, but women are still, today, denied unrestricted access to abortions. The ultimate decision still does not lie with us. The question of repealing the law and giving women the genuine right to choose continues.

Health feminists in the UK were mobilizing around different systemic issues in the 1970s. But they shared their US counterparts' mission to reclaim their body autonomy from medical authority. They, too, joined together in groups, networks, and collectives to tear down barriers of secrecy and shame around women's bodies and illnesses. They also created and distributed information and demystified the enigmatic authority of male-dominated medicine. In self-help clinics across the country, women were shown how to examine their vaginas and look at their cervixes. Volunteers also demonstrated the Del-Em technique. Many women's health groups provided urine testing for biological pregnancy detection for free or a few pence; home-testing kits were available from pharmacies, but they were expensive and often unreliable. The authority to officially determine a pregnancy lay, ultimately, with professional doctors and their laboratory tests—and these were not available on demand. Most doctors also refused to do pregnancy tests unless there was a medical reason. Results could take days to return from the lab. At self-help clinics, women could find out immediately, in the company of supportive women, and decide for themselves what they wanted to do next. Their pregnancy was something that was happening to them, to their bodies; it didn't begin as a medical event diagnosed under the judgmental glare of professional opinion.

UK feminist activists worked hard to draw attention to what women really needed from the NHS. All women should receive the treatment and care they wanted and deserved, "rather than having to accept the services the medical profession and government thinks we need." But from its very beginnings in the early 1970s, the movement was overwhelmingly white. There were only two Black women in the six-hundred-strong audience of the UK's first National Women's Liberation Conference at Oxford University in 1970. The issues spotlighted at the conference—on-demand access to contraception and abortion—were exceptionally important for Black and other ethnically diverse women. Black women particularly bore the brunt of Britain's eugenic legacy. They faced entrenched prejudice around their sexualities and reproductive rights. Community networks including the Black Women's Action Committee and the Brixton Women's group addressed how the stereotyping of Black women's bodies was impacting their health-care needs. Reproductive justice and birth control were crucial issues.

Throughout the 1970s, injections of Depo-Provera, a controversial three-month hormonal contraceptive, were disproportionately given to African, Caribbean, and Asian women in the UK. Black feminists protested that Depo—essentially temporary sterilization—was a eugenic procedure doled out by racist doctors to rob women of their freedom and fertility. Like the pill, Depo was effectively being tested on these women—the truth about its dangerous side effects was deliberately withheld. The Organisation of Women of African and Asian Descent (OWAAD), founded in 1978, also focused on raising public awareness about dehumanizing medical treatments. The Black feminist health movement raised consciousness at a public level about medical racism and inequality. But their advocacy and activism also created spaces for women to share information, gain knowledge, and speak for and about their individual body and health experiences. Dr. Jan McKenley, an activist with OWAAD and the National Abortion Campaign, remembered attending a radical health workshop at a retreat in rural Wiltshire in the late 1970s. "I'm lying in the arms of a woman who's supporting me, my legs are up and I've got a speculum inside of my vagina and another woman is holding a mirror so I can see my cervix and vagina and see how beautiful it is," she recalled. "Feminism gave me my body. It gave me my body back, and it just reminds you that in those days a lot of women felt their bodies weren't themselves, their bodies were not theirs. And that was really powerful and it was magic."

In 1981, Byllye Avery, the American health activist and reproductive justice advocate, launched the National Black Women's Health Project (NBWHP), initially as a pilot program with the National Women's Health Network. The US women's health movement had forced huge changes over the past decade. But, as in the UK, it was dominated by white organizers, white voices. Since 1974, Avery, with her peers Joan Edelson, Judy Levy, and Margaret Parrish, had been running a health center in Gainesville, Florida, providing services and referrals to women who needed them most. Low-income Black women in North Florida had a dire lack of access to safe abortions and reliable contraception, gynecological care, and preventative health measures. For Avery, who served on the board of the NWHN, Black women needed a grassroots health movement that centered on their experiences. Within two years, a network of self-help clinics, health projects, and peer-support communities had formed across the country under the banner of the NBWHP. And on June 24, 1983, over two thousand members gathered at Spelman College, America's oldest Black liberal arts women's college, for the first-ever national conference on Black women's health issues.

The words of Fannie Lou Hamer, the civil, political, and women's rights leader, were the conference's rallying cry. "I'm Sick and Tired of Being Sick and Tired," announced the conference program, each word translated into sign language under a silhouette frame. In 1961, Hamer was subjected to a radical hysterectomy, performed by a white male doctor, without her knowledge or consent at Sunflower County hospital in Mississippi, while undergoing surgery to remove a small tumor in her uterus. Hamer spoke of the violations of the "Mississippi appendectomy" at political rallies while she was leading the Mississippi Freedom Democratic Party. Sixty percent of Black women in Sunflower County had been covertly sterilized in the name of white greed, white social reform, and white knowledge. And the harrowing history of medicine's willful abuse of Black and other ethnically diverse women in the name of research, especially those who are vulnerable, and incarcerated, continues today. In September 2020, Dawn Wooten, a nurse at Irwin County Detention Center, a private Immigration and Customs Enforcement (ICE) facility in Georgia, alleged in a whistleblower complaint that an ob-gyn was performing "unwarranted" and often nonconsensual mass hysterectomies on detained women. According to Wooten, "Everybody he sees has a hysterectomy—just about everybody." Irwin County was likened to an "experimental concentration camp." "It was like they're experimenting with our bodies," stated one of the women at the facility. This doctor, whom Wooten referred to, chillingly, as "the uterus collector," has vehemently denied the allegation. But thanks to the incredible courage of Wooten, the medical exploitation of marginalized, silenced women has been brought to public and governmental attention.

Fannie Lou Hamer died in 1977. As the Black Women's Health Project conference literature explained, "the legacy she left" enabled Black women to "face the challenges and forge the campaigns necessary to walk in dignity and health." Black women in the early 1980s were dying young. They had higher rates of maternal and infant mortality; they suffered more severely with breast and cervical cancers, cardiovascular and kidney diseases, uterine fibroids, diabetes, and lupus. Medicine had acknowledged the higher rates of some of these diseases and conditions among Black women for decades. The prevalence of uterine fibroids, for instance, was discussed and theorized in medical literature in the 1930s. Although endocrinologists back then linked fibroids to increased estrogen—a theory still being explored today—they proposed that Black women had higher hormone levels, and therefore more fibroids, because they were more likely to contract pelvic inflammatory disease, an infection that can be sexually transmitted. Racist stereotyping of Black women's bodies and sexualities mired understanding of conditions like uterine fibroids. The NBWHP was forged to raise consciousness around the health disparities that medical science had ignored and to break down barriers of isolation and powerlessness that historically had hindered Black women from receiving vital care. The conference "acted like water to a thirsty seed, as the magnitude of the black community's critical health problems was brought to light."

"I arrived with 2000 black women, looking all the ways we look," remembered Felicia Ward, who attended the conference. "I'd never before experienced so many black women in one place at one time . . . Something was calling to me, and I ached, it was so familiar. I could feel myself waking up inside." Ward absorbed every moment of the workshops on living well and staying healthy, but one had a profound effect on her. On June 25, social justice advocate Lillie Pearl Allen led a workshop titled "Black and Female: What Is the Reality?" Hundreds of women crowded into the room, perched on tables, seated on the floor, sharing chairs. "Get as close as you can," Allen urged. "It's past time for holding back." Black women had internalized, over generations, messages that they should be tough, never cry, not show their pain. "For too long now we've been told to keep our business to ourselves," Allen said. "Well, the business of silence is killing us . . . We must begin to tell our stories. It's time to tell each other how it's been to be black and female." Ward listened to her sisters "telling what had to be told." "All the joys and sorrows of being black and female were revealed to me that day," she said. When Allen addressed how contained fear affected their bodies, Ward laughed with the others in relief and solidarity. "So, what happens?" asked Allen. "All that starts building up in us and we get aches and pains. Your body is not supposed to carry around all that junk."

Ward's memories revealed a truth medicine had yet to acknowledge: Black women were suffering and dying from chronic diseases because of medical and cultural perceptions of how they tolerated pain. In the 1980s, there were barely any studies of the ways gender and race intersected in the treatment of pain. Racist beliefs about differences in pain sensitivity were still very much ingrained. Until the first sociological investigations into racial bias in medicine were conducted in the 2000s, the impact of such pervasive attitudes on Black women's health care was anecdotal. Since the 1970s, data about disease prevalence showed that Black, Asian, and other ethnically diverse women were suffering disproportionately from poorly understood and under-researched chronic conditions. But as networks like NBWHP showed, the realities, especially of Black women's health needs, could never be reduced to a set of statistics or epidemiological data.

Structural racism had an enormous impact on the provision and access of adequate and consistent health and medical care. It also had a punitive effect on how Black women were treated—as "other" than white, a subgroup, an afterthought. Events like the 1983 conference showed that Black women didn't just suffer more; they suffered differently. As well as providing the "information, skills and resources" they needed to "live healthfully," the NBWHP wanted to enable them, individually and collectively, "to understand the concepts of emotional, mental, physical and spiritual health." The "interrelationship among these factors" was what medicine needed, urgently, to understand and address. By being empowered to tell their stories, speak for their own bodies, and share their histories, they could advocate for their own needs and "exercise control over their own lives." The NBWHP became the Black Women's Health Imperative (BWHI) in 2002. Since its inception in 1981, the organization has worked continuously to "address the massive challenges of racial and gender-based health disparities affecting Black women." By raising public awareness, delivering programs, developing policies, carrying out research, and publishing resources, the BWHI is leading change on "issues most critical to Black women's health" in the US, including "breast and cervical cancers, diabetes, HIV/AIDS, intimate partner violence and sexual assault, maternal health and reproductive health."

Chronic pain was—and still is—the most common symptom in many of the medically mysterious diseases affecting Black women, including lupus, sickle cell anemia, uterine fibroids, endometriosis, and postpartum heart conditions like cardiomyopathy. And, as Allen explained at her conference workshop in 1983, chronic pain is never merely a sign of illness. It is also a complex expression of personal, social, and historical trauma. Neurobiologists and neurologists across Europe and the US had been trying to figure out how women experienced, responded to, and expressed pain since the 1940s. After theories about the neurobiology of pain emerged in the mid-1960s, and the McGill Pain Questionnaire was developed in 1971, the question of how pain was influenced by psychosocial factors started to be explored. Beliefs that women were more sensitive to pain persisted well into the 1980s, as did those lazy assumptions that women's pain was primarily influenced by their emotions. Terms like "psychogenic," "functional," and "medically unexplained" cropped up often in the 1970s and 1980s, as ways of describing mysterious pain—particularly in women between the ages of twenty and forty, and especially if their pain happened to be in the abdomen, pelvis, uterus, or vulva. If no lesion, fibroid, or tumor could be found, then the origin of that pain was, all too often, assumed to be the patient's mind, not her body.

In a study of 188 patients—half of them women—at a New York State hospital pain unit in 1982, the clinical psychologist Dr. Dorothea Lack revealed that women had to wait, on average, around three years longer than men to be referred. They were also more frequently offered minor tranquilizers and antidepressants than further diagnostic tests. The men received more insurance compensation for pain treatment, and their clinical notes used validating language. "No emotional overlay is present," noted one physician of a man's pain. The women, however, were "complaining" of pain rather than "experiencing it," and they tended to be labeled as "hypochondrial." Despite "a decade of work by the women's movement" and the "growing assertiveness of women" against systemic sexism, the medical establishment was still dismissing women's pain as psychosomatic and their symptoms as emotional. The bias this demonstrated wasn't just delaying women's diagnoses; it was killing them.

Across medicine's history, physicians cried "hysteria" whenever a woman's symptoms confounded their understanding or exceeded their knowledge. By the mid-1980s, so many chronic "women's" diseases, including thyroid conditions like Hashimoto's and Graves'; rheumatic diseases like lupus, rheumatoid arthritis, and Sjögren's syndrome; and gastrointestinal disorders such as ulcerative colitis and Crohn's—were known to be autoimmune or immune-mediated. Most of these diseases overwhelmingly affected women. Medicine was beginning to consider that women had more active immune systems and higher antibody responses, making female biology more susceptible to autoimmunity. Diagnostic criteria had been laid down; there were batteries of tests available. But autoimmunity, as a biomedical concept, had only recently been accepted across the medical community. It flouted long-established logic about how bodies work and disease occurs. And many of these diseases had a long history of being deemed hysterical—especially neurological autoimmune diseases like multiple sclerosis and also myasthenia gravis. Novelty, controversy, and gender stigma create the perfect conditions for misdiagnosis and misconception to flourish.

In 1980, a new classification of "somatization disorder" appeared in the third edition of the *Diagnostic and Statistical Manual*, the standard-bearer for psychiatric diagnoses. Somatization neatly filled the space vacated by "hysteria" when it was removed as a stand-alone diagnosis in 1952. It became a way of classifying illnesses with physical symptoms but no identifiable organic or physiological cause. If a patient's pain persisted but her doctor couldn't account for it, they might assume it was a manifestation of "psychological factors or conflicts." Painful, irregular, and unusually heavy periods were three of the thirty-seven symptoms in the diagnostic criteria. Loss of interest in sex, pain during intercourse, and pain in the genitals, joints, stomach, and chest all made the list too. Women had to present with fourteen symptoms, men with twelve. But the criteria were spectacularly biased toward the telltale early signs and emotional effects of skepticism-clouded chronic diseases that mostly affected women, especially of the rheumatic, gastrointestinal, and gynecological kind.

To help physicians deal with their overly emotional, medically elusive cases, two American psychiatrists, in 1985, decided to simplify the criteria for "somatization" diagnoses. By studying 85 female psychiatric outpatients who all suffered from "multiple unexplained physical complaints" that began before they were thirty, the psychiatrists defined seven indicative symptoms as a "screening test" for somatization, which went by the acronym SDBLAVP. This stood for shortness of breath, dysmenorrhea, burning pain in sexual organs, lump in the throat, amnesia, vomiting, and painful extremities. And because most somatization sufferers were thought to be women, and the symptoms were so gendered, the psychiatrists came up with a maddeningly sexist mnemonic that they no doubt found rather witty: Somatization Disorder Besets Ladies and Vexes Physicians. "Ladies" beset with somatization, the psychiatrists claimed, believed they had been sick for a long time. They were intent on seeking diagnoses and treatments. They tended to be dramatic when describing their ailments. The typical sufferer, then, was hypochondriac, neurotic, and hysterical: the trifecta of medical slurs thrown at women for centuries.

Diagnoses like "somatization" were not meant to imply illnesses were feigned or imagined. But the startling range of feminized symptoms set a troubling precedent for misdiagnosis. It was far easier to conclude that the pain and bleeding of endometriosis, for instance, was psychological than to go to the trouble of actually diagnosing it. Somatization acknowledged the intricate ways that the mind can express itself through the body. But it clinically legitimized so many damaging myths—not only about women's excessive emotional relationship to illness but also about the unreliable, evasive, and unruly nature of female biology. So many of the chronic diseases obscured by "somatization" were poorly understood, shrouded in speculation, and under-researched.

In the absence of enough biomedical knowledge about the courses and causes of conditions like autoimmune diseases and endometriosis, physicians fell back on punitive gender stereotypes. And in the 1980s, oversights about women's illnesses were compounded by the exemption of almost all female subjects from clinical research trials and studies.

Since the 1940s, drugs to regulate the changeable and challenging aspects of female biology had been routinely rushed to market. And since the early 1960s, medicine had been waking up to the consequences of approving pharmaceutical substances before their side effects were understood. Thalidomide had been licensed since 1956 in Europe, Australia, and Canada as a treatment for anxiety, insomnia, and morning sickness. The drug was not authorized in the US because Frances Oldham Kelsey, a Canadian-born physician, pharmacologist, and reviewer for the FDA, rightly and courageously questioned the safety of a drug that had not been rigorously tested in clinical trials. Outside the US, thalidomide was declared safe for women to take during pregnancy because it was believed, at the time, that the drug could not cross the placenta's barrier and harm the fetus. The Distillers Company, which produced Distaval and other thalidomide brands, claimed from 1958 that it could "be given with complete safety to pregnant women and nursing mothers without adverse effect to mother or child." An ad from 1961 in the *Journal of the Pharmaceutical Society of Great Britain* claimed Distaval was so "outstandingly safe" that even if a small child accidently opened a bottle, they wouldn't be at risk of "harmful results."

Later that year, an Australian doctor alerted the medical community to a link between thalidomide and fetal development, which had been known about since the late 1950s. Into the early 1960s, in the forty-six countries that licensed thalidomide, more than ten thousand children were affected by the drug. Many had birth defects, including phocomelia, a malformation of the arms and legs, and thousands died months after they were born. In the wake of these devastating findings, the FDA issued in 1977 the guidance "General Considerations for the Clinical Evaluation of Drugs." It recommended that all women of "childbearing potential," between the ages of eighteen and forty-five, be excluded from early-phase clinical research. Even women who were on long-term contraception or whose male partners had had vasectomies were barred. Exceptions could be made only if a drug was being tested for a life-threatening condition.

Thalidomide was withdrawn from the UK in 1961. But another dangerous medication was still being prescribed to pregnant women—and in the US no less, which refused to license thalidomide. Since the late 1930s, diethylstilbestrol (DES), a synthetic estrogen, had been widely given to American women to prevent miscarriage and premature labor. Promoted as a "routine prophylaxis in ALL pregnancies," DES was deemed safe because its biochemist developers were certain it could not cross the placenta. But in the 1950s, two studies revealed that DES actually increased the risk of miscarriage. Regardless, it was still prescribed voraciously, "to make a normal pregnancy more normal," and for menopause symptoms. Many menopausal women taking DES suffered alarming symptoms, like bleeding and breast pain, but their concerns were dismissed out of hand. The FDA banned the use of DES as a growth stimulant for farmed poultry in 1959, because exposed male farmworkers were reporting impotence and breast growth. Shockingly, a drug considered too dangerous for chickens and men was somehow perfectly acceptable for women.

In 1971, researchers in Boston revealed that clear-cell adenocarcinoma, a rare form of vaginal cancer, had been found in girls as young as seven whose mothers had taken DES. Between five and ten million US women were thought to have taken DES since 1938, in pills, injections, and vaginal suppositories. The FDA issued a warning against prescribing DES to pregnant women in 1971, but the drug continued to be doled out as an emergency contraceptive—or "morning after" pill. Belita Cowan, a feminist health activist with the NWHN, had been researching DES since 1969. In 1972, she initiated a press conference in Washington, DC, in which she revealed that the claims for the drug were fraudulent and its side effects deliberately suppressed. In 1974, Cowan testified as an expert witness at Senate hearings on DES. She urged senators not to allow the FDA to approve DES as a contraceptive. The following December, Cowan testified before the House of Representatives, where she arranged for a childbirth advocate and two "DES

Daughters"—women who had been exposed to DES in utero—to share their stories. That month, hordes of protesters gathered at the steps of the FDA offices to protest "the indiscriminate use of DES, birth control pills, and estrogen replacement therapy in menopause." By then, DES had been identified as the cause of over three thousand cases of cancer in DES Daughters. "To this day," Cowan recalled in 1999, "the FDA has never approved DES as a morning-after pill, and I am very happy for that. I have always believed that one person, acting with passion, can make a difference."

The FDA research blackout was a wrongheaded reaction in so many ways. After all, the dangers of DES and thalidomide were unforeseen because they were not properly investigated in the first place. Understandably, the risks of trialing new drugs on vulnerable subjects—like pregnant women—should be mitigated. But barring *all* women from participating just because they could potentially give birth was not only downright sexist but shamefully myopic. It reinforced the paternalistic belief that medicine's duty was to protect women, even if that meant suppressing information from them. The ban also highlighted how female biology was regarded as reproductive first, human second. Absurdly, women were exempted on the grounds of biological difference, yet when it came to the effects of drugs not tested on them, they were assumed to be biologically the same as men. Situating the male body—usually white—as the standard in research about the clinical patterns of diseases also perpetuated some seriously exclusionist attitudes across the medical community. In the early 1980s, as the world faced a disturbing new epidemic, those blind spots of knowledge would prove to be catastrophic.

———

"Rare Cancer Seen in 41 Homosexuals," reported the *New York Times* in 1981. Of those forty-one men, all being treated in New York and San Francisco, eight had died within two years after first becoming ill. Dr. James Curran, spokesman for the CDC, told the *Times* that "no cases have been reported to date outside the homosexual community or in women." In August 1982, acquired immunodeficiency syndrome, AIDS, was named by the CDC. Before then, this terrifying disease was pejo-ratively called GRID—gay-related immune deficiency. AIDS was known, by 1982, to affect not only gay men but also intravenous drug users, hemophiliacs, and certain immigrant communities. Although cases were rarer, women were dying, often more quickly, of AIDS-related illnesses. But the need to research women as sufferers wasn't acknowledged or acted on. As well as being excluded from clinical defi-nitions of AIDS, women were automatically exempted from trials of preventative treatments and medications when the HIV virus was dis-covered in 1983.

Women were not being formally diagnosed, which left them unable to claim insurance and disability benefits. Some hospitals even re-fused to treat them. In 1985, Susan Blumenthal, a leading research sci-entist at the National Institutes of Health, led the workshop "Women and AIDS" to shine a spotlight on medicine's, and society's, ignorance. Blumenthal's work put pressure on the NIH to extend AIDS research to women. Over the next five years, protests and campaigns led by grass-roots groups including ACT UP (the AIDS Coalition to Unleash Power) lobbied the CDC and the NIH to include women and Black, Asian, and other ethnically diverse people, in all HIV/AIDS trials and research. As Blumenthal explained, the "omission of women as a focus of research, treatment and prevention efforts at the beginning of the epidemic re-sulted in the rapid rise in the number of cases of women with HIV/AIDS in America and worldwide."

That year, the US Public Health Service Task Force on Women's Health compiled a report stating that federally funded biomedical re-search must "ensure emphasis on conditions and diseases unique to, or more prevalent in, women of all ages." By examining how women's health problems were overlooked and underserved across the Public Health Service, the task force laid out a "blueprint" for change. The need for research, evaluation, public education, and information dissemina-tion, was unequivocal. The health conditions most affecting women's lives were those about which "little is known or for which appropriate therapies have not been determined." Women suffered from more long-term, chronic diseases than men did. They used medical services more often than men did. They had more need for preventative interventions, medication, and treatments than men did. But their health was being affected, every day, by lack of knowledge—especially about "devastating and debilitating diseases," including gynecological and breast cancers, lupus, thyroid conditions, diabetes, osteoporosis, and mental ill health—inadequate access to services, and a dearth of clinical data and large-scale studies. And all these impediments were magnified for Black and ethnically diverse women, older women, women who were economically disadvantaged, and women who were "physically and mentally disabled."

The absence of research drastically limited "understanding of the status of women's health, women's particular needs, and the services women require." As well as recommending that women were "adequately" represented in trials of drugs they might take, the report stressed how crucial it was for biomedical and medico-sociological studies to include participants of all ethnicities, ages, and social demographics. And it wasn't as if the expertise didn't exist. It was there at federal, state, local, and community levels, and "within women themselves." Data and analysis were, undeniably, urgently needed. But facts and figures alone couldn't shed light on what it meant to live as an unwell woman. Observations about how drugs metabolize wouldn't reveal the impact of gender expectations and sex-role behavior on women's feelings about themselves and their bodies. "Research should be undertaken to better understand those cultural conditions and socialization practices that affect women's health differently from that of men," the report recommended.

The women's health report prompted the NIH, in 1987, to recommend that women be included in all the trials and studies it supported. Two years later, the NIH stated that participant recruitment should always include women and minorities. If research teams failed to be inclusive, they had to have a clear rationale. Change was on the horizon, but there were still plenty of long-established attitudes and assumptions about how illnesses and diseases manifested in women that had to be put right. For decades, heart disease had been regarded as a male disease, primarily affecting men who played and worked too hard. "Sex-exclusive research" had "reinforced the myth" that myocardial infarction, angina, and chronic ischemic heart disease were "uniquely male" afflictions. The generated data about early-warning signs, screening tests including echocardiograms, indicative symptoms, and effective treatments were all based on men as the normative standard.

In the mid-1980s, it was revealed that women were more likely to die from heart diseases than men. Too often, this was because their diseases were misdiagnosed—and even completely overlooked. By 1989, heart diseases were the leading cause of women's deaths in the US and UK. And many were dying because they were not presenting the typical chest and left-arm pains of the male "Hollywood heart attack." Studies have since found that women often have no chest pain at all but rather referred pain in their stomachs, neck, and shoulders. The onset of a heart attack in women is often accompanied by nausea, fatigue, and breathlessness, symptoms that were historically dismissed as emotional and hysterical. Angina is more likely to be written off as "nonspecific chest pain" in women. Chest pain, by the way, along with palpitations, dizziness, and difficulty breathing, were all labeled "hysteric" in the early somatization criteria.

In 1991, Dr. Bernadine Healy, the American cardiologist and first female chair of the NIH, coined the term "Yentl syndrome" to describe how women received adequate medical attention only when their diseases mirrored male models. "Yentl," the heroine of a nineteenth-century short story in which a woman disguises herself as a man so she could study the Talmud, was immortalized in cinemas by Barbra Streisand in 1983. "Being 'just like a man' has historically been a price women have had to pay for equality," wrote Healy. "Being different from men has meant being second-class and less than equal for most of recorded time and throughout most of the world." Heart diseases were just one example of how "Yentl syndrome pervades medicine and medical research." Thanks to the careful thinking and intersectional intelligence of female researchers, policy makers, and health leaders, the world was finally waking up to some harsh truths about medicine's biases. It was time, Healy urged, for the medical community to "respond promptly" whenever it encountered the influence of Yentl syndrome. Although the NIH had loosened the research gender ban, Blumenthal and a group of scientists and advocates revealed in 1990 that the new guidelines had not been properly implemented and applied. The NIH had encouraged researchers to include women, but countless studies failed to analyze results according to gender differences.

Leading the charge for change, Healy launched the Women's Health Initiative (WHI) in 1991 to address the "major causes of death, disability and frailty among middle-aged and older women," including cardiovascular diseases, cancer, and osteoporosis. Only 13 percent of the NIH's budget was dedicated to women's health research. Over the next fifteen years, the WHI enrolled over 150,000 women in clinical trials and observational studies, which would finally show how the long-term use of hormone therapies was contributing to rising rates of breast, colon, and bowel cancers. The NIH changed its policy to "require, rather than recommend" the inclusion of women in funded research in 1991. In 1993, after the NIH Revitalization Act was passed in Congress, the law required all NIH-funded research to include women and minorities. The FDA followed suit, issuing guidelines about gender representation. With Blumenthal appointed deputy assistant secretary for women's health in the US Department of Health and Human Services and Healy at the helm of the WHI, the different-but-equal needs of unwell women were finally gaining the consideration, attention, and funding they desperately needed—and fundamentally deserved.

Back at the beginning of the feminist health movement, the Boston Women's Health Collective addressed how male-dominated medicine objectified women. In her essay in *Our Bodies, Ourselves*, Lucy Candib opposed the way that women, as patients, became "merely the vehicle which brings the disease to the interventionist." Doctors and health professionals need to focus on objective factors to piece together the puzzle of a person's illness. But for women, being objectified carries a dehumanizing and sometimes violating weight. Being reduced to symptoms, signs, and biological clues, Candib said, alienated women even further from their own bodies. Over the past two decades, women at grassroots, community, and governmental levels campaigned for female biology and physiology to be impartially understood. But they also fought for women to be *visible*, to be *seen*, to be treated as human beings and not just as vehicles or instruments. So much about being unwell could not be objectively measured. And so many illnesses and diseases— even ones that were acknowledged and understood—affected women's bodies and minds in ways that medicine couldn't or wouldn't recognize. Attitudes toward women in the early years of HIV/AIDS were object lessons in what happens when medicine comes up against its own ignorance. From the mid-1980s, as the medical community began to address its systemic failings and entrenched biases, a host of biologically baffling new afflictions and conditions—mostly affecting women—started to emerge. And medicine had to grapple with the fact that chronic illnesses, especially in women, were often more subjective than objective, more about feeling than previously defined clinical fact.

In the winter of 1984, a mysterious illness struck residents of Incline Village, an idyllic resort town on the north shore of Lake Tahoe, on the Nevada-California border. Around two hundred of the village's twenty-thousand-strong community developed fevers, swollen glands, sore throats, and aching muscles. But as their flulike symptoms retreated, crushing exhaustion set in—and it lasted for months. The afflicted were mostly white, wealthy women in their thirties and forties who were otherwise fit and healthy. One woman was sleeping for fifteen hours a day and counting; another said she felt like a "Raggedy Ann doll without the stuffing." Soon, many were experiencing other alarming symptoms: muscle weakness and pain, temporary paralysis, memory loss, blackouts, nightmares, and disorientation. By the following summer, the CDC had identified a possible cause. Ninety sufferers tested positive for an antibody to Epstein-Barr, the virus behind mononucleosis, or glandular fever. The press came to town, much to the chagrin of other residents and real-estate agents, who didn't want the resort's well-heeled reputation tarnished by contagion. A young mother with "both the illness and fresh good looks" told TV reporters she was afraid she would be "run out of town with a scarlet EBV" on her chest.

Many doctors doubted the Epstein-Barr verdict. News agencies from ABC to CBN ran stories on the "malaise of the '80s" and "Raggedy Ann syndrome" and "the yuppie plague." Other women with similar symptoms went to their doctors to request the test. Although they all complained of "flu-like illnesses followed by fatigue, persistent pain and neurological disturbances," most were testing negative. Skeptical doctors doubted the illness existed at all, dismissing chronic Epstein-Barr virus syndrome, as it was known, as a "vogue disease" and a "wastebasket diagnosis." But more outbreaks were being reported. In December 1985, it took out half the girls' basketball team at Incline High School. Virologists and immunologists across the US scrambled to figure out the real cause of this puzzling epidemic. Women were falling ill in the thousands with symptoms that were neither psychosomatic nor hypochondriac. But the press had already made its diagnosis. Chronic Epstein-Barr was caused by being well-off, bored, and almost certainly female. Here began the history of one of the most controversial and contested modern "women's" illnesses: myalgic encephalomyelitis, or chronic fatigue syndrome (ME/CFS).

Since the 1930s, outbreaks of suspiciously similar illnesses in groups of women had been recorded in the US, the UK, and Europe. The most common symptoms were persistent, relapsing fatigue, pain, and muscle weakness. Many sufferers also experienced symptoms of the more "nervous" variety: insomnia, emotional upsets, and sensory dysfunctions as well as cystitis and menstrual "derangements." In 1970, two physicians from the Department of Psychological Medicine at London's Middlesex Hospital reviewed fifteen outbreaks of a condition called benign myalgic encephalomyelitis recorded since 1934. Many occurred among female nurses treating infectious diseases including forms of polio. These women were exposed to infections before their own illnesses took hold. But no biological or viral evidence could be found. The psychologists concluded that the high instance among women and the lack of any identifiable cause meant these outbreaks were episodes of mass hysteria. They proposed that similar cases should be called myalgia nervosa—which basically means "emotional pain." And they chose this term specifically for its analogy with anorexia nervosa, the eating disorder and serious mental health condition that was associated, infuriatingly, with hysteria, hypochondria, and psychological delusions during the eighteenth and nineteenth centuries.

By the late 1980s, unexplained illnesses were rising, alarmingly, across the Western world in women between the ages of twenty and forty. By 1987, a condition that caused muscle tenderness, pain, and fatigue—mostly in women—was recognized by the American Medical Association. By 1990, this condition had a clinical criterion, laid down by the American College of Rheumatology, and an official name: fibromyalgia. To be diagnosed, a patient had to have tenderness in at least eleven of eighteen parts of her body when a doctor applied pressure. Many medical professionals, especially in the NHS, had a hard time accepting fibromyalgia was real. Unlike ME/CFS, there was no viral suspicion floating around it. But as with ME/CFS, fibromyalgia was quickly characterized as having no "organic etiology." The only clinical evidence was in a patient's reactions to, and descriptions of, pain. And when a cause for a woman's pain couldn't be identified in a lab or on a screen, then inevitably it was dismissed as emotional or pathologized as psychogenic.

In 1992, fibromyalgia and ME/CFS were lumped together in "affective spectrum disorder," a diagnostic category of overlapping physical and psychological conditions. This implied that debilitating pain and fatigue were primarily caused by mental ill-health conditions—including anxiety, depression, social phobia, and premenstrual dysphoria—that were decidedly feminized. Affective spectrum disorder recognized that physical symptoms exacerbated by the mind were very real for the sufferer. But undefined illnesses nevertheless invoked gendered stigma. A study of women treated for chronic fatigue at Boston's Brigham and Women's Hospital in 1992 showed that 90 percent had had their symptoms delegitimized by doctors. As one participant explained, doctors "try a whole bunch of things . . . and when everything fails, they just think you're nuts . . . They would say things like 'You can't be experiencing what you are experiencing. You need to see a psychologist. You're not as sick as you think you are.'" Many were disbelieved and patronized because "they 'don't look sick,'" while others had their symptoms trivialized as the discomforts of everyday life. After having an X-ray that showed "nothing wrong," one woman was pushed into taking antidepressants by her neurologist because "a lot of women . . . have a lot of trouble with depression that could cause other symptoms." Most of the women surveyed internalized these belittling, dismissive attitudes and began either to blame themselves or to believe that their illnesses must be imaginary. "I'd look in the mirror and think 'Are you crazy?' . . . Maybe it's all in your head."

"Medicine's focus on objective factors and its cultural stereotypes of women combine insidiously, leaving women at greater risk for inadequate pain relief and continued suffering," wrote Diane Hoffmann and Anita Tarzian, in their pathbreaking 2001 study "The Girl Who Cried Pain." Over the last decades, medicine's systemic prejudices against female pain had been spotlighted by the rise in unexplained, undefined, contested illnesses that all had one thing in common: pain. The galvanic energies of the feminist health movement had given voice to women's experiences of being doubted and distrusted. The frustratingly frequent response to women whose illnesses didn't conform to objective factors wasn't "I don't know," but "your suffering isn't real." But women were suffering in all-too-real ways that exceeded objective medical knowledge. By the time Hoffmann and Tarzian's study, subtitled "A Bias Against Women in the Treatment of Pain," was published, diagnoses of fibromyalgia and ME/CFS had risen to around thirty-five and fifteen, respectively, in every one hundred thousand patients in the UK. In the US, an estimated 2 to 5 percent of the population had fibromyalgia, and around 2.5 million had ME/CFS. Between 75 to 90 percent of fibromyalgia sufferers were women, and four times more women than men had ME/CFS.

Medical and cultural understandings of both these diseases have improved over the last decades. And this is thanks in part to voices like those of Jennifer Brea, the American filmmaker and activist who documented her illness experience in her award-winning film *Unrest* and spoke out about difficult-to-diagnose conditions in her popular 2017 TED Talk. And after revealing the pain of her recently diagnosed condition in her 2017 documentary *Five Foot Two*, Lady Gaga has become an awareness-raising advocate for the visibility and recognition of fibromyalgia. As both Brea and Gaga have shown, both diseases continue to be mired by misunderstanding, prejudice, and doubt. The legitimacy of ME/CFS and fibromyalgia is still contested by many members of the medical community. And those seeking diagnoses continue to be haunted by the hysterical perception that the only place women's pain and fatigue really exists is in their minds.

Hoffmann and Tarzian, who studied reports and data gathered since the 1970s, found that while women report chronic pain more frequently and intensely than men, their pain is statistically more likely to be dismissed as emotional or psychological. "The Girl Who Cried Pain" also showed how women's articulation of pain—through verbal and bodily languages, speech and gestures—affected how their pain was interpreted. If a woman was perceived as overly verbose or focusing too much on how her pain affected her personal life, then she was more likely to be suspected of exaggerating. For centuries, women who talked too much about their pain had been stigmatized as fusspots, time wasters, or attention seekers. Back in the nineteenth century, hysteria, neurosis, and nervous weakness were, indeed, wastebasket diagnoses for women whose illnesses couldn't be explained by any cause other than their gender. Surely medicine understood, by the twenty-first century, that diagnoses like these were discredited because they were fundamentally social and cultural—and worryingly divorced from science. And *surely* medicine must have learned, by then, that the specter of misdiagnosis and misconception haunted the clinical histories of all kinds of chronic conditions?

So many "women's" illnesses and diseases had been coaxed out from under the stone of hysteria by the biomedical advances of the last century. But even though many of these conditions have recognized diagnostic criteria, lists of clinical signs, and batteries of biological tests, women still endure arduous, humiliating struggles to be taken seriously. Diseases that historically were accused of being hysterical, including endometriosis, rheumatoid arthritis, multiple sclerosis, thyroid diseases including Graves', and ulcerative colitis, remain difficult to diagnose, complicated to treat, and—so far—impossible to cure. Medical bias against women means their pain, their hurt, is routinely invalidated— not only in diagnostic encounters but also during treatment. One of the most prevalent examples is the radical mastectomy, developed and perfected in the 1890s, which remained the standard surgical treatment for breast cancer for decades. Although its invention dramatically reduced cancer recurrence rates, this mutilating surgery, which removed the entire breast, chest-wall muscles, and lymph nodes in the armpits, could be unbelievably debilitating for survivors. Barely any attention was paid to the devastating ways such invasive surgery could affect women—psychologically as well as physically. It wasn't until more effective and less traumatic surgical interventions, which preserved chest muscles and nipples, were introduced in the early 1970s that women's quality of life—not just their survival—became a medical concern. And the last frontier in breast reconstruction, sensation, is still being advocated for by patient communities.

Medical gender bias, ingrained over centuries of misbelief, misconception, speculation, and assumption, has also contributed directly to the lack of knowledge about how to care for, treat, and support women with diseases that to this day mystify medicine. But there is nothing unexplained or uncertain about the suffering that millions of women across the world endure every day. And as medicine searches for answers, our diseases continue to flood our cells, grip our organs, attack our joints, and agitate our pain—and our numbers are rising. Around 4 percent of the world's population has an autoimmune disease, and nearly 80 percent of those are women. In 2010, approximately five million people worldwide were suffering from a form of lupus, one of the five most common autoimmune diseases. Most had systemic lupus erythematosus, and 90 percent were women. And I was one of them.

18

AUTOIMMUNE

In 2002, I started getting pains in my legs. Many mornings, I woke up with pain gripping me from hip to ankle. This went on for months. Sometimes, in the evenings, my ankles would swell up so much I couldn't walk. I missed days of work. I noted the pain in my diary, its intensity, its frequency, its quality. On a visit to my family GP, he felt around my blown-up ankles and feet and wondered aloud, "Mmm, I'm guessing you like a drink. This might be gout?" Gout is one of those old-timey diseases caused by too much cheese and booze. I didn't have gout. "Might I ask if an attractive young woman such as yourself might be pregnant?" I wasn't pregnant. Every morning I thumbed a tiny white pill out of a calendar packet and swallowed it down with the dregs of my tea. "I can see nothing wrong with you," he said, his eyes on the clock. "It's probably just your hormones."

The pain didn't let up. I went to homeopaths, osteopaths, physio-therapists. I slept with bandages wrapped tightly around my feet. I spent chunks of my temp-job wages at the health-food shop on arnica cream and vitamin complexes and sickly tinctures. Nothing helped. The fear of being in constant pain was so visceral that I felt it everywhere: in my head, in my throat, deep in my belly. I associated being away from home with being out of control. On the tube to work one morning, my vision blurred and everything began to spin. My pulse thudded deliri-ously in my temples. At Canary Wharf station, I begged a guard to let me use the private bathroom. That summer was the hottest on record in

London, and he was sure I was just overheated. I staggered into the morning sun, thrumming with adrenaline, and sat on a bench as my ragged breathing slowed and my heart rate stabilized. For the rest of that summer I was scared every day.

In the years that followed, I experienced pain, often first thing in the morning or last thing at night, but I pushed it aside. The doctors had told me nothing was wrong. In 2006, I married my husband in a museum of medieval musical instruments in the beautiful Wealden countryside. By October, I was pregnant. Our baby boy was born the following summer. He came into the world with huge brown eyes, a tiny tree-frog body, and a strange red rash on his head and face. "It's probably eczema," my health visitor told me, handing me a prescription for emollient cream and body wash. The rash persisted for months, then gradually disappeared. I forgot all about it.

When our son was sixteen months old, I was pregnant again. At twenty weeks, we went to the hospital for a routine sonogram. Our son was excited—he wanted a "brubba." Our new baby boy was perfect: a floating shadow made of sound and light. Suddenly, the sonographer turned the screen away. A rush of adrenaline flooded my body. "Is he OK?" I asked. "It's probably completely fine," she said, feigning a smile, "but we need to take another look and maybe talk to someone upstairs, OK? Nothing to worry about." Our baby was developing perfectly in every way except that his heart was beating far too slowly. I would be referred for another ultrasound, on the chambers and valves of his heart, with a specialist consultant at St. Thomas' Hospital in London.

Two weeks later, after lying in silence in the dark while one of the country's leading experts in fetal cardiac medicine pressed a Doppler onto my belly and delved into my baby's heart, I was told that he was suffering from a rare condition called congenital heart block. "Some kind of damage has occurred to the AV node, the part of the heart that controls electrical conduction," the consultant explained. "It's a bit like a signal box. The impulses are blocked, so the atria and ventricle are out of sync. This is causing his heart to slow down. It might right itself, but we can't be sure. We will monitor you every week, and if it doesn't improve, he will have to be born here. It's possible he might have to have surgery to install a pacemaker." I asked about the cause. "It might be hereditary, or it might be completely random," she said. "But tell me, have you ever had any problems with your eyes?" It seemed like a strange question; I wear glasses, but I knew that wasn't what she meant. She explained that if a mother has an underlying health condition, her blood might contain something that impacts the way their baby's heart develops. I told her no, there was nothing like that, nothing I could think of in my family either. I didn't think to mention my intermittent pain. I'd been told it didn't matter. "Just to be sure, we'll take some blood," she said. "When you come back next week, we'll have the results."

The consultant asked about my eyes because she wondered if I had Sjögren's syndrome, a disease where autoantibodies attack moisture-producing glands. Sjögren's is ten times more common in women than in men, and it shares many signs and symptoms with lupus. One of those is an antibody called anti-Ro, named in 1975 after the woman it was first found in, Mrs. Robair. She'd experienced years of nameless pain, like I had. Ten years later, anti-Ro was found in another woman, a twenty-eight-year-old who had suffered miscarriages and unexplained joint pain and rashes since she was a teenager. She had a son, aged two, who survived congenital heart block. Her blood tested positive for anti-Ro, just as mine did twenty-three years later, in a laboratory in South London. Today, 95 percent of congenital heart block cases occur in mothers with anti-Ro.

A week later, I returned to the clinic for a follow-up. My baby still had heart block. Anti-Ro had snuck across my placenta and bound to the cells of his developing heart, causing inflammation and slowing the heart muscle down. I could either hope the block went away on its own—which was unlikely, and potentially fatal—or take dexamethasone, a powerful steroid that would suppress my immune system. I decided to take it. I signed a form stating that I understood the risks this posed to my baby. Growth restriction. Adrenal damage. Preterm labor. Spontaneous abortion. Death. My notes from that appointment read, *She is stoical about the diagnosis of congenital heart block and has decided to go ahead with the steroids as advised.*

About four weeks before my due date, scans showed that my baby's heart was shifting into a more regular rhythm. The heart block was still there, but his pulse was gaining pace—87 beats per minute. Each week the interval lessened—102 beats per minute. Two weeks before he was due, the interval was barely detectable—127 beats per minute. "If I'd examined you for the first time now," the consultant said at our last appointment, "I wouldn't have noticed the heart block. Good luck to you." The steroids had worked.

Hal was born at home after a lightning-fast labor. For a moment after I pushed him into life, he didn't breathe. Dread swelled in my throat; seconds passed like centuries. At last he cried, and his skin got pink. The paramedics strapped me into a gurney, covered me with a blanket, and placed Hal in my arms. They took us away, blue lights flashing. When we arrived at the hospital, the midwife took Hal from my arms as I was wheeled to the operating theater. The speed and force of his birth had torn right through me, past my perineum. As the anesthesiologist administered the spinal block, the epidural, I held my breath. My legs were hoisted into stirrups. I gazed out the window at the waves crashing against the seawall. When the surgeon was done, they said, "Don't worry. I've sewn you up nice and tight." They hadn't asked if I wanted that extra stitch. That stitch mythologized in furtive waiting-room handshakes between husbands and obstetricians in the 1950s. That "husband stitch" sewn into me.

We stayed in the hospital for ten days. Hal needed antibiotics against a bacterial infection called Group B streptococcus that showed up in my blood tests early in pregnancy. Nobody mentioned the heart block or the weird antibody. My consultant hadn't attached the antibody to any disease in me. She was concerned with my baby's health, not mine. For nine months, my immune system was focused on my baby. What I didn't know, and none of my doctors knew, was that anti-Ro was crawling toward my own heart. But I'd fallen between the medical cracks, and no one thought to notice.

When the ache first crept into my back, between my shoulder blades, it was subtle enough to ignore. After a week it got worse, but I could tolerate it, so I didn't think it was worth mentioning. One night, pain woke me from sleep, clear and sharp like a stab. My heart was beating hard and fast, my breath was forced and shallow. I tried to walk to the bathroom, but my legs wouldn't let me. When I lay down, the pain was overwhelming. I bolstered pillows against the headboard and tried to calm my pulse. This is wrong, I thought. This is probably when you call an ambulance. But I didn't know how to form the words: *My body is breaking. It's broken.*

The next morning, after fitful sleep, I went to see my GP. He clipped a pulse monitor onto my finger, then told me to go immediately to the emergency room. I couldn't: I needed to feed my baby; I needed to be at home. "You must," he said. "This is an emergency." The triage nurse found me a bed and pulled the curtains round. She stuck electrodes on my chest and back and hooked me up to a monitor. I blew into a tube and held out my arm so that she could take samples of my blood. I listened to the whir of the monitor translate the contractions of my heart into lines and squiggles. I waited.

Hours passed before they wheeled me to the pit, where they put people who are too sick to leave but too well to stay. It's also where you go when your symptoms are a mystery. Through the night, I endured more blood work, an MRI scan, chest X-rays. My gown didn't do up properly, and after hours away from my baby, it was soaked with breast milk. I begged anyone who came near me for a breast pump. "I can't be here; I have a nine-week-old. He needs me. I have to feed him." Around 3:00 a.m. two doctors arrived, wheeling an ancient-looking computer on a trolley. They needed to look at my heart. I lay on my side and a female doctor moved a Doppler across my back and under my left arm. The membrane surrounding my heart, the pericardium, was inflamed. The fluid around it, which the heart needs to function properly, was engulfing my pericardial cavity. My heart was drowning. At 9:00 a.m. a young male doctor came to see me. I asked how long I'd have to stay. "You can go home this morning," he said wearily. "Ibuprofen, four times a day, should reduce the inflammation. Rest, and go see your GP if the symptoms don't improve." My diagnosis was acute pericardial effusion, increased fluid around the heart. On my discharge notes, the doctor wrote, *Her anxiety about feeding her baby outweighs her anxiety about her own health.*

I was still weak and in pain. I couldn't walk or breathe properly. My skin was gray, my ribs protruded beneath my skin. Back home, cosseted in blankets, I held my baby tight. I couldn't feed him because of the contrast medium they'd injected so that my organs would glow on the MRI. I pumped chemical-spoiled milk from my breasts and cried as I poured it down the sink. Two days later, I was rushed back to hospital with a resting heart rate of 198 beats per minute. I was wheeled straight to a bed and seen by a female doctor, a specialist in pregnancy-related heart conditions. "I know it's shit," she said, as I wept on her, "but your baby needs you healthy. You're no use to him dead, are you?"

This time, the doctors knew what was happening in my body, but what they couldn't explain was why. I was given a tentative diagnosis of peripartum cardiomyopathy (PPCM), a rare form of heart disease that affects only one in five thousand to ten thousand women up to six months after giving birth. On my chart, a doctor wrote, *PPCM—Idiopathic*. Idiopathic is a classification given to diseases of unknown cause. From the ancient Greek, it translates as "one's own suffering." In the late 1970s, an autoimmune reaction was identified as a trigger for idiopathic heart disease after pregnancy. One of my doctors discovered clues in my blood. He'd tested for an autoantibody called rheumatoid factor, first discovered in 1949, by a female biologist named Elizabeth Price, who had rheumatoid arthritis. My whole body, not just my heart, was inflamed. The doctor ordered more blood tests. I carried other autoantibodies too, called antinuclear antibodies, which were damaging the nuclei of my cells.

Rudolf Virchow was one of the first physicians to observe heart inflammation during autopsies on women who had died in the postpartum months. Some speculated that the stresses of carrying and delivering children were the cause; others believed that pregnancy exacerbated underlying heart conditions. In 1907, the British obstetric physician G. F. Blacker argued that women with such complaints should be banned from marrying, bearing children, and nursing them. PPCM wasn't documented until 1937, when a study published in the *New Orleans Medical and Surgical Journal* described seven patients with severe heart failure, four of whom died. A follow-up study in 1938 presented cases of eighty women with pregnancy-related heart dysfunction. Nearly all of them were of African heritage.

The term "toxic postpartum heart disease" was used until 1971, when the term PPCM was first coined and a diagnostic criterion was laid down. In the earliest clinical paper, cardiologists noted that much of the existing literature described PPCM in Black women. Since then, cases have appeared all over the world, but especially in Nigeria, Jamaica, and Johannesburg. The prevalence of PPCM in African and in Black women was clearly not just because those cases emanated "from hospitals dealing with predominantly black populations." Today, PPCM is known to affect Black women disproportionally. They suffer more severe symptoms, have longer recovery times, and have a much higher mortality rate than white women. Medicine still does not understand why this is. It might be a combination of genetic and socioeconomic factors or a question of access to medical care. Not enough research has been dedicated to finding out.

The doctor passed my notes to a consultant rheumatologist. He strode into my room one evening and announced, "We think you have systemic lupus erythematosus. Near as damn it." After I'd suffered for seven years with flares of pain, swelling, and other symptoms that had been overlooked, ignored, and dismissed, what had been happening in my body now had a name. The doctors explained that it was very likely I'd had lupus for a long time and that pregnancy had probably triggered this severe flare. He told me that the estrogen flooding back through my blood after my baby was born might have set it off. He said that Hal's heart block was a form of neonatal lupus, in which unborn babies are affected by their mothers' autoantibodies. Hal was unlucky; most babies born to lupus mothers just get benign rashes. That was what my first baby had. If only I had known. I was experiencing a serious flare caused by my antibodies attacking my tissues. By treating the inflammation and suppressing my immune system, my symptoms would gradually retreat, and my disease, hopefully, would go into remission. "After this, you might be well for years," he said. "But lupus is unpredictable; there's no way to know for sure. There's no cure, but we can manage the symptoms. We'll have to keep a close eye on you from now on."

I knew nothing about this disease called lupus, this disease that had made me a medical subject, a patient to be scrutinized and surveilled. I soon learned that most diagnoses are made in women between the ages of eighteen and forty-five, and predominantly more Black, Asian, and ethnically diverse women are affected. The most common factor in the occurrence of lupus is being female. Despite years of research, the reasons are still not known. Lupus manifests completely differently from sufferer to sufferer. It begins with vague symptoms, like pain and tiredness, that are often overlooked as nothing serious. Those symptoms can wax and wane unpredictably. And like many autoimmune diseases, a diagnosis can be very difficult to obtain. In the UK, the average length of time between first reporting symptoms and receiving a diagnosis is three years. In the US, it is 4.6 years. In one sense, I had been lucky. My baby's heart condition hastened my diagnosis. Without it, I might have still been waiting, after seven years and counting, for an explanation of my nameless pain.

My lupus diagnosis was devastating, but it was also a relief. I had experienced the frustration and humiliation of having my symptoms dismissed since my early twenties. Countless times I tried to explain my persistent pain and swollen joints to doctors, only to have them written off as hormonal, psychological, and even a possible pregnancy. I'd been on the receiving end of withering glances, eye rolls, smirks, and heavy sighs. I was young and full of feelings. I started to believe I must have been making it up, that the pain was all in my mind. Guilt and shame gnawed at me until I didn't trust my body anymore.

The realization that lupus had lurked undetected inside me for years was revelatory. Over the last ten years, I have stitched the history of my body, and my life, back together with this new thread of knowledge. I understand now that who I have become is indelibly intertwined with my disease. This hidden disease had shaped my relationship to my body and, with it, the way I exist as a woman in the world. But as I have learned to live as an unwell woman, I have also realized that my history is a shared history. Written into the history of my disease are the histories of women whose suffering led to the formation of the medical knowledge that saved my life. The medical science that helped me heal would not exist without those women who, for centuries, struggled to have their pain recognized, valued, legitimized. The history of medicine is the history of unwell women, of their bodies, minds, and lives. I owe them everything.

BELIEVE US

Medicine saved my life. The medication I take every day, and have taken for ten years, tempers my autoantibodies, but it will never completely disarm my immune system. I have been in the hospital many times over the last ten years: for suspected blood clots, for pneumonia when antibodies flooded my lungs, for X-rays and MRIs and blood tests and checkups. Luckily, serious flares have been rare, but my disease is always there, agitating my joints, wearing me out mentally and physically. I can't bear bright lights, and if I party or work too hard, my body makes me pay. Sometimes when I wash my hair, fistfuls of strands come away. There are days when my thoughts cloud and I can't remember anything. I've been sternly advised to never get pregnant again.

I visit the lupus clinic at Guy's Hospital in London every six months. I can call them whenever I need to. My diagnosis is all over my notes. But even so, my experience has shown me that if you are a woman, especially one who has a disease medicine doesn't fully understand and requires you to go to the GP often, you will encounter the kinds of gender biases that have been ingrained in medical culture and practice for centuries. I've been told I look too well to be ill. I've been told my symptoms have nothing to do with lupus and are probably to do with stress. I've been laughed at by harried, time-poor emergency doctors when I reel off my latest inflammation results and immune blood work markers. I've had flares dismissed as chest infections and had depression provoked by my illness put down to "not breathing deeply enough." I've argued with GPs about the necessity of my medicine. I've been sent away from doctors' offices in tears and told to "see how you get on." Like so many women who live every day with unpredictable, inexplicable symptoms, I find it's impossible to separate the issue of my gender from the sense that my disease is not perceived as legitimate.

I was diagnosed with lupus at the beginning of the third wave of feminist health activism. Over the last ten years I have read countless stories by women with diseases like mine: chronic, incurable diseases that medicine doesn't understand, finds difficult to diagnose, and all too frequently dismisses. Unwell women are exposing the extent to which medical mystification permeates the quality of our care and treatment, and how the degree of impact depends on our gender, skin color, and socioeconomic status. Unwell women are building a knowledge base where medicine has failed to; they are bringing to light the experiences, feelings, and realities lived every day that medicine can't, or won't, accommodate.

Illness is so much more than the name of a disease, a list of blood test results and biomarkers, or a prescription torn from a pad. It's the human condition to suffer at some stage. Illness always bleeds beyond the borders of doctors' appointments, hospital visits, courses of treatment, medication doses, diagnostic tests, clinical observations, and data. Illness is stitched into our bodies and our lives in ways that simply can't be measured in a laboratory or read from a screen. Our symptoms are the reality of our illnesses. We mystify medicine because medicine isn't looking for answers in the right places. We mystify medicine because medicine isn't paying the right kind of attention. We mystify medicine because medicine needs unassailable facts. I know so many women who have been told that their symptoms are feigned, imagined, or exaggerated. A gulf opens up between a woman's lived experience of her illness and medicine's comprehension of her disease, between her intimate knowledge of her own body and medicine's requirement of objective proof. But we can't do that work ourselves: believing and responding to individual testimony is the only way to start.

If medicine is to solve our medical mysteries, it needs, urgently, to deliver policies, support research, and increase funding on local, national, and global scales. And the tide is beginning to turn. Since 2010, the World Health Organization has been committed to changing international policy related to the "global epidemic" of "silent killers," which are estimated to be killing eighteen million women every year. For women outside the Western world, socioeconomic, cultural, and geographical barriers to even basic health care and medical treatment are thought to be contributing directly to entrenched poverty and gender inequality. The WHO notes that women have very different health-care needs than men do and that for too long research has not accommodated the different ways that women are affected by chronic, noncommunicable diseases. A 2014 report in the journal *Global Health Action* suggested that neglect—in medical research and funding—is directly responsible for the epidemic of delayed diagnosis, severe disease progression, and premature death in women all over the globe.

Now, more than ever, we need medicine to face up to its history. Medicine has inherited a troubling legacy of gaps and omissions that it is trying to redress. But gender bias in medicine is not only scientific or biomedical. It is cultural, it is social, it is political. Whether medicine likes to admit it or not, centuries-old ideas about how women's pain is emotional rather than physiological are being internalized by doctors today in their responses to women self-reporting their symptoms. Knowledge about *why* a person's gender impacts the perceived legibility of their illness is essential if the culture is to be changed. By learning how implicit and explicit bias is at play in the doctor's office and emergency room, unwell women can begin to advocate for their own health, question their care, and break down the barriers of authority that have historically silenced and undermined them. And now, more than ever, the legacy of unwell women who have bravely testified to medicine's systemic failings resounds powerfully.

Through the work of feminist trailblazers like Charlotte Perkins Gilman and pathbreaking writers and philosophers including Audre Lorde, Susan Sontag, and Anne Boyer, chronic ill-health experiences emerge as a source of extraordinary strength, insight, creativity, and activism. Serena Williams, who courageously shared her experience of suffering a life-threatening pulmonary embolism after giving birth to her daughter by cesarean section in 2017, shone a light on the ways that systemic racism still impacts the care and treatment of Black women during childbirth. The activist, author, and actor Gabrielle Union brought attention to the frequently misdiagnosed and poorly understood condition uterine adenomyosis, a rare form of endometriosis, when she spoke out about her long battle with miscarriage and infertility in 2017. The actor Tia Mowry, diagnosed with endometriosis when she was thirty, is now a leading campaigner for endo awareness who spotlights the diagnostic challenges and disease differences experienced by Black women. When the actor Selma Blair attended an Oscar after-party in 2019, her beautiful gown accessorized with a patent-leather walking cane, she opened up about finally being diagnosed with multiple sclerosis after enduring undiagnosed symptoms for seven years. After revealing that she had been diagnosed with lupus in 2015 and undergoing a kidney transplant in 2017, actor Selena Gomez has raised consciousness around the physical and mental health challenges of living with this complex, incurable disease. And when the singer-songwriter FKA twigs wrote a letter to her fans in 2017 about her ordeal of undergoing laparoscopic surgery to remove six uterine fibroids, she told fellow sufferers of this painful and still unexplained condition to remember "that you are amazing warriors and that you are not alone."

Thanks to the activism of celebrities, writers, artists, filmmakers, bloggers, and journalists, the cultural geography of women's chronic ill health is shifting. As more women use their platforms and influence to speak up about the realities of chronic ill health, unwell women are being empowered to find their voices. To be an unwell woman today is to fight against ingrained injustices against women's bodies, minds, and lives; but we no longer have to live in silence and shame. Empowering unwell women to advocate for themselves is crucial, but we also need change to be facilitated within the medical establishment itself. Although there is so much work to be done, meaningful strides, thankfully, are being made.

Since I was diagnosed with lupus, biomedical research projects all over the world have been advancing new theories about the prevalence of chronic, unexplained diseases in women. As autoimmune diseases increase, and medicine still can't explain why, stem-cell researchers have been working on ways to regenerate immunity so that a person's immune system relearns not to attack its own cells. Endocrinologists have recently identified that estrogen stimulates autoimmunity, and geneticists have found that a gene expressed on the X chromosome, of which most biological females have two, influences the production of autoantibodies. Tests on mice have also showed that estrogen triggers immune responses against females' own tissues, whereas testosterone works protectively. A blood test to diagnose endometriosis is being developed, and researchers are addressing the need for reliable, noninvasive biological marker tests. In 2011, in the US, a team of eighty researchers gathered to discuss the possible causes, best diagnostic methods, and ideal treatments for vulvodynia, with all agreeing that the disease remains a mystery because it has been historically stigmatized and underresearched. Recent studies into vaginismus have shown how medicine has always focused solely on the way it impedes penetrative sex, and that women with the condition need multidisciplinary care from gynecologists, physical therapists, and psychologists.

Unwell women need medicine to understand what it means to negotiate an establishment that we so urgently depend on, and which can be so hostile and challenging to us. Our mysterious diseases are acknowledged as difficult to diagnose, manage, and treat. But the truth about our illnesses is in our own bodies. Medicine has to let us translate the languages they are trying to speak. For centuries, our bodies have been demonized and demeaned until we feared them, felt shame because of them, were humiliated by them. Medicine has historically pathologized what it means to be a woman, and what it is to live in a female body, to such a degree that being unwell has been normalized in society and culture, while a woman's rights over her own body remain contested even today. But over the centuries of medicine's long history, women—as doctors, researchers, activists, rebels, campaigners, and, most of all, patients—have continuously challenged the medical orthodoxy that has insidiously controlled our lives. Medicine's history has always been, and is still being, rewritten by women's resistance, strength, intelligence, and incredible courage. To echo Jan McKenley's words, feminism has given us our bodies back. We need medicine to understand how hard it has been for us to get to a place where we are able to speak up about how it feels and where it hurts. We are the most reliable narrators of what is happening in our own bodies. The lives of unwell women depend on medicine learning to listen. To paraphrase the great Maya Angelou, when a woman tells you she is in pain, believe her the first time.

ACKNOWLEDGMENTS

I owe thanks to many people without whose efforts and care this book would not exist. First and foremost, my wonderful agent, Emma Finn, for sharing and inspiring my vision from the very beginning. I will always be grateful for your intelligence, insight, and unwavering support. Thank you to Kate Burton, and everyone at C&W Agency, for working so hard to bring this book into the world, and for your warmth and encouragement. I am incredibly grateful to Amelia Atlas at ICM for finding the perfect home for this book in the US.

To my editors, Maya Ziv and Maddy Price (UK). Thank you for everything you have done, individually and as a team, to shape this book so beautifully. It has been an honor to bring *Unwell Women* to life through your expert eyes. Thank you for believing in me, for propelling me on, for challenging and supporting me. Huge thanks to Emily Canders, Natalie Church, Hannah Feeney, Claire Sullivan, and everyone at Dutton for your tireless efforts behind the scenes. Thank you, Maureen Klier, for such elegant and meticulous copyediting.

I am immeasurably grateful to my loved ones, family, and friends for providing me with the strength and space to write this book. Special thanks to Cecilia Aldarondo for sharing the moment, for the spa and karaoke cure, for knowing when to put it in the oven; Kate Bayman, my good witch, for always being there; Thea Downie, comrade and confidant, you make joy my heart. And to my oldest and best, Dorothy Lehane, deepest thanks and love. Without you I wouldn't have found meaning in being unwell. Thank you to Matt for the gift of time to think and write, and to my children, Oscar and Hallam, who amaze me every day. You three are my home.

I am indebted to the generations of historians, theorists, researchers, and activists who have mined the rich history of women, medicine, and medical culture before me. Thank you for enabling me to contribute to, and continue, this crucial conversation. A few months after I began writing this book, the COVID-19 pandemic made it impossible for me to do the physical research I had planned. But thanks to the skill and dedication of digital archivists and librarians, I have been able to access a wealth of historical and contemporary source material during lockdown. Particular thanks to the staff at the library of the Wellcome Collection, London, for making thousands of years of medical and health history freely available to members for remote use.

Finally, thank you to all the unwell women throughout history, who have made history. It has been such a privilege to share your stories and experiences. I am in awe of your suffering, courage, and resilience. To the community of unwell women journeying through ill health today, solidarity always.

SELECTED BIBLIOGRAPHY
AND FURTHER READING

A NOTE ON SOURCE MATERIAL

In this bibliography, I have included a selection of modern and contemporary books on medical culture, the social history of women, and feminist writings on health, bodies, and medicine. Articles, essays, clinical papers, and online sources are referenced in the endnotes. The majority of my historical sources, especially up to the early twentieth century, were accessed through the digital library of the Wellcome Collection in London, one of the world's major resources for medical history and science. Original material related to women's suffrage in the UK was sourced from the Women's Rights Collection of the London School of Economics' digital library. Resources on Margaret Sanger were found through the Margaret Sanger Papers' Project, hosted by the Division of Libraries at New York University and formed by Dr. Esther Katz in 1985. Other historical texts and books have been sourced through digitized and open-access archives, including the Internet Archive, Project Gutenberg, and Hathi Trust. Many clinical papers have been accessed through PubMed, and essays on historical aspects of medicine and society through JSTOR, the digital library of academic and scholarly journals, which extended its free access during the COVID-19 pandemic. I am incredibly grateful to all the organizations, publications, archivists, librarians, volunteers, and historians who have aided my research.

Appignanesi, Lisa. *Mad, Bad, and Sad: A History of Women and the Mind Doctors from 1800 to the Present.* London: Virago, 2008.
Bliss, Eula. *On Immunity: An Inoculation.* London: Fitzcarraldo Editions, 2015.
Bourke, Joanna. *The Story of Pain: From Prayer to Painkillers.* Oxford: Oxford University Press, 2014.
Boyer, Anne. *The Undying.* New York: Farrar, Straus and Giroux, 2019.
Bryan, Beverley, Stella Dadzie, and Suzanne Scafe. *Heart of the Race: Black Women's Lives in Britain.* 2nd ed. London: Verso, 2018.
Chen, Constance M. *"The Sex Side of Life": Mary Ware Dennett's Pioneering Battle for Birth Control and Sex Education.* New York: New Press, 1996.
Cooper Owens, Deirdre. *Medical Bondage: Race, Gender, and the Origins of American Gynecology.* Athens: University of Georgia Press, 2017.

Criado-Perez, Caroline. *Invisible Women: Exposing Data Bias in a World Designed for Men*. London: Vintage, 2019.

Dean-Jones, Lesley Ann. *Women's Bodies in Classical Greek Science*. Oxford: Clarendon Press, 2010.

Dionne, Evette. *Lifting as We Climb: Black Women's Battle for the Ballot Box*. New York: Viking, 2020.

Dudley-Shotwell, Hannah. *Revolutionizing Women's Healthcare: The Feminist Self-Help Movement in America*. New Brunswick, NJ: Rutgers University Press, 2020.

Ehrenreich, Barbara, and Deirdre English. *Witches, Midwives, and Nurses: A History of Women Healers*. 2nd ed. New York: Feminist Press, 2010.

Federici, Silvia. *Caliban and the Witch: Women, the Body, and Primitive Accumulation*. Brooklyn: Autonomedia, 2004.

———. *Witches, Witch-Hunting and Women*. PM Press, 2018.

Fine, Cordelia. *Testosterone Rex: Unmaking the Myths of Our Gendered Minds*. London: Icon Books, 2017.

Frampton, Sally. *Belly Rippers: Surgical Innovation and the Ovariotomy Controversy*. London: Palgrave Macmillan, 2019.

Friedan, Betty. *The Feminine Mystique*. London: Penguin, 1965.

Green, Monica, ed. and trans. *The Trotula: An English Translation of the Medieval Compendium of Women's Medicine*. Philadelphia: University of Pennsylvania Press, 2002.

Hill, Sarah E. *How the Pill Changes Everything: Your Brain on Birth Control*. New York: Avery, 2019.

hooks, bell. *Feminist Theory: From Margin to Center*. 2nd edition. London: Pluto Press, 2000.

Houck, Judith A. *Hot and Bothered: Women, Medicine, and the Menopause in Modern America*. Cambridge, MA: Harvard University Press, 2006.

Hustvedt, Ari. *Medical Muses: Hysteria in Nineteenth-Century Paris*. London: Bloomsbury, 2011.

Kenner, Charmian. *No Time for Women: Exploring Women's Health in the 1930s and Today*. London: Pandora Press, 1985.

King, Helen. *Hippocrates Woman: Reading the Female Body in Ancient Greece*. London: Routledge, 1998.

Lorde, Audre. *The Cancer Journals*. Special ed. San Francisco: Aunt Lute Books, 1997.

Löwy, Ilana. *A Woman's Disease: The History of Cervical Cancer*. Oxford: Oxford University Press, 2011.

Mangham, Andrew, and Greta Depledge, eds. *The Female Body in Medicine and Literature*. Liverpool: Liverpool University Press, 2011.

Martin, Emily. *The Woman in the Body*. Milton Keynes: Open University Press, 1987.

Morgen, Sandra. *Into Our Own Hands: The Women's Health Movement in the United States, 1969–1990*. New Brunswick, NJ: Rutgers University Press, 2002.

Moscucci, Ornella. *The Science of Women: Gynaecology and Gender in England, 1800–1929*. Cambridge: Cambridge University Press, 1990.

Oakley, Ann. *The Captured Womb: A History of the Medical Care of Pregnant Women*. New York: Blackwell, 1984.

Oudshoorn, Nelly. *Beyond the Natural Body: An Archeology of Sex Hormones*. London: Routledge, 1994.

Park, Katharine. *Secrets of Women: Gender, Generation, and the Origins of Human Dissection*. New York: Zone Books, 2010.

Perkins Gilman, Charlotte. *The Man-Made World*. New York: Cosimo Classics, 2007.
———. *The Yellow Wallpaper*. London: Penguin Classics, 1995.
Rich, Adrienne. *Of Woman Born: Motherhood as Experience and Institution*. London: Virago, 1977.
Rippon, Gina. *The Gendered Brain: The New Neuroscience That Shatters the Myth of the Female Brain*. London: The Bodley Head, 2019.
Roberts, Dorothy. *Killing the Black Body: Race, Reproduction, and the Meaning of Liberty*. 20th anniversary ed. New York: Vintage, 2017.
Rodnite Lemay, Helen. *Women's Secrets: A Translation of Pseudo-Albertus Magnus' "De Secretis Mulierum" with Commentaries*. Albany: State University of New York Press, 1992.
Rowbotham, Sheila. *Hidden from History: 300 Years of Women's Oppression and the Fight Against It*. London: Pluto Press, 1973.
Seaman, Barbara. *The Doctor's Case Against the Pill*. 25th anniversary updated ed. Alameda, CA: Hunter House, 1995.
Showalter, Elaine. *The Female Malady: Women, Madness, and English Culture, 1830–1980*. London: Virago, 1987.
———. *Hystories: Hysterical Epidemics and Modern Culture*. London: Picador, 1997.
Smith, Susan L. *Sick and Tired of Being Sick and Tired: Black Women's Health Activism in America, 1890–1950*. Philadelphia: University of Pennsylvania Press, 1995.
Sontag, Susan. *Illness as Metaphor*. New York: Farrar, Straus and Giroux, 1978.
Spearing, Sinéad. *A History of Women in Medicine: Cunning Women, Physicians, Witches*. Barnsley: Pen and Sword, 2019.
Sterling, Dorothy, ed. *We Are Your Sisters: Black Women in the Nineteenth Century*. New York: W. W. Norton, 1997.
Walzer Leavitt, Judith, ed. *Women and Health in America*. 2nd ed. Madison: University of Wisconsin Press, 1999.
Washington, Harriet A. *Medical Apartheid: The Dark History of Medical Experimentation on Black Americans from Colonial Times to the Present*. New York: Anchor, 2006.
Watkins, Elizabeth Seigel. *The Estrogen Elixir: A History of Hormone Replacement Therapy in America*. Baltimore: Johns Hopkins University Press, 2007.
———. *On the Pill: A Social History of Oral Contraceptives, 1950–1970*. Baltimore: Johns Hopkins University Press, 2001.

NOTES

INTRODUCTION

4   **22 percent of Black women in the United States:** National Partnership for Women and Families, "Black Women's Maternal Health: A Multifaceted Approach to Addressing Persistent and Dire Health Disparities," April 2018, https://www.nationalpartnership.org /our-work /health /reports/black-womens -maternal-health.html.

4   **"less sensitive nerve endings":** Kelly M. Hoffman, Sophie Trawalter, Jordan R. Axt, and M. Norman Oliver, "Racial Bias in Pain Assessment and Treatment Recommendations, and False Beliefs About Biological Differences Between Blacks and Whites," *Proceedings of the National Academy of Sciences of the United States of America* 113, no. 16 (2016): 4296–301.

4   **birth complications . . . Black women:** Jamila Taylor, Cristina Novoa, Katie Hamm, and Shilpa Phadke, "Eliminating Racial Disparities in Maternal and Infant Mortality: A Comprehensive Policy Blueprint," Center for American Progress, May 2, 2019, https://www.americanprogress.org/issues/women/reports /2019/05/02/469186/eliminating-racial-disparities-maternal-infant-mortality/.

7   **more severe growth of endometrial tissue:** G. H. Shade, M. Lane, and M. P. Diamond, "Endometriosis in the African American Woman—Racially, a Different Entity?," *Gynecological Surgery* 9 (2012): 59–62.

8   **"male perspectives [and] standards":** Carolyn Hibbs, "Androcentrism," in *Encyclopedia of Critical Psychology*, ed. T. Teo (New York: Springer, 2014), https:// doi.org/10:1007/978-1-4614-5583-7_16.

8   **dissecting "androcentric culture":** Charlotte Perkins Gilman, *The Man-Made World* (1911; New York: Cosimo Classics, 2007).

8   **"a subspecies told off for reproduction only":** Gilman quoting an unnamed "English Scientist" from 1888, in *The Man-Made World*, p. 5.

12 **virus is devastating:** See Jo Bibby, "Will COVID-19 Be a Watershed Moment for Health Inequalities?," Health Foundation, May 7, 2020, https://www .health.org.uk/publications/long-reads/will-covid-19-be-a-watershed-moment -for-health-inequalities; and Angela Saini, "The Data Was There—So Why Did It Take Coronavirus to Wake Us Up to Racial Health Inequalities?," *The Guardian*, June 11, 2020, https://www.theguardian.com/uk-news/2020/jun/11/the

-data -was -there-so-why-did-it-take-coronavirus-to-wake-us-up-to-racial-hea
lth-inequalities.

12 **"... makes us think about hormones":** Roni Caryn Rabin, "Can Estrogen and Other 'Sex' Hormones Help Men Survive Covid-19?," *New York Times*, updated May 7, 2020, https://www.nytimes.com/2020/04/27/health/coronavirus -estrogen-men.html.

13 **"... social factors first, not biology":** Heather Shattuck-Heidorn, Meredith W. Reiches, and Sarah S. Richardson, "What's Really Behind the Gender Gap in Covid-19 Deaths?," *New York Times*, June 24, 2020, https://www.nytimes.com /2020/06/24/opinion/sex-differences-covid.html.

1: WANDERING WOMBS

19 **pregnancy would make her healthy:** Hippocrates, Rebecca Flemming, and Ann Ellis Hanson, "Hippocrates' *Peri Partheniôn* (*Diseases of Young Girls*): Text and Translation," *Early Science and Medicine* 3, no. 3 (1998): 241–52.

20 **spared this misery:** See Hippocrates, *Diseases of Women 1*, in *Hippocrates: Volume XI*, ed. and trans. Paul Potter, Loeb Classical Library 538 (London: Harvard University Press, 2018), 33–35.

20 **like "diseases in men":** Hippocrates, *Diseases of Women 1*, 131.

22 **"... a woman who has not borne children":** Hippocrates, *Diseases of Women 1*, 9.

22 **the world, the universe, and everything in it:** See Lesley Ann Dean-Jones, *Women's Bodies in Classical Greek Science* (Oxford: Clarendon Press, 2010), 70; and Mark J. Adair, "Plato's View of the 'Wandering Uterus,'" *Classical Journal* 91, no. 2 (1995): 153–63.

22 **"an animal within an animal":** Aretaeus, *The Extant Works of Aretaeus, the Cappadocian*, ed. and trans. Francis Adams (London: Sydenham Society, 1856), 286–87.

23 **sickness of the world on Pandora:** See Helen King, *Hippocrates Woman: Reading the Female Body in Ancient Greece* (London: Routledge, 1998), 23–39, for discussion of the way the myth of Pandora influenced and shaped Hippocratic gynecology.

24 **"manifold and diverse" forces of the womb:** Preface to *De passionibus mulierum*, Version B, from Paris, Bibliothèque Nationale de France (1075–1100, Italy), trans. and quoted in Monica H. Green, "From 'Diseases of Women' to 'Secrets of Women': The Transformation of Gynecological Literature in the Later Middle Ages," *Journal of Medieval and Early Modern Studies* 30, no. 1 (Winter 2000): 9.

24 **view of human health:** Dean-Jones, *Women's Bodies in Classical Greek Science*, 23–24.

24 **"... does not issue forth like an animal":** Soranus, "On Hysterical Suffocation," book 3, in *Soranus Gynecology*, trans. Owsei Tempkin (Baltimore: Johns Hopkins University Press, 1956), 153.

25 **encouraged restoring her health:** Soranus, "On Hysterical Suffocation," 152.

25 **gynecological complaints as "her disgrace":** Green, "From 'Diseases of Women' to 'Secrets of Women,'" 9.

26 **"... ashamed to tell even if they know":** Ann Ellis Hanson, "Hippocrates: 'Diseases of Women 1,'" *Signs* 1, no. 2 (Winter 1975): 567–84.

26 **testimony ... taken more seriously:** Elaine Wainwright, *Women Healing / Healing Women: The Genderization of Healing in Early Christianity* (New York: Routledge, 2006), 46.

26 **teaching of women's medicine:** See Monica H. Green's discussion of medicine in Salerno in her introduction to *The Trotula: An English Translation of the*

Medieval Compendium of Women's Medicine (Philadelphia: University of Pennsylvania Press, 2002), 9–14.

27 **"...anguish of their diseases":** Green, "Book of the Conditions of Women," in *The Trotula*, 65.

28 **"to consume the windiness":** Green, "Book of the Conditions of Women," in *The Trotula*, 94.

2: POSSESSED AND POLLUTING

29 **championed on their own terms:** Christine de Pizan, *The Book of the City of Ladies*, trans. Rosalind Brown-Grant (London: Penguin, 1999).

30 **"he got what he deserved":** De Pizan, *The Book of the City of Ladies*, 21.

30 **"...female body is inherently flawed":** De Pizan, *The Book of the City of Ladies*, 21.

31 **"...secret things about the nature of women":** Helen Rodnite Lemay, *Women's Secrets: A Translation of Pseudo-Albertus Magnus' "De Secretis Mulierum" with Commentaries* (Albany: State University of New York Press, 1992), 59.

32 **mortally wound his penis:** Rodnite Lemay, *Women's Secrets*, 89.

32 **Eve's snack of choice:** Rodnite Lemay, *Women's Secrets*, 142.

32 **"...other evidence than your own body":** De Pizan, *The Book of the City of Ladies*, 21–22.

33 **"...more suitable that a woman":** Jacqueline Félice de Almania, *Chartularium universitatis pariseinsis*, ed. E. Chatelin and H. Denifle and trans. Emilie Amt (Paris: Delalain, 1891), 111, cited in Franklin J. Griffen, "The Healthcare Needs of Medieval Women," *Ex Posto Facto* 20 (2011), 90–91.

34 **"venom doesn't act on itself...":** Rodnite Lemay, *Women's Secrets*, 130.

35 **scrutinized, regulated, surveilled, and controlled:** See Silvia Federici, *Caliban and the Witch: Women, the Body, and Primitive Accumulation* (Brooklyn: Autonomedia, 2014), especially "The Great Witch-Hunt in Europe," 163–218.

36 **she must have used sorcery—"love magic":** Sigrid Brauner, *Fearless Wives and Frightened Shrews: The Construction of the Witch in Early Modern Germany*, ed. Robert H. Brown (Amherst: University of Massachusetts Press, 1995), 46–49.

36 **"all witches have been slaves from a young age...":** Hans Peter Broedel, *The Malleus Maleficarum and the Construction of Witchcraft* (Manchester: Manchester University Press, 2003), 2.

37 **"...with regard to male organs":** *Malleus maleficarium*, trans. Rev. Montague Summers (London: Pushkin Press, 1928), 58.

37 **"cast some glamour" over his penis:** *Malleus maleficarium*, 119.

37 **some witches collected penises:** *Malleus maleficarium*, 121.

38 **"...Catholic faith than midwives":** *Malleus maleficarium*, 66.

38 **"surpass all other witches...":** *Malleus maleficarium*, 269.

39 **"And why did you touch the child before it got sick?":** *Malleus maleficarium*, 213.

39 **"sentence her to flames":** *Malleus maleficarium*, 248.

39 **appeared in the late fifteenth century:** See Nachman Ben-Yehuda, "The European Witch Craze of the 14th to 17th Centuries: A Sociologist's Perspective," *American Journal of Sociology* 86, no. 1 (July 1980): 10.

39–40 **During the sixteenth and seventeeth centuries:** For insight into the extent of the witch hunt in early modern Europe, and estimated figures for prosecution and execution of people for witchcraft, see Brian P. Levack, *The Witch-Hunt in Early Modern Europe*, fourth edition (New York: Routledge: 2016), 19–22.

40 **a threat, a hazard, a scourge:** See Federici, *Caliban and the Witch*, 184, for a brilliant passage on the association of aspects of "female personality"—namely displayed by "the women who exercised her sexuality outside the bonds of marriage and procreation"—and witchcraft accusations.

41 **"Act Against Conjuration, Witchcraft . . .":** 1604: 1 James 1 c.12: "An Act against Conjuration, Witchcraft and dealing with evil and wicked Spirits," Statutes Project: Putting Historic British Law Online, https://statutes.org.uk /site/the-statutes/seventeenth-century/1604-1-james-1-c-12-an-act-against-witch craft.

41 **75 percent of whom were women:** Julian Goodare, "A Royal Obsession with Black Magic Started Europe's Most Brutal Witch Hunts," *National Geographic*, October 17, 2019, https://www.nationalgeographic.co.uk/history-and -civilization/2019/10/royal-obsession-black-magic-started-europes-most-brutal -witch.

41 **In England, around five hundred people were executed:** "Witchcraft," UK Parliament, https://www.parliament.uk/about/living-heritage/transformingso ciety/private-lives/religion/overview/witchcraft.

41 **forty-four-year-old woman was accused:** *Great news from the west of England: being a true account of two young persons lately bewitch'd in the town of Beckenton in Somerset-shire . . .* (London: T. M., 1689), Wellcome Library, https://wellcom ecollection.org/works/fmt4x878.

43 **Jackson then "rayled at her . . .":** "A brief and sincere Narration of Mary Glover's late wofull affliction . . ." (1602), in *Witchcraft and Hysteria in Early Modern London: Edward Jorden and the Mary Glover Case*, ed. Michael MacDonald (London: Routledge, 1991), 3.

43 **afflicted woman was possessed:** Edward Jorden, *A Briefe Discourse of a Disease Called the Suffocation of the Mother* (London, 1603), 1.

44 **"The passive condition of womankind":** Jorden, *A Briefe Discourse*, 1.

3: UNDER HER SKIN

46 **descriptions of "womb suffocation":** Edward Jorden, *A Briefe Discourse of a Disease called the Suffocation of the Mother* (London, 1603), 14–15.

46 **send up poisonous vapors:** Jorden, *A Briefe Discourse*, 15.

46 **"womb suffocation" was "easily overcome":** Jorden, *A Briefe Discourse*, 26.

46 **"metaphysical" or "demonical" intervention:** Jorden, *A Briefe Discourse*, 2.

46 **"rareness and strangeness" of the uterus:** Jorden, *A Briefe Discourse*, 2.

47 **woven network of nerves:** *Principles of Anatomy According to the Opinion of Galen by Johann Guinter and Andreas Vesalius*, ed. Vivian Nutton (London: Routledge, 2017), 94–96.

47 **the *Disease Woman*:** Rachel Wertheim, "The 'Disease Woman' of the Wellcome Apocalypse," Wellcome Library blog, December 20, 2015, http://blog .wellcomelibrary.org/2015/12/the-disease-woman-of-the-wellcome-apocalypse. The Wellcome Apocalypse is a miscellany of medical drawings and texts from fifteenth-century Germany, which includes the "disease woman," an illustration of the "physician's imaginative conception of the internal workings of the female body," identified by historian Monica H. Green. The illustration served as a practical guide for "the pathology and physiology of the pregnant female body." As Wertheim writes, "The 'disease woman' presented a way in which that body

could be contained, classified and controlled within the safe context of a masculinised medical framework."

48 **lover of a monk:** Andreas Vesalius, *Fabrica*, quoted in Katharine Park, *Secrets of Women: Gender, Generation, and the Origins of Human Dissection* (New York: Zone Books, 2010), 215, 216.

48 **"removed all her skin . . .":** Park, *Secrets of Women*, 216.

48 **sex workers or women condemned:** Maurits Biesbrouck and Omer Steeno, "Andreas Vesalius' Corpses," *Acta medico-historica adriatica* 12, no. 1 (2014): 25.

48 **after an accused woman had given birth:** Katherine Eggert, *Disknowledge: Literature, Alchemy, and the End of Humanism in Renaissance Italy* (Philadelphia: University of Pennsylvania Press, 2015), 169.

48 **Vesalius stated that she was very tall:** Park, *Secrets of Women*, 211.

49 **physiology of menstruation:** Andreas Vesalius, *Fabrica*, quoted in Park, *Secrets of Women*, 219.

49 **claimed he was the first man to discover:** Mark D. Stringer and Ines Becker, "Colombo and the Clitoris," *European Journal of Obstetrics and Gynecology and Reproductive Biology* 151 (2010): 131.

49 **"the love" or "sweetness" of Venus:** Stringer and Becker, "Colombo and the Clitoris," 131.

50 **flowed "forth in all directions . . .":** Stringer and Becker, "Colombo and the Clitoris," 131.

50 **described a female patient:** Realdo Colombo, "'On Those Things Rarely Found in Anatomy': An Annotated Translation from the 'De Re Anatomica'" (1559), Robert J. Moes and C. D. O'Malley, *Bulletin of the History of Medicine* 34, no. 6 (November–December 1960): 527–28.

50 **considered his patient "wretched":** Colombo, "'On Those Things Rarely Found in Anatomy,'" 527.

50 **"processes and working" of the clitoris:** Stringer and Becker, "Colombo and the Clitoris," 131–32.

50 **hitherto overlooked female pleasure organ:** Stringer and Becker, "Colombo and the Clitoris," 132.

51 **might possess a "tiny phallus":** Andreas Vesalius, *Observationum anatomicarum Gabrielis Fallopii examen* (Venice: Francesco de'Franceschi da Siena, 1564), 43, quoted in Katharine Park, "The Rediscovery of the Clitoris: French Medicine and the Tribade, 1570–1620," in *The Body in Parts: Fantasies of Corporeality in Early Modern Europe*, ed. Carla Mazzio and David Hillman (New York: Routledge, 1997), 177.

51 **". . . to healthy women":** Vesalius, quoted in Park, "The Rediscovery of the Clitoris," 177.

51 **nomenclature was as undefined:** Helen E. O'Connell, Kalavampara V. Sanjeevan, and John M. Hutson, "Anatomy of the Clitoris," *Journal of Urology* 174 (October 2005): 1192.

51 **glans makes up only about a fifth:** O'Connell, Sanjeevan, and Hutson, "Anatomy of the Clitoris"; Sharon Mascall, "Time to Rethink the Clitoris," BBC News, June 11, 2006, http://news.bbc.co.uk/1/hi/health/5013866.stm; and Naomi Russell, "The Still-Misunderstood Shape of the Clitoris," *The Atlantic*, March 9, 2017, https://www.theatlantic.com/health/archive/2017/03/3d-clitoris/518991.

52 **sensation-restoring surgeries:** Rachel E. Gross, "The Clitoris, Uncovered: An Intimate History," *Scientific American*, March 4, 2020, https://www.scientificamerican.com/article/the-clitoris-uncovered-an-intimate-history.

52 **trans people undergoing gender affirmation:** Vojkan Vukadinovic, Borko Stojanovic, Marko Majstorovic, and Aleksandar Milosevic, "The Role of Clitoral Anatomy in Female to Male Sex Reassignment Surgery," *Scientific World Journal* (2014), https://www.researchgate.net/publication/263548196_The_Role_of_Clitoral_Anatomy_in_Female_to_Male_Sex_Reassignment_Surgery.

52 **parable of culture:** O'Connell, Sanjeevan, and Hutson, "Anatomy of the Clitoris," 1194.

53 **". . . vayle of Nature's secrets . . .":** John Banister (1578), *The Historie of Man*, quoted in Lauren Kassell, "Medical Understandings of the Body, *c.* 1500–1750," in *The Routledge History of Sex and the Body, 1500 to the Present*, ed. Sarah Toulalan and Kate Fisher (London: Routledge, 2013), 66.

53 ***Mikrokosmographia* was published:** Jillian Linster, "When 'Nothing' Goes Missing: The Impotent Censorship of Helkiah Crooke's *Mikrokosmographia*," *The Crooke Book: Adventures in Early Modern Anatomy*, accessed November 12, 2020, https://crookebook.files.wordpress.com/2013/03/crooke-images-paper-3-10-13.pdf.

4: ON HER NERVES

55 **making "amorous enticements":** Richard Watkins, *News from the Dead; or, A True and Exact Narration of the miraculous deliverance of Anne Greene* (Oxford: Leonard Litchfield, 1651), 1.

55 **sent to Oxford jail:** Watkins, *News from the Dead*, 1.

55 **"to avoid their shame . . .":** James I, cap. 27, *Statutes at Large from Magna Charta to the End of the Eleventh Parliament of Great Britain, Anno 1761*, 8 volumes, ed. Danby Pickering (Cambridge: Joseph Bentham, 1763), 7, 298, quoted in Susan C. Staub, "Surveilling the Secrets of the Female Body: The Contest for Reproductive Authority in the Popular Press of the Seventeenth Century," in *The Female Body in Medicine and Literature*, ed. Andrew Mangham and Greta Depledge (Liverpool: Liverpool University Press, 2011), 53–54.

57 **writ large in mid-seventeenth-century:** Susan C. Staub discusses how Watkins's *News from the Dead*, a "popular pamphlet," "vividly illustrates the intersection of the two types of knowledge vying for authority over the female body in the period: the intuitive 'amateur' knowledge of midwives and matrons and the 'professional,' scientific knowledge of male physicians." Staub, "Surveilling the Secrets of the Female Body," 52.

57 **baby was not "vital":** Staub, "Surveilling the Secrets of the Female Body," 57.

58 **men . . . claimed authority:** See Monica H. Greene, "Gendering the History of Women's Healthcare," *Gender and History* 20, no. 3 (November 2008): 487–518; see also Staub, "Surveilling the Secrets of the Female Body," 57–58.

58 **remove signs of life:** Edward Jorden stated that suffocation of the mother could suspend "sense, motion, breath, heat, or any sign of life at all." Deprived of "vital influence," a woman's pulse became faint, her lungs stopped working, and she would sink "like a dead corpse." Jorden suggested not burying any seemingly dead womb-suffocated woman for at least three days. Edward Jorden, *A Briefe Discourse of a Disease Called the Suffocation of the Mother* (London, 1603), 9.

59 **"restoring . . . a living one":** Watkins, *News from the Dead*, 8.

59 **". . . though she's dead":** Verse by Rob. Sharrock, fellow of New College, in Watkins, *News from the Dead*, 18.

59 **hard to know how many women:** See Greene, "Gendering the History of Women's Healthcare," 495; and Jennifer Richards, "Reading and Hearing *The Womans Booke* in Early Modern England," *Bulletin of the History of Medicine* 89 (2015): 434–62.

60 **". . . which yee women . . .":** John Sadler, *The Sicke Woman's Private Looking-Glasse* (London: Anne Griffin, 1636; Ann Arbor: Text Creation Partnership, 2011), https://quod.lib.umich.edu/e/eebo/A11278:0001:001/1:4?rgn=div1;view =fulltext.

60 **". . . ill affected wombe":** Sadler, *The Sicke Woman's Private Looking-Glasse.*

60 **". . . cure of uterine diseases":** Sadler, *The Sicke Woman's Private Looking-Glasse.*

61 **Seventeen women, including Mary Spencer:** Mildred Tongue, "The Lancashire Witches: 1612 and 1634," *Transactions of the Historical Society of Lancashire and Cheshire* 83 (1932): 157–69, Historical Society of Lancashire and Cheshire, *Transactions* digital archive, https://www.hslc.org.uk/wp-content /uploads/2017/06/83-7-Tonge.pdf.

62 **appeared to be hysteric:** See Carl Zimmer's discussion of Willis's 1650 casebook in *Soul Made Flesh: The Discovery of the Brain—and How It Changed the World* (New York: Simon & Schuster: 2005), 103–6.

63 **organs and muscles:** Zimmer, *Soul Made Flesh*, 174–82.

64 **eventually death:** Thomas Willis, *An Essay of the Pathology of the Brain and Nervous Stock: In Which Convulsive Diseases Are Treated of*, trans. Samuel Pordage (London: J. B. for T. Dring, 1681), 86.

64 **behemoth that was hysteria:** See Willis, *An Essay of the Pathology of the Brain*, 76–77.

65 **". . . species of this disorder":** Thomas Sydenham, "An Epistle from Dr. Thomas Sydenham to Dr. Wm. Cole; Treating of the Smallpox and Hysteric Diseases" (1681–82), in *The Works of Thomas Sydenham, M.D., on Acute and Chronic Diseases, with Their Histories and Modes of Cure*, ed. Benjamin Rush (Philadelphia: Benjamin and Thomas Kite, 1809), 272.

65 **"the pleasure of men":** Sydenham, "Treating of the Smallpox and Hysteric Diseases," 277.

65 **"such male subjects as lead a sedentary . . .":** Sydenham, "An Epistolary Dissertation to Dr. Cole," in *The Works of Thomas Sydenham, translated from the Latin edition of Dr. Greenhill . . . by R. G. Latham M.D.* (London: The Sydenham Society, 1848/1850), 85.

65 **". . . disturbance of mind":** Sydenham, "Treating of the Smallpox and Hysteric Diseases," 277.

65–66 **Hysteric women, he believed:** Sydenham, "Treating of the Smallpox and Hysteric Diseases," 275.

66 **"weak and wretched":** Mary Wollstonecraft, *A Vindication of the Rights of Women* (1792; London: Vintage Books, 2015), 1.

67 **"Taught from infancy . . .":** Wollstonecraft, *A Vindication of the Rights of Women*, 31.

67 **the sisters fled:** Claire Tomalin, "Eliza," chap. 3, in *The Life and Death of Mary Wollstonecraft* (London: Penguin Books, 1974).

68 **"Weak minds fall a prey . . .":** Mary Wollstonecraft, *Thoughts on the Education of Daughters, with Reflections on Female Conduct in the More Important Duties of Life* (1787; Cambridge: Cambridge University Press, 2014), 159.

68 **Mystery and misconception:** Christine Hallett, "The Attempt to Understand Puerperal Fever in the Eighteenth and Early Nineteenth Centuries: The Influence of Inflammation Theory," *Medical History* 49, no. 1 (2005): 1–28.

68 **Some believed the fever:** Nicholas Kadar, "Ignaz Semmelweis: 'The Savior of Mothers,'" *American Journal of Obstetrics and Gynecology*, December 2018, 520.

68 **handwashing prevented physicians:** See Kadar, "Ignaz Semmelweis," 519–22; M. Best and D. Neuhauser, "Ignaz Semmelweis and the Birth of Infection Control," *BMJ Quality and Safety* 13 (2004): 233–34; Safiya Shaikh and Daniella Caudle, "Ignaz Philipp Semmelweis (1818–1865)," *Embryo Project Encyclopedia*, April 6, 2017.

68 **revolutionizing antiseptic techniques:** "Joseph Lister's Antisepsis System," Science Museum, October 14, 2018, https://www.sciencemuseum.org.uk /objects-and-stories/medicine/listers-antisepsis-system.

68 **"... her equal in the world":** William Godwin, letter to playwright Thomas Holcroft, September 10, 1797, quoted in Richard Holmes, "How a Husband's Loving Biography Ruined His Wife's Reputation: On William Godwin's Scrupulously Honest Life of Mary Wollstonecraft," *Literary Hub*, March 21, 2017, https:// lithub.com/how-a-husbands-loving-biography-ruined-his-wifes-reputation/.

5: FEELING PAIN

70 **"hysterical affection":** John Rutter, "Case of Hysteralgia," *Edinburgh Medical and Surgical Journal* 4, no. 14 (April 1808): 168.

71 **"mistaken in her belief":** Rutter, "Case of Hysteralgia," 174.

71 **"If this pain . . .":** Rutter, "Case of Hysteralgia," 175.

71 **J.S. had also been subject:** Rutter, "Case of Hysteralgia," 169.

71 **her "horrid pain":** Rutter, "Case of Hysteralgia," 174.

72 **Sauvages's sixteen "species":** "Hysteralgia," in Abraham Bees, *The Cyclopaedia; or, Universal Dictionary of Arts, in Thirty-Nine Volumes*, vol. 18 (London: Longman, Hurst, Rees, Orme, and Brown, 1819), 8.

72 **many sufferers are misdiagnosed:** "Pelvic Pain," National Health Service, October 2018, https://www.nhs.uk/conditions/pelvic-pain; Yun Sung Jo et al., "A Misdiagnosed Cause of Chronic Pelvic Pain: Abscess with Foreign Body," *Pain Medicine* 15, no. 9 (September 2014): 1637–39; L. M. Speer, S. Mushkbar, and T. Erbele, "Chronic Pelvic Pain in Women," *American Family Physician* 93, no. 5 (March 2016): 380–87.

72 **depression or anxiety:** See Vânia Meira e Siqueira-Campos et al., "Anxiety and Depression in Women with and Without Chronic Pelvic Pain: Prevalence and Associated Factors," *Journal of Pain Research* 12 (April 16, 2019): 1223–33.

73 **"... annoyed by a small pain":** Frances Burney, "Journal Letter to Esther Burney, 22 March–June 1812," in *Frances Burney: Journals and Letters*, ed. Peter Sabor and Lars E. Troide (London: Penguin Books, 2001), 431.

73 **"glitter of polished steel":** Burney, "Journal Letter to Esther Burney," 441.

73 **"... edges of the wound":** Burney, "Journal Letter to Esther Burney," 442. A "poniard" is a long, thin dagger.

73 **she "never moved . . .":** Burney, "Journal Letter to Esther Burney," 442.

74 **"... tolerated with great courage":** Official medical report of Burney's procedure, translated and quoted in Julia L. Epstein, "Writing the Unspeakable: Fanny Burney's Mastectomy and the Fictive Body," *Representations*, no. 16 (1986): 150–51.

74 **"They reflect upon . . .":** John Rodman, *A Practical Explanation of Cancer in the Female Breast, with the Method of Cure and Cases of Illustration* (London: Paisley, 1815), 56.

74 **"sharpened by sympathy":** Rodman, *A Practical Explanation of Cancer in the Female Breast,* 58.

74 **". . . distempered her frame . . .":** Rodman, *A Practical Explanation of Cancer in the Female Breast,* 65.

75 **Rodman "gained ascendancy . . .":** Rodman, *A Practical Explanation of Cancer in the Female Breast,* 70.

75 **"dispositions of mind":** Rodman, *A Practical Explanation of Cancer in the Female Breast,* 2.

75 **"airs and duplicities":** Thomas Trotter, *A View of the Nervous Temperament* (New York: Wright, Goodenow, and Stockwell, 1808), 25.

76 **"savage" women's pain:** Trotter, *A View of the Nervous Temperament,* 27.

76 **"will bear cutting . . .":** Henry James Johnson, "Extirpation of an Ovarium", *The Medico-chirurgical Review, and Journal of Practical Medicine* 5, no. 10 (1827): 620, cited in Deirdre Cooper Owens, *Medical Bondage: Race, Gender, and the Origins of American Gynecology* (Athens: University of Georgia Press, 2017), 30–31.

77 **Sims told Westcott:** J. Marion Sims, *The Story of My Life,* ed. H. Marion Sims (New York: D. Appleton, 1849), 227.

77 **repulsed by their "soft parts":** Sims, *The Story of My Life,* 231.

77 **"not charge a cent . . .":** Sims, *The Story of My Life,* 236.

78 **". . . they must live and suffer":** Sims, *The Story of My Life,* 240.

78 **". . . relief of human suffering":** Sims, *The Story of My Life,* 246.

79 **"pain of parturition":** Charles D. Meigs, *Lecture on Some of the Distinctive Characteristics of the Female: Delivered Before the Class of the Jefferson Medical College, January 5, 1847* (Philadelphia: T. K and P. G. Collins, 1847), 18–19.

79 **her daughter Anesthesia:** See P. M. Dunn, "Sir James Young Simpson (1811–1870) and Obstetric Anesthesia," *Archives of Disease in Childhood—Fetal and Neonatal Edition* 83, no. 3 (2002); and Ray J. Defalque and Amos J. Wright, "The Myth of Baby 'Anesthesia,'" *Anesthesiology* 111, no. 3 (2009): 682.

80 **according to Meigs's calculations:** Charles D. Meigs, *Obstetrics: The Science and the Art* (Philadelphia: Lea and Blanchard, 1849), 316. See also A. D. Farr, "Early Opposition to Obstetric Anesthesia," *Anesthesia* 35 (1980): 901.

80 **Chloroform, he claimed:** J. Y. Simpson, *Anesthesia; or, the Employment of Chloroform and Ether in Surgery, Midwifery, etc.* (Philadelphia: Lindsay and Blakiston, 1849), 186.

80 **an intimate occasion:** Farr, "Early Opposition to Obstetric Anesthesia," 903–4.

80–81 **". . . that blessed Chloroform . . .'":** Queen Victoria's Journals, Friday, April 22, 1853, http://www.queenvictoriasjournals.org.

6: CONTAGIOUS PLEASURES

82 **this offensive procedure:** Marshall Hall, "On a New and Lamentable Form of Hysteria," *The Lancet* 55, no. 1396 (June 1850): 660–61.

83 **doctor-patient boundaries:** See Margarete Sandelowski, "This Most Dangerous Instrument: Propriety, Power, and the Vaginal Speculum," *Journal of Obstetric, Gynecologic and Neonatal Nursing* 29, no. 1 (January 2000): 75.

83 **Hall gravely declared:** Hall, "On a New and Lamentable Form of Hysteria," 661.

83 **superstitions of the past:** William Jones, *Practical Observations on Diseases of Women* (London: H. Bailliere, 1839), 1.

84 **"vague information" women imparted:** Jones, quoting physician, surgeon, and writer on "diseases of women" Sir Charles Mansfield Clarke, in *Practical Observations on Diseases of Women*, 33.

84 **advantage of the speculum:** Jones, *Practical Observations on Diseases of Women*, 33.

85 **"revolting attachment . . .":** Hall, "On a New and Lamentable Form of Hysteria," 661.

86 **"some obscure uterine mischief":** Thomas Litchfield, "On the Use and Abuse of the Speculum," letter to the editor, *The Lancet* 55, no. 1397 (June 1850): 705.

86 **glance down the throat:** Charles Locock, quoted in the Proceedings of the Royal Medical and Chirurgical Society meeting, *The Lancet* 55, no. 1397 (June 1850): 702.

86 **"measure of medical police":** Philippe Ricord, *A Practical Treatise on Venereal Diseases*, trans. A. Sidney Doane (New York: J. S. Redfield, Clinton Hall, 1848), 216.

87 **"under the dominion":** Robert Brudenell Carter, *On the Pathology and Treatment of Hysteria* (London: John Churchill, 1853), 33.

87 **women conceal such feelings:** Brudenell Carter, *On the Pathology and Treatment of Hysteria*, 47.

87 **their "prurient desires":** Brudenell Carter, *On the Pathology and Treatment of Hysteria*, 69.

88 **". . . practice of solitary vice":** Brudenell Carter, *On the Pathology and Treatment of Hysteria*, 83.

88 **"subdues every feeling of modesty . . .":** Samuel Ashwell, *A Practical Treatise on the Diseases Peculiar to Women* (Philadelphia: Lee and Blanchard, 1844), 500.

88 **". . . enlarged, and sensitive clitoris":** Ashwell, *A Practical Treatise on the Diseases Peculiar to Women*, 500.

89 **served as chief obstetrician:** E. A. Heaman, *St. Mary's: A History of a London Teaching Hospital* (Canada: McGill–Queens University Press, 2003), 47–48.

89 **ovariotomy was needlessly performed:** Robert Lee, *Clinical Reports of Ovarian and Uterine Diseases, with Commentaries* (London: John Churchill, 1853).

89 **her body emaciated:** Isaac Baker Brown, *On Surgical Diseases of Women* (London: John W. Davies, 1861), 384–92.

91 **considered his clitoridectomy:** Isaac Baker Brown, *On the Curability of Certain Forms of Insanity, Epilepsy, Catalepsy and Hysteria in Females* (London: Robert Hardwicke, 1866), 37.

92 **"naturally prone" to:** Brown, *On the Curability of Certain Forms of Insanity*, 58.

92 **". . . and licentious profligates":** L. Larmont, *Medical Adviser and Marriage Guide: Representing All the Diseases of the Genital Organs of the Male and Female*, 8th ed. (Paris: E. Warner, 1864), 339.

92 **". . . the whole human race":** Brown, *On the Curability of Certain Forms of Insanity*, 13.

93 **women of their parish:** Elisabeth A. Sheehan, "Victorian Clitoridectomy: Isaac Baker Brown and His Harmless Operative Procedure," in *The Gender/Sexuality Reader: Culture, History, Political Economy*, ed. Roger N. Lancaster and Micaela di Leonardo (New York: Routledge, 1997), 329.

93   **family drawing rooms:** Sheehan, "Victorian Clitoridectomy," 330.

93   **"... half the woman gone ...":** William Acton, *Prostitution, Considered in Its Moral, Social, and Sanitary Aspects, in London and Other Large Cities and Garrison Towns, with Proposals for the Mitigation and Prevention of Its Attendant Evils* (London: John Churchill and Sons, 1857), 166.

93   **"... towel over your face":** Josephine Butler relaying the words of "violated women" in a letter to James John Garth Wilkinson, in Wilkinson, *The Forcible Introspection of Women for the Army and Navy by the Oligarchy, Considered Physically* (London: F. Pitman, 1870), 23.

94   **"... at our mercy":** Seymour Haden, quoted in "Meeting to Consider the Proposition of the Council for the Removal of Mr. I. B. Brown," *British Medical Journal* 1, no. 327 (April 1867): 396.

94   **"... if she would consent":** Dr. Henry Oldham, quoted in "Meeting to Consider the Proposition of the Council for the removal of Mr. I. B. Brown," 408.

94   **strong majority vote:** "Meeting to Consider the Proposition of the Council for the Removal of Mr. I. B. Brown," 409.

95   **"... I know my own make":** Butler quoted in Wilkinson, *The Forcible Introspection of Women*, 22.

95   **"... for *our* bodies":** Butler to Joseph Edmondson, March 28, 1872, quoted and cited in Brian Harrison, "Women's Health and the Women's Movement," *Biology, Medicine and Society, 1840–1940*, ed. Charles Webster (1981; Cambridge: Cambridge University Press, 2002), 45.

7: BLEEDING MAD

98   **"Britain's First Female Medical Students":** Aya Riad, "The Surgeon's Hall Riots: A Turning Point," *Edinburgh Medicine Timeline*, University of Edinburgh, June 3, 2020, https://blogs.ed.ac.uk/edmedtimeline/2020/03/06/the-surgeons-hall-riot-a-turning-point.

98   **"... of preventable suffering":** Sophia Jex-Blake, "Medicine as a Profession for Women," in *Women's Work and Women's Culture*, ed. Josephine Butler (London: Macmillan, 1869), 106.

98   **"... of mind and body":** Jex-Blake, "Medicine as a Profession for Women," 108.

99   **felt about menstruating:** Elaine Showalter, "Victorian Women and Menstruation," *Victorian Studies* 14, no. 1, "The Victorian Woman" (September 1970): 83–89; see also Julie-Marie Strange, "Menstrual Fictions: Languages of Medicine and Menstruation, c. 1850–1930," *Women's History Review* 9, no. 3 (2000): 607–28.

99   **fall foul of "hysterics":** "The Menstrual Discharge," in *Dr. Buchan's Domestic Medicine; or, a Treatise on the Prevention and Cure of Diseases by Regimen and Simple Medicines* (Philadelphia: Claxton, Remsen, and Haffelfinger, 1871), 398. William Buchan, a Scottish physician, first published *Domestic Medicine* in 1769. It remained one of the most popular "lay" medical manuals in Europe, the colonies, and the United States for nearly a century, selling over eighty thousand copies.

99   **losing her mind:** Buchan, *Domestic Medicine*, 398–400.

100 **grounds of "menstrual insanity":** "Trial of Martha Brixey" (May 12, 1845), Proceedings of Old Bailey online, https://www.oldbaileyonline.org/print.jsp?div=t18450512-1180.

100 "... ovaries of prostitutes ...": Edward John Tilt, *On Diseases of Menstruation and Ovarian Inflammation* (New York: Samuel S. and William Wood, 1851), 54.

101 "... impulse of unsatisfied desires": Tilt, *On Diseases of Menstruation*, 55.

101 inevitably turn hysteric: Tilt, *On Diseases of Menstruation*, 55–58.

101 "... they have beards": Thomas K. Chambers, "Clinical Lecture on Hysteria" (St. Mary's, November 7, 1861), *British Medical Journal*, December 21, 1861, 651.

101 "... has thwarted them": Chambers, "Clinical Lecture on Hysteria," 651.

102 Chambers diagnosed "hysteria ...": Chambers, "Clinical Lecture on Hysteria," 652.

103 "... trials of life": Edward Tilt, "On Hysteria and Its Interpreters," *British Medical Journal* 2, no. 572 (December 1871): 690–92.

103 dilated Omberg's cervix: Interview with Robert Battey in David W. Wandell and Eley McClellan, *Battey's Operation* (Louisville, KY: Morton, 1875), 5.

103 "... sensitive and retiring girl": Robert Battey, "Normal Ovariotomy," *Atlanta Medical and Surgical Journal* 10, no. 6 (September 1872; Atlanta: Plantation Publishing Company's Press, 1872): 323.

104 "... overshadowed her life": Battey, "Normal Ovariotomy," 324.

104 "... in unsuitable cases": T. Spencer Wells, *Diseases of the Ovaries; Their Diagnosis and Treatment* (London: John Churchill and Sons, 1864), xiv.

104 "invaded the hidden recesses ...": Battey, "Normal Ovariotomy" (paper read before the Georgia Medical Association; Atlanta, Herald Publishing Company's Steam Presses, April 1873), 3.

105 English surgeons objected: See Lawrence D. Longo, "The Rise and Fall of Battey's Operation: A Fashion in Surgery," *Bulletin of the History of Medicine* 53, no. 2 (Summer 1979): 244–45.

105 "... grace of thankfulness": See Curtis Tyrone, "Certain Aspects of Gynecologic Practice in the Late Nineteenth Century" (paper read at the meeting of the History of Medicine Society, Tulane University of Louisiana School of Medicine, November 1950), *American Journal of Surgery* 84 (1952): 95–106.

106 her symptoms forged forth: Mills's patient's account appears in Charles K. Mills, "A Case of Nymphomania, with Hystero-epilepsy and Peculiar Mental Perversions—the Result of Clitoridectomy and Oophorectomy; the Patient's History as Told by Herself," reported by William H. Morrison, Philadelphia Hospital, *Medical Times and Register*, April 18, 1885, 534–40.

8: REST AND RESISTANCE

107 "... we hold women ...": Frederick Douglass, "The Rights of Women," *The North Star*, (July 1948). https://www.census.gov/programs-surveys/sis/resources/historical-documents/north-star.html

108 only Black voice: Evette Dionne, *Lifting as We Climb: Black Women's Battle for the Ballot Box* (New York: Viking, 2020), 8–9, 34–35.

108 "... man toward woman": Report of the Women's Rights Convention, Seneca Falls, New York, July 19–29, 1848; original text included in "Women's Rights," National Historical Park New York, https://www.nps.gov/wori/learn/history-culture/report-of-the-womans-rights-convention.htm.

108 Douglass's *North Star* press: *Report of the Woman's Rights Convention, Held at Seneca Falls, N.Y., July 19th and 20th, 1848* (Rochester, NY: North Star Printing Office, 1848). The pamphlet can be viewed online at New York Heritage Digital

Collections, "Seneca Falls Historical Society," https://cdm16694.contentdm
.oclc.org/digital/collection/p16694coll96/id/52.

The papers of the *Declaration of Sentiments* signed at Seneca Falls are now lost,
so the *North Star* publication remains, at present, the only original copy. The
papers, taken to Douglass's *North Star* p rinting office, might have been destroyed
in a fire at Douglass's home in 1872. See Liz Robbins and Sam Roberts, "Early
Feminists Issued a Declaration of Independence. Where Is It Now?," *New York
Times*, February 9, 2019, https://www.nytimes.com/interactive/2019/02/09/nyreg
ion/declaration-of-sentiments-and-resolution-feminism.html.

108   "...a thorough education": "Report of the Women's Rights Convention," Na-
       tional Park Service, https://www.nps.gov/wori/learn/historyculture/report-of
       -the-womans-rights-convention.htm.

110   "...relation of the sexes...": Edward Hammond Clarke, *Sex in Education; or,
       A Fair Chance for Girls* (1873; Boston: Houghton Mifflin, 1884), 12, 13.

110   classrooms and colleges: Clarke, *Sex in Education*, 117.

110   "Nature punishes disobedience": Clarke, *Sex in Education*, 72, 60.

110   "the true womanly standard": Julia Ward Howe, "Sex and Education," in *Sex
       and Education: A Reply to Dr. E. H. Clarke's "Sex in Education,"* ed. Howe (Bos-
       ton: Roberts Brothers, 1874), 14.

110   "trans-atlantic homes": Clarke, *Sex in Education*, 63.

111   "...effects upon female health": Henry Maudsley, "Sex in Mind and Educa-
       tion," *Popular Science Monthly* 5 (June 1874): 198–215.

112   Garrett Anderson wrote: Elizabeth Garrett Anderson, "Sex in Education: A
       Reply," *Fortnightly Review*, 1874, excerpted in *Free and Ennobled: Source Read-
       ings in the Development of Victorian Feminism*, ed. Carol Bauer and Lawrence
       Ritt (Oxford: Pergamon Press, 1979), 269–71.

113   "No woman could publish...": Howe, "Sex and Education," 7.

113   embarked on womanhood: Howe, "Sex and Education," 28.

113   "...become without exception": Howe, "Sex and Education," 16.

113   "...*nothing else to do*": Eliza Bisbee Duffey, *No Sex in Education; or, An Equal
       Chance for Both Boys and Girls* (Philadelphia: J. M. Stoddart, 1874), 85. Italics in
       original.

114   Putnam Jacobi left home: Rachel Swaby, "The Godmother of American Med-
       icine," *The Atlantic*, April 8, 2015, https://www.theatlantic.com/technology
       /archive/2015/04/getting-educated-does-not-make-women-infertile-and-other
       -discoveries-made-in-the-1880s/389922.

114   "...rest during menstruation": See Carla Jean Bittel, *Mary Putnam Jacobi and
       the Politics of Medicine in Nineteenth-Century America* (Chapel Hill: University
       of North Carolina Press, 2009), 126–28.

114   Putnam Jacobi submitted: Mary Putnam Jacobi, "Do Women Require Mental
       and Bodily Rest During Menstruation?" (1875), in Putnam Jacobi, *The Question
       of Rest for Women During Menstruation* (New York: G. P. Putnam's Sons, 1877).

114   "constantly returning debility...": Putnam Jacobi, *The Question of Rest for
       Women During Menstruation*, 15.

115   made experimental analyzes: Putnam Jacobi, "Experimental," in *The Question
       of Rest for Women During Menstruation*, 115–61. See also Bittel, *Mary Putnam
       Jacobi and the Politics of Medicine*, 130–33.

115   periods was established: Bittel, *Mary Putnam Jacobi and the Politics of Medicine*,
       130–31.

115 **"easily become injurious"**: Putnam Jacobi, *The Question of Rest for Women During Menstruation*, 227.

115 **"... women whose nutrition ..."**: Putnam Jacobi, *The Question of Rest for Women During Menstruation*, 227.

115 **"... obstetrical practice at menstrual periods"**: Edward Tilt, "The Relations of Women to Obstetric Practice" (extract from the president's address, delivered at the Obstetrical Society on January 7, 1874), *British Medical Journal*, January 16, 1874, 73.

116 **"future womanly usefulness"**: S. Weir Mitchell, *Wear and Tear; or, Hints for the Overworked* (Philadelphia: J. B. Lippincott, 1871), 33.

117 **their biological destiny**: See Suzanne Poirier, "The Weir Mitchell Rest Cure: Doctors and Patients," *Women's Studies* 10 (1983): 17–18.

117 **"a rather nervous temperament"**: S. Weir Mitchell, *Lectures on Diseases of the Nervous System, Especially in Women* (Philadelphia: Henry C. Lea's Son, 1881), 55, quoted in Poirier, "The Weir Mitchell Rest Cure," 18.

117 **"... drama of hysteria"**: S. Weir Mitchell, *Fat and Blood: And How to Make Them* (Philadelphia: J. B. Lippincott, 1877), 27–28.

117 **"One or two scoldings ..."**: Mitchell, *Lectures on Diseases of the Nervous System*, 27.

118 **"... to treat hysteria"**: Mitchell, *Lectures on Diseases of the Nervous System*, 30.

118 *New England Magazine*: Charlotte Perkins Gilman, "The Yellow Wallpaper," *New England Magazine* 11, no. 5 (January 1892): 647–57.

118 **"... images of distress"**: Charlotte Perkins Gilman, *The Living of Charlotte Perkins Gilman: An Autobiography* (New York: D. Appleton-Century, 1935; Madison: University of Wisconsin Press, 1990), 90.

119 **"... but you will know"**: Charlotte Perkins Gilman to S. Weir Mitchell (April 19, 1897), appended in Denise D. Knight "'All the Facts of the Case': Gilman's Lost Letter to Dr. S. Weir Mitchell," *American Literary Realism* 37, no. 3 (Spring 2005): 274.

119 **"... as long as you live"**: Gilman, *The Living of Charlotte Perkins Gilman*, 96.

119 **"... wade in glue"**: Gilman, *The Living of Charlotte Perkins Gilman*, 102.

119 **with constant rest**: See Mary Putnam Jacobi, "Some Considerations on Hysteria," in *Essays on Hysteria, Brain-Tumor, and Some Other Cases of Nervous Disease* (New York: G. P. Putnam's Sons, 1881), 1–80.

120 **"... helped me much"**: Gilman, *The Living of Charlotte Perkins Gilman*, 291.

120 **"... measure of power"**: Charlotte Perkins Gilman, "Why I Wrote *The Yellow Wallpaper*," *Forerunner Magazine*, October 1913.

120 **"... its hazy boundaries"**: S. Weir Mitchell, "Rest in Nervous Disease: Its Use and Abuse," in *A Series of American Clinical Lectures* 1, no. 4, ed. E. G. Seguin (New York: G. P. Putnam's Sons, 1875), 94.

120 **"... in the evening"**: F. C. Skey, *Hysteria: Remote Causes of Disease in General; Treatment of Disease by Tonic Agency; Local or Surgical Forms of Hysteria, etc. Six Lectures Delivered to Students of St. Bartholomew's Hospital, 1866* (London: Longmans, Green, Reader and Dyer, 1867), 47.

120 **"'will-o'-the-wisp'"**: Edward Tilt, *A Handbook of Uterine Therapeutics, and of Diseases of Women*, 4th ed. (1869; New York: William Wood, 1881), 85.

121 **their own terms**: For a fascinating investigation into the relationship between women and the alienists, neurologists, psychologists, and psychiatrists of the nineteenth and early twentieth centuries, including Charcot and Freud, see Lisa

Appignanesi's brilliant *Mad, Bad, and Sad: A History of Women and the Mind Doctors from 1800 to the Present* (London: Virago, 2008). See also Elaine Showalter's masterful *The Female Malady: Women, Madness and English Culture, 1830–1980* (London: Virago, 1987), particularly her chapter "Feminism and Hysteria: The Daughter's Disease," 145–64.

121 **hysteric "queens":** To learn about the lives of Charcot's most famous hysteric patients, his "queens" Marie "Blanche" Wittmann, Louise "Augustine" Gleizes, and Geneviève Basile Legrand, see Asti Hustvedt's beautiful, rich archival exploration *Medical Muses: Hysteria in Nineteenth-Century Paris* (New York: Bloomsbury, 2011).

9: SUFFRAGE AND SUPPRESSION

125 **social, legal, and political rights:** See Dale E. Miller, "Harriet Taylor Mill," *The Stanford Encyclopedia of Philosophy* (Spring 2019 edition), ed. Edward N. Zalta, https://plato.stanford.edu/archives/spr2019/entries/harriet-mill; Jo Ellen Jacobs, "'The Lot of Gifted Ladies Is Hard': A Study of Harriet Taylor Mill Criticism," *Hypatia* 9, no. 3 (Summer, 1994): 132–62; Janet A. Seiz and Michèle A. Pujol, "Harriet Taylor Mill," *American Economic Review* 90, no. 2 (May 2000): 476–79.

126 **"... male citizens of the community":** Harriet Taylor Mill, *Enfranchisement of Women: An Essay by Mrs. John Stuart Mill* (1851; reprinted from the *Westminster and Foreign Quarterly Review*; Missouri Woman's Suffrage Association, 1868), 3.

126 **"Women have never...":** Taylor Mill, *Enfranchisement of Women*, 6.

126 **faced the criticism:** See Jacobs, "'The Lot of Gifted Ladies Is Hard,'" 132–62.

126 **women had "shown fitness...":** Taylor Mill, *Enfranchisement of Women*, 10.

127 **before Seneca Falls:** See Evette Dionne, "Abolitionist Women Embrace the Fight," in *Lifting as We Climb: Black Women's Fight for the Ballot Box* (New York: Viking, 2020), 6–28.

127 **"Ain't I a Woman?":** Sojourner Truth's speech was transcribed faithfully by Marius Robinson and published in the *Anti-Slavery Bugle* in 1851. Another version, with most of the words changed and a "southern slave dialect" attributed to Truth, was constructed by Frances Dana Gage and published twelve years later in the *New York Independent*. It is Gage's version, with the addition of the resounding phrase "Ar'n't I a woman?," that has become the most common and popular reading. Both versions of Truth's speech can be read on the website of the Sojourner Truth Project, created by Leslie Podell (California College of the Arts, San Francisco), https://www.thesojournertruthproject.com/compare-the-speeches.

To read more about Truth's life, see her book *Narrative of Sojourner Truth* (1850; 1884), which is included with *Book of Life*, a collection of letters and sketches about Truth's life written subsequent to the original 1850 publication of the *Narrative* in a volume published by Penguin Random House in 1998, https://www.penguinrandomhouse.com/books/296530/narrative-of-sojourner-truth-by-sojourner-truth.

128 **"... ice is cracked":** Sojourner Truth's speech to the American Equal Rights Association, May 9, 1867, *New Frame*, August 15, 2019, https://www.newframe.com/from-the-archive-speech-to-the-american-equal-rights-association%EF%BB%BF.

128 **"... and not the woman"**: Dionne, *Lifting as We Climb*, 46.

128 **"... mattered to black women"**: Dionne, *Lifting as We Climb*, 54.

128 **Black activists, writers, and educators:** See Evette Dionne, "The Rise of Black Women's Suffrage Clubs," in Dionne, *Lifting as We Climb*, 56–75.

129 **women's "legal subordination"**: John Stuart Mill, *The Subjection of Women* (London: Longmans, Green, Reader, and Dyer, 1869), 1.

129 **"... differences between men and women ..."**: J. Crichton-Browne, "The Annual Oration on Sex in Education" (delivered before the Medical Society of London), *British Medical Journal* (May 7, 1892), 1636.

130 **females' lower position:** For a brilliant discussion of the influence of Darwinian evolutionary theory on the gendered beliefs of Victorian psychologists, psychiatrists, and neurologists about female insanity, see Elaine Showalter, "Nervous Women: Sex Roles and Sick Roles," in *The Feminine Malady: Women, Madness, and English Culture* (London: Virago, 1987), 121–129.

130 **"the great mass of women ..."**: Mr. Wadleigh, "Report (to accompany bill S. resolution 12)," Report 523, 45th Cong., 2d Sess., June 14, 1878, https://www.senate.gov/artandhistory/history/People/Women/Nineteenth_Amendment_Vertical_Timeline.htm.

131 **"... her by ignorance"**: Senator Joseph Dolph, *Congressional State Record*, US Senate (January 25, 1887), 985.

131 **Senate also considered:** *Arguments Before the Select Committee on Woman Suffrage*, US Senate, March 7, 1884, in Cong. Rec. (January 25, 1887), 992–1002.

132 **"... her entire nature"**: Mary Putnam Jacobi, *Common Sense Applied to Woman Suffrage: A statement of the reasons which justify the demand to extend the suffrage to women, with consideration of the arguments against such enfranchisement, and with special reference to the issues presented to the New York State Convention of 1894* (New York: G. P. Putnam and Sons, 1894), 85.

132 **"differentiation of the sexes"**: Putnam Jacobi, *Common Sense Applied to Woman Suffrage*, 108.

132 **"... What a mournful disillusion!"**: Putnam Jacobi, *Common Sense Applied to Woman Suffrage*, 108.

133 **"... question of the suffrage ..."**: "Opposed to Woman Suffrage—Anti-Suffrage Association Gives Reasons to Congress of Women," *New York Times*, July 2, 1899, 18.

133 **"... certainty injure women"**: Miss Katherine E. Conway, "Nature's Stern Barriers," *The Remonstrance* (Boston, January 1908), 3, from the Massachusetts Association Opposed to the Further Extension of Suffrage to Women Records, Massachusetts Historical Society Collections online, accessed November 16, 2020, https://www.masshist.org/database/3381.

134 **"... immediate action in the matter"**: *Votes for Women* 2, no. 40 (December 10, 1908). The archives of *Votes for Women* have been digitized as part of London School of Economics Women's Rights Collection. To browse this incredible collection of suffragist literature, journals, pamphlets, and reports, visit https://digital.library.lse.ac.uk/collections/suffrage.

134 **"... offered them a stone"**: "At the Albert Hall," *Votes for Women*, December 10, 1908.

134 **"with great violence"**: Helen Ogston, "Why I Used the Dog-Whip," *Votes for Women*, December 10, 1908.

135 "... against injustice heard": "Extraordinary Violence," *Votes for Women*, December 10, 1908.

136 "... are suffering from hysteria ...": "Hysterical Enthusiasm," *The London Times*, December 11, 1908.

136 "... literature of the question": "Some Suffering from Hysteria," *New York Times*, December 13, 1908.

136 "The sensation is most painful": "Forcible Feeding: A Statement by Mary Leigh to Her Solicitor," *Votes for Women*, October 15, 1909.

137 decried "forced feeding": Louisa Garrett Anderson, "Fasting Prisoners and Compulsory Feeding," *British Medical Journal* (October 1, 1909), 1099.

137 "That's my business": Statement by Mary Richardson on forcible feeding, February 6, 1914, "Suffragettes on File," National Archives (catalog ref: HO 144/1305/248506), https://www.nationalarchives.gov.uk/education/resources/suffragettes-on-file/mary-richardson.

138 "violent resistance": Agnes Savill and Victor Horsley, "Preliminary Report on the Forcible Feeding of Suffrage Prisoners," *British Medical Journal*, August 31, 1912, 505.

138 rectum and vagina: Historian June Purvis writes, "Although the word 'rape' is not used in the personal accounts of force-fed victims, the instrumental invasion of the body, accompanied by overpowering physical force, great suffering and humiliation was akin to it, especially so for women fed through the rectum or vagina." Purvis, "The Prison Experiences of the Suffragettes in Edwardian Britain," *Women's History Review* 4, no. 1 (1995): 123. Purvis includes the testimony of Fanny Parker, who went by the pseudonym Janet Arthur, who was fed in this way in Scotland's Perth prison in 1914. She was fed though the rectum "in a cruel way" that caused her "great pain." A subsequent feeding, through the vagina, "proved to be a grosser and more indecent outrage, which could not have been done for any other purpose than torture. It was followed by soreness, which lasted several days." See "Another Prison Infamy," *Votes for Women*, August 7, 1914.

138 dangerous pathology: British physician and mental illness specialist Thomas Claye Shaw, for example, believed the militant suffragists were exhibiting a new manifestation of female insanity. Suffrage, he wrote in *The Lancet*, had revealed elements of women's "emotional strength" and "intense concentrated ideism" that were "hitherto unknown ... for we are having practical displays of revenge, spite, and all the embodiments of what is generally called 'devilry.'" Claye Shaw, "The Psychology of the Militant Suffragette," *The Lancet*, May 17, 1913, 1415. For the pioneering bacteriologist Almroth Wright, militant suffrage was a symptom of menopausal insanity. Wright claimed the movement was led by "sexually embittered" older women whose mental state had become disordered thanks to their empty wombs and atrophied ovaries. Wright, *The Unexpurgated Case Against Woman Suffrage* (London: Constable, 1913), and *Suffrage Fallacies: Sir Almroth Wright on "Militant Hysteria"; a Letter Reprinted from "The Times" of Thursday, March 28, 1912* (London: John Parkinson Bland, 1912).

10: BIRTH CONTROL

143 "... bound and helpless": Marguerite Tracy and Mary Boyd, *Painless Childbirth: A General Survey on All Painless Methods with Special Stress on*

"Twilight Sleep" and Its Extension to America (New York: Frederick A. Stokes, 1915), 8.

143 **"not a trace of a memory"**: Tracy and Boyd, *Painless Childbirth*, 9.

143 **". . . not felt by the woman . . ."**: Bernhard Krönig, "Painless Delivery in Dämmerschlaf" (1908), trans. Tracy and Boyd, appendix 1, in *Painless Childbirth*, 212.

144 **45.5 percent of all women's deaths:** Bureau of the Census, *Mortality Statistics: 1910*, Bulletin 109, United States Department of Commerce and Labor (Washington, DC: United States Government Printing Office, 1912), 25.

144 **Protracted and difficult labors:** Judith Walzer Leavitt, "Under the Shadow of Maternity: American Women's Responses to Death and Debility Fears in Nineteenth-Century Childbirth," *Feminist Studies* 12, no. 1 (Spring 1986): 136–38.

145 **"Am I not almost a savage?":** Elizabeth Cady Stanton, letter to Lucretia Mott, October 22, 1852, quoted in Joanna Bourke, *The Story of Pain: From Prayer to Painkillers* (Oxford: Oxford University Press, 2014), 209–10.

145 **"to an alarming extent":** Krönig, "Painless Delivery in Dämmerschlaf"; and Tracy and Boyd, *Painless Childbirth*, 205–6.

147 **". . . put away like the dead":** "Mrs. Mark Boyd's Story," in Tracy and Boyd, *Painless Childbirth*, 195.

147 **". . . by my own efforts":** "Mrs. Mark Boyd's Story," in Tracy and Boyd, *Painless Childbirth*, 196.

148 **"the Painless Childbirth propaganda":** "Mrs. Francis Carmody's Story," Tracy and Boyd, *Painless Childbirth*, 200.

148 **". . . curse of their sex":** "Twilight Sleep: Miss Tracy and Mrs. Boyd's Survey of New Methods," *New York Times*, April 11, 1915.

149 **". . . new era has dawned . . .":** "Twilight Sleep Is Subject of a New Investigation," *New York Times*, January 31, 1915.

150 **". . . doctors are opposed to it":** Judith Walzer Leavitt, *Brought to Bed: Childbearing in America, 1750–1950* (Oxford: Oxford University Press, 1986), 131.

150 **". . . Women have torn away . . .":** Hanna Rion, *The Truth About Twilight Sleep* (New York: McBride, Nast, 1915), 55–56.

151 **". . . neurologist to elucidate":** J. H. Salisbury, "The Twilight Sleep in Obstetrics," *Journal of American Medicine* 63, no. 16 (1914): 1410. Also cited in L. MacIvor Thompson, "The Politics of Female Pain: Women's Citizenship, Twilight Sleep and the Early Birth Control Movement," *Medical Humanities* 45 (2019): 67–74.

152 **end of the bed:** Bertha Van Hoosen, *Scopolamine-Morphine Anesthesia* (Chicago: House of Manz, 1915), 41–42.

153 **". . . be called normal?":** Joseph B. DeLee, *The Principles and Practice of Obstetrics* (Philadelphia: W. B. Saunders, 1914), xii–xiii.

153 **episiotomy site tightly stitched:** See Judith Walzer Leavitt, "Joseph B. DeLee and the Practice of Preventative Obstetrics," *American Journal of Public Health* 78, no. 10 (October 1988): 1354.

153 **". . . as she was before":** Joseph B. DeLee, "The Prophylactic Forceps Operation," *American Journal of Obstetrics and Gynecology* 1 (1920): 41.

153 **"the wretchedness of unwilling parenthood":** Mary Ware Dennett, "Speech at the Meeting Which Organized the National Birth Control League" (March 1915), Papers of Mary Ware Dennett and the Voluntary Parenthood League,

Schlesinger Library, Radcliffe Institute, Harvard University, http://jackiewhit
ing.net/Women/Mother/DennettBC.htm.

153 **she needed surgery:** See Constance M. Chen, *The Sex Side of Life: Mary Ware Dennett's Pioneering Battle for Birth Control* (New York: New Press, 1996), 49–56.

154 **"... the Right to live":** *The Woman Rebel* 1, no. 1 (March 1914): 3, https://libcom .org/files/The%20Woman%20Rebel%20v1.n01.pdf.

155 **"... strongest will-power":** Margaret H. Sanger, *Family Limitation*, rev. 6th ed. (1917), 6, Michigan State University Libraries, https://archive.lib.msu.edu /DMC/AmRad/familylimitations.pdf.

155 **sex "is not desired ...":** Sanger, *Family Limitation*, 6.

155 **"physiological, emotional, and spiritual":** Dennett, "Speech at the Meeting Which Organized the National Birth Control League."

156 **love "can't be bought":** Dennett, *The Sex Side of Life: An Explanation for Young People* (New York, 1919), 16.

156 **"... there is hunger":** Margaret Sanger, "What Every Girl Should Know: Part III—Some Consequences of Ignorance and Silence," *New York Call*, March 2, 1913, 15; Public Writings and Speeches of Margaret Sanger, *New York University*, https://www.nyu.edu/projects/sanger/webedition/app/documents/show .php?sangerDoc=304928.xml.

157 **"... unhappiness and worry":** Margaret H. Sanger, "Abortion in the United States," *The Woman Rebel* 1, no. 3 (May 1914): 24, https://libcom.org/files/The %20Woman%20Rebel%20v1.n03.pdf.

158 **weakened her pulse:** "Mrs. Byrne Now Fed by Force," *New York Times*, January 28, 1917.

158 **She was so unwell:** "Mrs. Byrne Pardoned; Pledged to Obey Law," *New York Times*, February 2, 1917.

158 **"... asylums and premature graves":** Sanger, *Family Limitation*, 3.

159 **"... normal male organ":** Lesley Hall, "'The Subject Is Obscene: No Lady Would Dream of Alluding to It': Marie Stopes and Her Courtroom Dramas," *Women's History Review* 22, no. 2 (2013): 257.

159 **"a service to humanity":** Marie Carmichael Stopes, *Married Love, or Love in Marriage* (London: Critic and Guide, 1918), xiii.

160 **"horrible and criminal abortion":** Stopes, *Married Love*, 89–90.

161 **the "Racial Cap":** Rubber Vault Cap (with the "Racial" trademark), 1915–1925, Marie Stopes Memorial Foundation, Obstetrics, Gynecology and Contraception collections, Science Museum, http://brought tolife.sciencemuseum.org.uk /brought tolife/objects/display?id=92331.

162 **"... physically and mentally tainted":** Marie Carmichael Stopes, *Radiant Motherhood: A Book for Those Who Are Creating the Future* (London: G. P. Putnam's Sons; and Toronto: Musson Book Company, 1918), 212.

162 **"... structure of racial betterment":** Margaret H. Sanger, "Birth Control and Racial Betterment," *Birth Control Review* (February 1919), the Public Writings and Speeches of Margaret Sanger, https://www.nyu.edu/projects/sanger /webedition/app/documents/show.php?sangerDoc=143449.xml.

163 **fitness of "the black race":** W. E. B. DuBois, "Black Folk and Birth Control," *Birth Control Review* 16, no. 6 (June 1932): 166–67, document 17B, "Women and Social Movements," Alexander Street, https://documents.alexanderstreet.com /d/1000670632.

164   **young, impoverished women:** See "The Supreme Court and the Sterilization of Carrie Buck," Facing History and Ourselves, https://www.facinghistory.org /resource-library/supreme-court-and-sterilization-carrie-buck.

164   **pejorative and dehumanizing:** See "The Sanger-Hitler Equation," Newsletter 32 (Winter 2002–2003), Margaret Sanger Papers Project, New York University, https://www.nyu.edu/projects/sanger/articles/sanger-hitler_equation.php.

165   **". . . safeguard their lives":** Margaret H. Sanger, "My Way to Peace," January 17, 1932, Margaret Sanger Papers Project, New York University, https://www .nyu.edu/projects/sanger/webedition/app/documents/show.php?sangerDoc=1290 37.xml.

11: FEMININE RADIANCE

168   **". . . diseases and physical disabilities of women . . .":** In her first book, *The Evolution of Woman*, published in 1894 by G. P. Putnam's Sons, New York, Eliza Burt Gamble inaugurated her feminist critique of Darwinian concepts of gender difference by arguing that patriarchal society, and not evolutionary factors, was responsible for forcing women into inferior social roles and positions. Gamble wrote her book, which the *Chicago Tribune* called "an ingenious plea for the superiority and supremacy of the female sex," after spending a year studying evolutionary and anthropological theory at the Library of Congress, in Washington, DC, in 1885. *The Sexes in Science and History*, Gamble's third book, was a reexamination and republication of her research and work in *The Evolution of Women*. See "The Evolution of Eliza Burt Gamble: Her Life, Works and Influence," *Women in Science*, Michigan State University Archives, http://womenin science.history.msu.edu/Biography/C-4A-2/eliza-burt-gamble.

168   **"The diseases peculiar to the female constitution . . .":** Eliza Burt Gamble, *The Sexes in Science and History: An Inquiry into the Dogma of Women's Inferiority to Men* (New York: G. P. Putnam's Sons, 1916), 54.

169   **". . . materially injured her constitution":** Gamble, *The Sexes in Science and History*, 54.

169   **". . . equipped male mate":** Gamble, *The Sexes in Science and History*, 99.

170   **this expanding discipline:** See Ornella Moscucci on Blair Bell as the pioneer of gynecological endocrinology in *The Science of Women: Gynecology and Gender in England 1800–1929* (Cambridge: Cambridge University Press, 1990), 206.

170   **"femininity and its causes":** William Blair Bell, *The Sex Complex: A Study of the Relationships of the Internal Secretions to the Female Characteristics and Functions in Health and Disease* (London: Baillière, Tindall and Cox, 1916), 2.

170   **". . . consequence of the ovary":** Rudolf Virchow, "The Puerperal State: Woman and the Cell," lecture to the Berlin Obstetrical Society, January 11, 1848, quoted in Mary Putnam Jacobi, *The Question of Rest for Women During Menstruation* (New York: G. P. Putnam's Sons, 1877), 109–10.

170   **". . . the mystery of sex":** Blair Bell, *The Sex Complex*, 2.

171   **". . . on all the internal secretions":** Blair Bell, *The Sex Complex*, 5. Italics in original.

171   **neurological and vascular disturbances:** Chandak Sengoopta, "The Modern Ovary: Constructions, Meanings, Uses," *History of Science* 38, no. 4 (2000): 442.

171   **confined to a sanatorium:** Carlo Bonomi, "The Castration of Women and Girls," in *The Cut in the Building of Psychoanalysis*, vol. 1, *Sigmund Freud and Emma Eckstein* (Routledge, 2015), 39.

172   **fed either raw or cooked:** J. Lindholm and P. Laurberg, "Hypothyroidism and Thyroid Substitution: Historical Aspects," *Journal of Thyroid Research* (2011), doi:10:4061/2011/809341.

172   **"mild and genial climates":** Robert Alex Lundie, "The Treatment of Myxoedema," *Transactions of the Medical and Chirurgical Society of Edinburgh* 12 (1893): 134.

172   **she had no thyroid:** Lindholm and Laurberg, "Hypothyroidism and Thyroid Substitution."

172   **"oppressed by the weight . . .":** Lundie, "The Treatment of Myxoedema," 135–36.

172   **"difficult to believe they were sisters . . .":** Lundie, "The Treatment of Myxoedema," 136.

173   **". . . where magic potions . . .":** Lundie, "The Treatment of Myxoedema," 136.

173   **placebo of "scraped meat":** Emil Novak, "An Appraisal of Ovarian Therapy" (6th annual scientific session of the Association for the Study of Internal Secretions, St. Louis, Missouri, May 22, 1922), *Endocrinology* 6, no. 5 (September 1, 1922): 600.

173   **tissues of cow ovaries:** Thomas Schlich, "Reconstructing Women: Ovarian Transplants," in *The Origins of Organ Transplantation: Surgery and Laboratory Science, 1880–1930* (Rochester, NY: University of Rochester Press, 2010), 87.

174   **these proved successful:** Elizabeth A. McAninch and Antonio C. Bianco, "The History and Future of Treatment of Hypothyroidism," *Annals of Internal Medicine* 164, no. 1 (2016): 50–56.

174   **ovarian tissue being absorbed:** Sengoopta, "The Modern Ovary," 443–44.

174   **". . . rest of the genital system":** Josef Halban (1899), quoted in Chandak Sengoopta, "The Modern Ovary," 445.

174   **". . . airplanes and woman students":** W. J. O'Connor, *British Physiologists 1885–1914: A Biographical Dictionary* (Manchester: Manchester University Press, 1991), 42.

175   **". . . functions known to womanhood":** Dr. Arthur Johnstone, *New York Medical News* (October 6, 1900), quoted in "The Internal Secretion of the Ovary," *Hospital and Health Review* 29, no. 734 (October 20, 1900): 47.

175   **Only if the ovaries:** A. Louise McIlroy, "The Physiological Influence of Ovarian Secretions," *Proceedings of the Royal Society of Medicine* 5 (July 1, 1912): 342.

176   **Her surgical brilliance:** "Dame Anne Louise McIlroy, 1877–1968," Royal College of Physicians, https://history.rcplondon.ac.uk/inspiring-physicians /dame-anne-louise-mcilroy.

176   **one hundred volunteer women doctors:** "Dr. Louise McIlroy," First World War Glasgow, https://www.firstworldwarglasgow.co.uk/index.aspx?articleid =11526; Marlène Cornelis, "'My dears, if you are successful over this work, you will have carried women's profession forward a hundred years': The Case of the Scottish Women's Hospital for Foreign Service" (thesis, University of Glasgow, September 2018), https://nvmg.nl/app/uploads/2019/04/Dissertation -Appendix-1.pdf.

176   **". . . men's uncontrollable desires":** McIlroy quoted in Lesley A. Hall, "A Suitable Job for a Woman: Women Doctors and Birth Control to the Inception of the NHS," in *Women and Modern Medicine*, ed. Lawrence Conrad and Anne Hardy (New York: Ropodi, 2001), 129.

177   **"seize upon the evident differentiations":** Blair Bell, *The Sex Complex*, 121.

178 "... flooding her mind": Blair Bell, *The Sex Complex*, 208.

179 "no longer be a woman...": Blair Bell, *The Sex Complex*, 115.

179 dismissed as useless: See Judith A. Houck, *Hot and Bothered: Women, Medicine, and the Menopause in Modern America* (Cambridge, MA: Harvard University Press, 2006), 27–28.

180 "... menopause has been built up": Andrew F. Currier, *The Menopause: A Consideration of the Phenomena Which Occur to Women at the Close of the Child-Bearing Period* (New York: D. Appleton, 1897), quoted and discussed in Houck, *Hot and Bothered*, 14.

180 weather nature's storm: See Houck, *Hot and Bothered*, 44.

180 "... specific physical disorders": Walter M. Gallichan, *The Critical Age of Women* (London: T. Werner Laurie, 1927), 7–8.

180 "... without some general disturbances": William Blair Bell, *The Principles of Gynecology: A Manual for Students and Practitioners*, 3rd ed. (1910; New York: W. Wood, 1919), 116.

181 lexicon of lack and failure: Emily Martin, "Medical Metaphors of Women's Bodies," in *The Woman in the Body: A Cultural Analysis of Reproduction* (Milton Keynes: Open University Press, 1989), 42–46.

181 misdiagnosed—especially as depression and anxiety: Louise R. Newson, "My Personal Experience of Menopause," *British Journal of General Practice: The Journal of the Royal College of General Practitioners* 67, no. 656 (2017): 125.

182 more "violent derangements": Blair Bell, *The Sex Complex*, 206.

182 restore fertility in "sterile" women: Virgil Coblentz, *The Newer Remedies: A Reference Book for Physicians, Pharmacists, and Students* (Philadelphia: P. Blakiston's Son, 1899), 97, 98, 100.

184 Pinkham's compound "restored me...": "Testimony of Five Women Proves That Lydia E. Pinkham's Vegetable Compound Is Reliable," *Lompoc Journal*, no. 11 (July 27, 1912), California Digital Newspaper Collection, UCR Center for Bibliographical Studies and Research, https://cdnc.ucr.edu/cgi-bin/cdnc?a=d&d=LJ19120727.2.46&e=-------en--20--1--txt-txIN-------1.

184 providing radiation therapy: John B. Nanninga, *The Gland Illusion: Early Attempts at Rejuvenation Through Male Hormone Therapy* (Jefferson, NC: McFarland, 2017), 87–88.

185 "... hormones into the bloodstream": Gertrude Atherton, "Introduction," *Black Oxen* by Gertrude Atherton, ed. Melanie V. Dawson (Broadview, 2012), 22.

185 "wrote steadily for four hours": Atherton, "Introduction", *Black Oxen*, 22–23.

185 "a future menaced with utter fatigue": Gertrude Atherton, *Adventures of a Novelist* (London, 1932), 542, quoted in Sengoopta, "The Modern Ovary," 462.

185 "... women's road to the goal of rejuvenation...": John Kindred on "Rejuvenation in Women," during "Rejuvenation of the Bodily and Sexual Powers of Men and Women," Cong. Rec. (House, 1927), https://www.govinfo.gov/content/pkg/GPO-CRECB-1927-pt2-v68/pdf/GPO-CRECB-1927-pt2-v68-11-2.pdf.

187 "its biological counterparts, maleness and femaleness": H. Benjamin, "The Transexual Phenomenon," *Transactions of the New York Academy of Sciences* 29, no. 4, series 2 (1967): 428.

187 Progynon pills promised: "Glass Bottle for Progynon Pills, 1928–1948," Science Museum, London, Wellcome Trust, https://wellcomecollection.org/works/zzzx2g6s.

187   **product called Emmenin:** S. R. Davis, I. Dinatale, L. Rivera-Woll, and
       S. Davison, "Postmenopausal Hormone Therapy: From Monkey Glands to
       Transdermal Patches," *Journal of Endocrinology* 185 (2005): 207–22.

189   **relief for many women:** Judith A. Houck, "How to Treat a Menopausal Woman:
       A History, 1900–2000," *Current Women's Health Reports* 2, no. 5 (October
       2002): 351.

189   **poorly tested synthetic estrogens:** Patricia A. Jansen, "Menopause and His-
       torical Constructions of Cancer Risk," *Canadian Bulletin of Medical History* 28,
       1 (2011): 51–52.

12: LIFTING THE CURSE

190   **"none of them did . . . any good":** Patient testimony in Clelia Duel Mosher, "A
       Physiologic Treatment of Congestive Dysmenorrhea and Kindred Disorders
       Associated with the Menstrual Function," *Journal of the American Medical As-
       sociation* 62, no. 17 (1914): 1297–1301.

191   **"pain, cramps or any bad effects":** Patient testimony in Mosher, *A Physiologic
       Treatment,* 10.

191   **ambitions to become a doctor:** Katharine R. Parker, "Clelia Duel Mosher and
       the Change in Women's Sexuality," in *The Human Tradition in the Gilded Age and
       Progressive Era,* ed. Ballard C. Campbell (Wilmington, DE: Scholarly Resources
       Inc., 2000): 119–20; see also Klara Platoni's biography of Mosher in "The Sex
       Scholar," *Stanford Magazine* (March–April 2010), https://stanfordmag.org/con
       tents/the-sex-scholar.

192   **assumed they must be "abnormal":** Clelia Duel Mosher, "Functional Periodic-
       ity in Women and Some of the Modifying Factors," *California State Journal of
       Medicine* 9, no. 1 (1911): 4–5.

192   **Mosher was a solitary person:** Parker, "Clelia Duel Mosher and the Change in
       Women's Sexuality," 132–33.

193   **ties and simple brimmed hats:** Parker, "Clelia Duel Mosher and the Change in
       Women's Sexuality," 122.

193   **". . . misery can scarcely be measured":** Mosher, "Functional Periodicity in
       Women," 7.

193   **evolved "costal" breathing:** Henry Sewell and Myra E. Pollard, "On the Rela-
       tions of Diaphragmatic and Costal Respiration, with Particular Reference to
       Phonation," *Journal of Physiology* 11, no. 3 (1890): 159–69.

194   **constrictive clothing and medical speculations:** Clelia Duel Mosher,
       "Strength of Women," *Proceedings of the International Conference of Women Physi-
       cians* (New York: Woman's Press, 1920), 17.

194   **"Health is the birthright . . .":** Clelia Duel Mosher, *Women's Physical Freedom*
       (New York: Woman's Press, 1923), 89.

194   **all healthy and vigorous:** Mosher, *A Physiologic Treatment* (1914), 12–13.

195   **". . . at one time in my life":** J. P. Pratt and Edgar Allen, "Clinical Tests of the
       Ovarian Follicular Hormone," *Journal of the American Medical Association* 86, no.
       26 (1926): 1967.

195   **"central idea" of women's lives:** Mosher, "Functional Periodicity in Women
       and Some of the Modifying Factors," 4–5.

195   **". . . during the menopause and afterward":** Discussion, Mosher, "Strength of
       Women," 20.

196 **rare in women over twenty-five:** G. Herman, "Discussion on the Causes and Treatment of Dysmenorrhoea," *British Medical Journal* 2, no. 2599 (1910): 1211.

196 **"be relieved of menstruation and its sufferings":** Herman, "Discussion on the Causes and Treatment of Dysmenorrhoea," 1212.

196 **"neurasthenia" . . . "hysteria":** Herman, "Discussion on the Causes and Treatment of Dysmenorrhoea," 1212.

197 **"prevented convenient coitus":** Sir John Bland-Sutton, *Fibroids of the Uterus: Their Pathology, Diagnosis, and Treatment* (London: Science Reviews, 1913), 61.

197 **". . . a *woman*, and not a thing":** H. H. Hahn, "Electricity in Gynecology: Based on an Experience of Over One Thousand Applications," *Journal of American Medicine* 20 (1893): 328, quoted and discussed in Lawrence D. Longo, "Electrotherapy in Gynecology: The American Experience," *Bulletin of the History of Medicine* 60, no. 3 (1986): 351.

197 **"Hysterectomy for fibroids is unrivaled . . .":** Bland-Sutton, preface, *Fibroids of the Uterus* (1913), 61.

197–98 **might become malignant:** Ornella Moscucci, "The 'Ineffable Freemasonry of Sex': Feminist Surgeons and the Establishment of Radiotherapy in Early Twentieth-Century Britain," *Bulletin of the History of Medicine* 81 (2007): 141–42.

198 **"post-operative insanity":** Alban H. Doran, *The Present Position of Our Knowledge with Regard to the Treatment of Uterine Fibroids* (London: Royal College of Surgeons, 1903), 13.

198 **two to three times more likely to be affected:** Linda Goler Blount, "It's Not Normal: Black Women, Stop Suffering from Fibroids," Black Women's Health Imperative, April 3, 2019, https://bwhi.org/2019/04/03/its-not-normal-black-women-stop-suffering-from-fibroids.

198 **have a hysterectomy:** All-Party Parliamentary Group on Women's Health, *Informed Choice? Giving Women Control of Their Healthcare*, report on treatment of endometriosis and fibroids, based on a survey of 2,600 women treated at NHS trusts in the UK, 2017, http://www.appgwomenshealth.org/inquiry2017.

199 **seventy hysterectomies during their residencies:** See "The 'Madness' of Unnecessary Hysterectomy Has to Stop," Lown Institute, April 12, 2019, https://lowninstitute.org/guest-post-the-madness-of-unnecessary-hysterectomy-has-to-stop. The author refers, and links to, obstetrics and gynecology case-log minimums laid down by the Accreditation Council for Graduate Medical Education (US) in 2018, https://www.acgme.org/Portals/0/PFAssets/ProgramResources/220_Ob_Gyn_Minimum_Numbers_Announcement.pdf?ver=2018-06-25-104354-993.

199 **And in the UK:** All-Party Parliamentary Group on Women's Health, *Informed Choice?*, 16, 21.

199 **"the treatment *deluxe*":** Louisa Martindale, "The Treatment of Thirty-Seven Cases of Uterine Fibromyomata by Intensive X-Ray Therapy," *British Medical Journal* 538 (October 9, 1920): 539.

199 **". . . free from any mortality":** Martindale, "The Treatment of Thirty-Seven Cases of Uterine Fibromyomata," 539.

200 **woman doctors to bravely lead:** Louisa Martindale, "The Woman Doctor's Future," in *The Woman Doctor* (London: Mills and Boon, 1922), 133–53.

201 **"for the radiological treatment of women . . .":** Robert J. Dickson, "The Marie Curie Hospital 1925–1968," *British Medical Journal* (November 16, 1968): 444.

201 **private donations and public organizations:** See Dickson, "The Marie Curie Hospital 1925–1968"; and Ornella Moscucci, "The 'Ineffable Freemasonry of Sex.'"

201 **all cancer clinics worldwide:** "The Marie Curie Hospital," *British Medical Journal* 2 (December 15, 1934): 1105.

201 **13,802 cases of cancer:** Dickson, "The Marie Curie Hospital 1925–1968," 446.

202 **illness that "greatly handicapped (women)...":** "The Economics of Menstruation," *British Medical Journal* (April 7, 1928): 606.

202 **pursued research projects:** Barbara Brookes, "'The Glands of Destiny': Hygiene, Hormones and English Women Doctors in the First Half of the 20th Century," *Canadian Bulletin of Medical History* 23, no. 1 (2006): 55–57.

203 **"... greater sense of proportion":** Alice E. Sanderson Clow, opening paper, "Discussion on Dysmenorrhea in Young Women: Its Incidence, Prevention, and Treatment" (British Medical Association Proceedings of the Annual Meeting, Bradford, 1924, Section of Obstetrics and Gynecology), *British Medical Journal* (September 27, 1924): 558–61, 564–66.

203 **"... normal healthy women":** "The Economics of Menstruation," *British Medical Journal* (April 7, 1928): 606.

203 **"normal" bleeding woman:** T. G. Stevens, in the textbook *The Diseases of Women* (1931), claimed "that 'very few women' could be said to be 'normal, mentally or physically, during menstruation.'" Brookes, "The Glands of Destiny," 60.

204 **Her "nervous disturbance":** Robert T. Frank, "Case 3," in "The Hormonal Causes of Premenstrual Tension" (read at a meeting of the Section of Neurology and Psychiatry, New York Academy of Medicine, February 10, 1931), *Archives of Neurology and Psychiatry* 26, no. 5 (1931): 1054–55.

204 **"foolish ..." and "reprehensible actions":** Frank, "The Hormonal Causes of Premenstrual Tension," 1054.

205 **many "obscure diseases":** Robert T. Frank and M. A. Goldberger, "Clinical Data Obtained with the Female Sex Hormone Blood Test," *Journal of the American Medical Association* 90 (January 14, 1928): 106.

205 **connecting PMT to conflicts:** Karen Horney, "Premenstrual Tension," *Feminine Psychology* (1931; New York: W. W. Norton, 1967), 99–106.

206 **"a servant of the species":** Paul Roazen, *Helene Deutsch: A Psychoanalyst's Life* (New Brunswick: Transaction, 1992), 234, 340; David S. Janowsky, "Menstrual and Premenstrual Mood Disorders" (Psychodynamic Hypotheses), in *Phenomenology and Treatment of Psychophysiological Disorders*, ed. W. E. Fann et al. (New York: Spectrum Publications, 1982), 112–13.

206 **period blood triggered "phantasies":** Mary Chadwick, *The Psychological Effects of Menstruation* (New York: Nervous and Mental Disease Publishing, 1932).

206 **"distinctive biological characteristics":** Emil Novak, *The Woman Asks the Doctor*, 2nd ed. (1935; Baltimore: Williams and Wilkins, 1944), vii.

206 **"... cobwebbery of mystery":** Novak, *The Woman Asks the Doctor*, 14.

207 **watershed moment for menstrual health:** Rainey Horwitz, "Menstrual Tampon," *Embryo Project Encyclopedia* (May 25, 2020), http://embryo.asu.edu/handle/10776/13151. See also Sarah Kowalski, "Welcome to This New Day for Womanhood! Tampons in American History," December 1999, https://www.sccs.swarthmore.edu/users/01/sarahk/hers/school/tampon.html.

208 **"highly useful to gynecologists":** See Johanna Goldberg "'Solving Woman's Oldest Hygienic Problem in a New Way': A History of Period Products," Books, Health and History, New York Academy of Medicine, March 4, 2016,

https://nyamcenterforhistory.org/2016/03/04/solving-womans-oldest-hygienic -problem-in-a-new-way-a-history-of-period-products; and Ashley Fetters, "The Tampon: A History," *The Atlantic*, June 1, 2015, https://www.theatlantic.com /health/archive/2015/06/history-of-the-tampon/394334.

208 **"strenuous struggle for freedom"**: Tampax advertisement, "Women Are Winning the War—of Freedom" (UK, 1942), reprinted in Sophie Elmhurst, "Tampon Wars: The Battle to Overthrow the Tampax Empire," *The Guardian*, February 11, 2020.

13: DUTIFUL AND DISCIPLINED

211 **". . . health remains for her"**: Margery Spring Rice, *Working-Class Wives: Their Health and Conditions* (1939; London: Virago, 1981), 85–86.

211 **". . . ignoring obvious symptoms"**: "Maternal Mortality and Morbidity: Final Report of Departmental Committee," *British Medical Journal* 2, no. 3736 (August 13, 1932): 328. See also Ann Oakley, "Blaming the Victim?," in *The Captured Womb: A History of the Medical Care of Pregnant Women* (Oxford: Blackwell, 1984), 72–74.

211 **". . . resulting from childbirth"**: Spring Rice, *Working-Class Wives*, 19.

212 **". . . inseparable from maternity"**: "Maternal Mortality and Morbidity," *British Medical Journal*, 329.

212 **". . . expert study and care"**: Spring Rice, *Working-Class Wives*, 19.

213 **housewife's "health and happiness"**: Spring Rice, *Working-Class Wives*, 14, 18.

213 **". . . explain it to a doctor"**: Spring Rice, *Working-Class Wives*, 69.

214 **"our bodies are our own"**: F. W. Stella Browne, "Cooperative Women Demand Legalization of Abortion," *New Generation*, July 1934, Wellcome Collection, https://wellcomecollection.org/works/jd48925c.

215 **couldn't afford "female pills"**: Kate Fisher, *Birth Control, Sex, and Marriage in Britain, 1918–1960* (Oxford & New York: Oxford University Press: 2006), 159–63; and Stephen Brooke, *Sexual Politics: Sexuality, Family Planning, and the British Left from the 1880s to the Present Day* (Oxford & New York: Oxford University Press, 2011), 94.

215 **life-threatening sepsis:** Garson Romalis, "Why I Do Abortions" (speech to the Morgentaler Symposium, Toronto, January 25, 2008), *Reproductive Health Matters* 16, no. 31, supplement (2008): 66.

215 **the "masculine mythology"**: Lesley A. Hall, "'I Have Never Met a Normal Woman': Stella Browne and the Politics of Womanhood," *Women's History Review* 6, no. 2 (2006): 171–72.

215 **abstinence was dehumanizing:** F. W. Stella Browne quoted in Vicky Igliowski-Broad, "The Inter-Departmental Committee on Abortion," National Archives, October 26, 2017, https://blog.nationalarchives.gov.uk/inter -departmental-committee-abortion.

215 **improve the "existing situation"**: Deputation from the National Council of Women of Great Britain, Tuesday, February 11, 1936, at 11:00 a.m., National Archives. See Igliowski-Broad, "The Inter-Departmental Committee on Abortion."

216 **". . . girls always lead men on"**: "Charge of Procuring Abortion: *Rex v. Bourne*," *British Medical Journal* 2, no. 4046 (July 23, 1938): 199.

216 **". . . case of this sort"**: Letter from Dr. Joan Malleson to Mr. Bourne, May 21, 1938, "Charge of Procuring Abortion: *Rex v. Bourne*," 199.

217   **found not guilty:** "Charge of Procuring Abortion: Acquittal," *British Medical Journal* 2, no. 4046 (July 23, 1938): 204–5.

217   **"... conduct among young girls":** "The Abortion Report: Legal, Medical and Sociological Aspects—Clarification of Law Recommended," *British Medical Journal* 1, no. 4093 (June 17, 1939): 1250.

218   **"an ordinary decent girl ...":** "The Judge's Summing-Up," in "Charge of Procuring Abortion: *Rex v. Bourne*," 204.

218   **"... no concern of his":** "Charge of Procuring Abortion: *Rex v. Bourne*," 202.

218   **"... dead on the floor":** *Rex v. Bourne*, Central Criminal Court, J. Macnaghten, July 18–19, 1938, Women's Link Worldwide, https://www.womenslinkworld wide.org/files/2769/gjo-reinounido-1939-en-pdf.pdf.

218   **"predatory harpy":** See Kate Gleeson's discussion of the *Bourne* case and the authority of the medical establishment "over both women's abortion decisions and the procedure's legitimacy" in "The Strange Case of the Invisible Woman in Abortion-Law Reform," *Gender, Sexualities and Law*, ed. Jackie Jones et al. (New York: Routledge, 2011), 219. Gleeson writes, "At this time, the female lay-abortionist was frequently demonized as a 'predatory harpy' and, unsurprisingly, the overwhelming majority of those arrested for procuring abortion were women."

220   **"... those who can pay for it":** Leaflet, Workers' Birth Control Group (1927), Trades Union Congress archive, Warwick Digital Collections, https://wdc .contentdm.oclc.org/digital/collection/health/id/1716.

220   **condoms in the post:** Dr. Mary Caldwell's statements to the Birkett Committee, quoted in Madeleine Simms, "The Compulsory Pregnancy Lobby—Then and Now," Marie Stopes Memorial Lecture 1975, *Journal of the Royal College of General Practitioners* 25 (1975), 714–15.

220   **"counsel of despair":** Dorothy Thurtle, "The Minority Report," in "The Abortion Report: Legal, Medical and Sociological Aspects," 1251.

222   **"... guards the Kitchen Front":** Lord Woolton, BBC broadcast, April 8, 1940, quoted in Angela Davis, "Wartime Women Giving Birth: Narratives of Pregnancy and Childbirth, Britain c.1939–1960," *Studies in History and Philosophy of Biological and Biomedical Sciences* 47 (2014): 258.

222   **MOF declared in 1943:** Ann Oakley, *The Captured Womb: A History of the Medical Care of Pregnant Women* (Oxford: Blackwell, 1984), 122–25.

223   **person who didn't submit:** Gisela Bock, "Racism and Sexism in Nazi Germany: Motherhood, Compulsory Sterilization, and the State," *Signs*, no. 3, "Women and Violence" (Spring 1983): 411–15.

224   **admitted just to be sterilized:** "California" file in "Eugenics: Compulsory Sterilization in 50 American States," "Disability as Deviance" honors course students, ed. Lutz Kaelber, University of Vermont, 2009, http://www.uvm.edu /%7Elkaelber/eugenics/CA/CA.html. See also Dorothy Roberts, *Killing the Black Body: Race, Reproduction, and the Meaning of Liberty* (1997; New York: Vintage, 2017), 69–70.

225   **"hyperfertile" and "criminally inclined":** Sarah Zhang, "A Long-Lost Data Trove Uncovers California's Sterilization Program," *The Atlantic*, January 3, 2017, https://www.theatlantic.com/health/archive/2017/01/california -sterilization-records/511718/; Courtney Hutchison, "Sterilizing the Sick, Poor to Cut Welfare Costs," ABC News, July 18, 2011, https://abcnews.go.com /Health/WomensHealth/sterilizing-sick-poor-cut-welfare-costs-north-carolinas /story?id=14093458; and Alexandra Minna Stern, "Sterilized in the Name of

Public Health: Race, Immigration, and Reproductive Control in Modern California," *American Journal of Public Health* 95, no. 7 (2005): 1128–38.

225 **"high moron level":** Sterilization Order, Pacific Colony, Spadra, 1936, Sterilization and Social Justice Lab, University of Michigan, and California State Archives, https://www.ssjlab.org, included in Natalie Lira, "Latinos and the Consequences of Eugenics," PBS, October 16, 2018, https://www.pbs.org/wgbh/americanexperience/features/eugenics-latinos-and-the-consequences-of-eugenics.

225 **"Mississippi appendectomy":** Mississippi and North Carolina files in "Eugenics: Compulsory Sterilization in 50 American States."

226 **help run the Harlem clinic:** Roberts, *Killing the Black Body*, 87.

226 **battery-operated lamps:** George Davis, "A Healing Hand in Harlem," including an interview with May Chinn, *New York Times*, April 22, 1979, https://www.nytimes.com/1979/04/22/archives/a-healing-hand-in-harlem.html.

226 **clinic employed Black nurses:** Roberts, *Killing the Black Body*, 87–88.

226 **". . . relations between Blacks and whites":** Roberts, *Killing the Black Body*, 86.

227 **for health preservation only:** Lakshmeeramya Malladi, "United States v. One Package of Japanese Pessaries (1936)," Embryo Project Encyclopedia, May 24, 2017, https://embryo.asu.edu/pages/united-states-v-one-package-japanese-pessaries-1936.

227 **"recognize the need":** Margaret Sanger (1929), quoted in Roberts, *Killing the Black Body*, 88.

227 **Harlem Clinic closed:** Roberts, *Killing the Black Body*, 88.

227 **". . . lower living conditions":** National Emergency Council, *Report on the Economic Conditions of the South* (Washington, DC: United States Government Printing Office, 1938), 29.

228 **". . . spring from these conditions":** Mary Rinehardt [*sic*] and Margaret Sanger for the Birth Control Federation of America, "Birth Control and the Negro," draft proposal (July 1939), quoted in Joyce C. Follet, "The Negro Project," in *Making Democracy Real: African American Women, Birth Control, and Social Justice, 1910–1960*, Smith College (2019), https://sophia.smith.edu/making-democracy-real/the-Negro-project.

228 **"We do not want word to go . . .":** Margaret Sanger to Gamble, December 10, 1939, quoted and discussed in Roberts, *Killing the Black Body*, 77–78.

228 **". . . physicians in the country":** Dorothy Boulding Ferebee, "Planned Parenthood as a Public Health Measure for the Negro Race," presented at the symposium Planned Parenthood in Public Health and Welfare Programs, Thursday, January 29, 1942; Florence Rose Papers, Sophia Smith Collection, Smith College, Smith Libraries Exhibits, https://libex.smith.edu/omeka/items/show/447.

228 **"dried up female fanatic":** "Birth Control or Race Control? Sanger and the Negro Project," newsletter no. 28 (Fall 2001), Margaret Sanger Papers Project, New York University, https://www.nyu.edu/projects/sanger/articles/bc_or_race_control.php.

229 **". . . mothers and babies of this country":** Ferebee, "Planned Parenthood as a Public Health Measure for the Negro Race."

229 **". . . 'duty' for the poor":** Angela Davis, "Racism, Birth Control, and Reproductive Rights," in *From Abortion to Reproductive Freedom: Transforming a Movement*, ed. Marlene Gerber Fried (Boston: South End Press, 1990), 15, 20, quoted in Roberts, *Killing the Black Body*, 58.

230 "...economic circumstances justify": Peter Engelman, "Planned Parenthood," in *A History of the Birth Control Movement in America* (Santa Barbara: Praeger, 2011), 178; and Sarah Laskow, "What Planned Parenthood Taught WWII Veterans About Birth Control," *Atlas Obscura*, September 26, 2017, https://www.atlas obscura.com/articles/planned-parenthood-pamphlets-wwii-baby-boom-family -planning.

14: CONTROL AND PUNISH

231 **"denied any sexual exposure":** John R. Haserick and Roland Long, Case 3, "Systemic Lupus Erythematosus Preceded by False-Positive Serologic Tests for Syphilis: Presentation of Five Cases," presented at Midwest Regional Meeting of American College of Physicians in Columbus, Ohio, October 13, 1951, *Annals of Internal Medicine* 37, no. 3 (1952): 561.

232 **curb the rise of syphilis:** See Louis G. Iasili, "The Pre-marital Blood Test Law," *St. John's Law Review* 13, no. 1 (November 1938): 199–205.

232 **perpetuated racist misbeliefs:** For a discussion of the history of racist medical and biological misbeliefs about syphilis, see Harriet A. Washington's chapter "'A Notoriously Syphilis-Soaked Race': What *Really* Happened in Tuskegee?," in her brilliant book *Medical Apartheid: The Dark History of Medical Experimentation on Black Americans from Colonial Times to the Present* (New York: Anchor Books, 2006), 157–85.

233 **$40 and $50 million every year:** Allan M. Brandt, "'Shadow on the Land': Thomas Parran and the New Deal," in *No Magic Bullet: A Social History of Venereal Disease in the United States Since 1880*, expanded edition (New York: Oxford University Press, 1987), 129–130, 133–134.

233 **"unmentionable moral scourge . . .":** Iasili, "The Pre-marital Blood Test Law," 199.

233 **this "great plague":** "The Next Great Plague to Go" was the title of Parran's article on syphilis, which included infographics and statistics on disease rates and social costs, published in the progressive periodical *Survey Graphic* in 1936. The article reached the public widely through reprints in *Reader's Digest*, excerpts in newspaper articles, and health awareness posters. See Erin Wuebker's Venereal Disease Visual Culture Archive, "a project to present and make available visual culture materials related to syphilis and gonorrhea from the first half of the twentieth century," at https://vdarchive.newmedialab.cuny.edu/about.

233 **"... transmission from parent to child":** Iasili, "The Pre-marital Blood Test Law," 199.

233 **to their "progeny":** J. K. Shafer, "Premarital Health Examination Legislation: History and Analysis," *Public Health Reports* 69, no. 5 (1954): 487.

234 **responsibility of sexual health:** Shayla Love, "Why Aren't Straight Men Told to Get Regular STD Tests?," *Vice*, October 13, 2017, https://www.vice.com/en /article/xwgbma/straight-men-std-test-recommendations.

235 **"... protection for herself and humanity":** "The Mother's Charter," poster of the American Committee on Maternal Welfare, published in *Public Health Nursing* 33 (1941), 727, reprinted in Elizabeth Temkin, "Driving Through: Postpartum Care During World War II," *American Journal of Public Health* 89, no. 4 (April 1999): 588.

235 **"... Not for the Diseased":** "Happiness Ahead—for the Healthy but Not for the Diseased," c. 1942–1944, Venereal Disease Visual History Archive, https:// vdarchive.newmedialab.cuny.edu/items/show/215.

235   **women the perpetrators:** See Venereal Disease Visual Culture Archive; and
      Elizabeth Gettelman and Mark Murrmann, "The Enemy in Your Pants: The
      Military's Decades-Long War Against STDs," *Mother Jones* (May–June 2010),
      https://www.motherjones.com/media/2010/05/us-military-std-posters/.

235   **"hazards . . . of venereal diseases":** Eliot Ness, statement on the function of the
      Social Protection Division, issued by the Office of Defense, Health and Welfare
      Services (1941), quoted in Marylin E. Hegarty, *Victory Girls, Khaki-Wackies and
      Patriotes: The Regulation of Female Sexuality During World War II* (New York:
      New York University Press, 2008), 19.

235   **rapid detection centers:** J. Parascandola, "Quarantining Women: Venereal
      Disease and Rapid Treatment Centers in World War II America," *Bulletin of the
      History of Medicine* 83, no. 3 (Fall 2009): 431–59.

236   **". . . sexually delinquent women":** Statement issued by the Office of Defense
      Health and Welfare Services (1941), quoted in Hegarty, *Victory Girls, Khaki-
      Wackies and Patriotes*, 19.

236   **preservation of public health:** Erin Weubker, "Taking the Venereal Out of
      Venereal Disease: The 1930s Public Health Campaign Against Syphilis and
      Gonorrhea," *Notches: (Re)marks on the History of Sexuality*, May 31, 2016, http://
      notchesblog.com/2016/05/31/taking-the-venereal-out-of-venereal-disease-the
      -1930s-public-health-campaign-against-syphilis-and-gonorrhea; and Cari
      Romm, "During World War II, Sex Was a National-Security Threat," *The
      Atlantic*, October 8, 2015, https://www.theatlantic.com/health/archive/2015/10
      /during-world-war-ii-sexually-active-women-were-a-national-security-threat/40
      9555.

237   **Endo began to be recognized:** For a fascinating historical overview of endo-
      metriosis, see Camran Nezhat, Farr Nezhat, and Ceana Nezhat, "Endometrio-
      sis: Ancient Disease, Ancient Treatments," *Fertility and Sterility* 98, no. 65
      (December 2012), https://www.fertstert.org/article/S0015-0282(12)01955-3
      /fulltext#sec8:5.3.

237   **"endometriosis" in 1927:** See John A. Sampson, "Peritoneal Endometriosis
      Due to the Menstrual Dissemination of Endometriosis into the Peritoneal Cav-
      ity," *American Journal of Obstetrics and Gynecology* 14, no. 4 (1927), 422–69.

237   **"a riddle of etiology":** Walter R. Holmes, "Endometriosis," *American Journal
      of Obstetrics and Gynecology* 43, no. 2 (1942): 263.

238   **"put off child-bearing . . .":** Joe Vincent Meigs, "Endometriosis: Its Signifi-
      cance," *Annals of Surgery* 114, no. 5 (1941): 866–74.

238   **throughout the 1940s:** See Kate Seear, *The Making of a Modern Epidemic: En-
      dometriosis, Gender and Politics* (London: Routledge, 2016), 36–37.

240   **"career woman's disease":** Carolyn Carpan, "Representations of Endometriosis
      in the Popular Press: 'The Career Woman's Disease,'" *Atlantis* 27, no. 2 (Spring–
      Summer 2003): 32–40.

240   **obeying "nature's rules":** Meigs (1948), quoted in Seear, *The Making of a Modern
      Epidemic*, 36.

241   **figures of its prevalence:** David E. Hailman (1941), "The Prevalence of Dis-
      abling Illness Among Male and Female Workers and Housewives," based on
      data from the National Health Survey, in *Illness and Medical Care Among
      2,500,000 Persons in 83 Cities, with Special Reference to Socio-Economic Factors*
      (a collection of 27 reprints), Federal Security Agency, US Public Health Service
      (Washington, DC: United States Government Printing Office, 1945).

15: PUBLIC HEALTH, PRIVATE PAIN

245   "... worries in times of illness": "The New National Health Service," Ministry of Health and the Central Office of Information (February 24, 1948), Socialist Health Association, https://www.sochealth.co.uk/national-health-service /the-sma-and-the-foundation-of-the-national-health-service-dr-leslie-hilliard -1980/the-start-of-the-nhs-1948.

246   "... for the rest of my life": Sylvia Diggory, quoted in Denis Campbell, "Nye Bevan's Dream: A History of the NHS," *The Guardian*, January 18, 2016, https:// www.theguardian.com/society/2016/jan/18/nye-bevan-history-of-nhs-national -health-service.

246   "choose your doctor now": *Read the Leaflet* (1948) and *Choose Your Doctor* (1948), trailer films about the National Health Service, British Pathé Historical Collection, https://www.britishpathe.com/video/choose-your-doctor-trailer and https://www.britishpathe.com/video/trailer-read-the-leaflet-english.

247   "It was such a relief . . .": Mary Dowlding quoted in "The NHS: 'One of the Greatest Achievements in History,'" BBC News, July 1, 1998, http://news.bbc .co.uk/1/hi/events/nhs_at_50/special_report/123511.stm.

247   subject to medical scrutiny: For a fascinating in-depth analysis of the way the NHS shifted medical culture and practice around postnatal care and childbirth, see Ann Oakley, "The Doctor's Dilemma," in *The Captured Womb: A History of the Medical Care of Pregnant Women* (Oxford: Blackwell, 1984), 132–51.

248   "... achieve and enjoy good health": President Truman, "Special Message to Congress Recommending Comprehensive Health Program," November 19, 1945, Healthcare-Now, https://www.healthcare-now.org/legislation/presi dent-trumans-special-message-to-the-congress-recommending-a-comprehensive -health-program.

248   pregnancy, birth, and the postnatal period: Elizabeth Temkin, "Driving Through: Post-Partum Care During World War II," *American Journal of Public Health* 89, no. 4 (April 1999): 587–89.

249   She died at home: John R. Haserick and Roland Long, "Systemic Lupus Erythematosus Preceded by False-Positive Serologic Tests for Syphilis: Presentation of Five Cases," *Annals of Internal Medicine* 37, no. 3 (1952): 561.

250   autoimmunity was plausible: For a comprehensive and fascinating account of the clinical, biomedical, and social histories of autoimmunity, as well as the lived illness experiences of sufferers, see Warwick Anderson and Ian R. Mackay, *Intolerant Bodies: A Short History of Autoimmunity* (Baltimore: Johns Hopkins University Press, 2014).

251   "major clinical manifestations" of lupus: Joseph Earle Moore, Laurence E. Shulman, and James T. Scott, "The Natural History of Systemic Lupus Erythematosus: An Approach to Its Study Through Chronic Biologic False Positive Reactors: Interim Report" (presented at the 69th annual meeting of the American Clinical and Climatological Association, November 2, 1956), *Journal of Chronic Diseases* 5, no. 3 (March 1957): 61.

251   suffered some "emotional instability": Moore, Shulman, and Scott, "The Natural History of Systemic Lupus Erythematosus," table 4 (white, 21-year-old female), 65.

252   modern psychosomatic medicine: Helen Flanders Dunbar, *Emotions and Bodily Changes* (New York: Columbia University Press, 1935); Constance M. McGovern, "Helen Flanders Dunbar: Pioneer in Psychosomatic Medicine,"

Women in Medicine Magazine, December 11, 2016, http://www.womeninmedi cinemagazine.com/profile-of-women-in-medicine/helen-flanders-dunbar-pion eer-in-psychosomatic-medicine.

253 **"Holy Seven":** Franz Alexander, "The Development of Psychosomatic Medicine," *Psychosomatic Medicine* 24, no. 1 (January 1962), 20. See also Chase Patterson Kimball, "Diagnosing Psychosomatic Situations," in *Clinical Diagnosis of Mental Disorders*, ed. B. B. Wolman (Boston: Springer, 1978), 677–708.

253 **after the procedure:** Walter Freeman and James W. Watts, "Psychosurgery During 1936–1946," *Archives of Neurology and Psychiatry* 58, no. 4 (1947): 421.

253 **75 percent of the patients . . . were women:** Andrea Tone and Mary Koziol, "(F)ailing Women in Psychiatry: Lessons from a Painful Past," *Canadian Medical Association Journal* 190, no. 20 (2018): E625.

254 **"agitated," "anxious," or "obsessive" women:** Freeman and Watts, "Psychosurgery During 1936–1946," 420.

254 **"Easier than curing a toothache":** "My Lobotomy," *All Things Considered*, NPR, November 16, 2005, https://www.npr.org/2005/11/16/5014080/my-lobotomy -howard-dullys-journey?t=1603796908094. Also referenced by Lyz Lenz, "The Secret Lobotomy of Rosemary Kennedy," *Marie Claire*, March 31, 2017, https:// www.marieclaire.com/celebrity/a26261/secret-lobotomy-rosemary-kennedy.

254 **"full of don't-give-a-damness":** Walter Freeman and James Watts, *Psychosurgery in the Treatment of Mental Disorders and Intractable Pain*, 2nd ed. (Oxford: Blackwell Scientific Publishers, 1950), 187.

255 **Her lobotomy was kept secret:** Katie Serena, "The Little-Known History of Rosemary Kennedy, Who Was Lobotomized So That JFK Could Succeed," All That's Interesting, November 6, 2017, updated March 6, 2020, https://allthatsin teresting.com/rosemary-kennedy-lobotomy.

255 **". . . greater than the pain":** Freeman and Watts, "Psychosurgery During 1936–1946," 422.

256 **". . . situations in everyday life":** Richard W. Levy et al., "Experiences with Prefrontal Lobotomy for Intractable Ulcerative Colitis," *Journal of American Medicine* 160 (1956): 1277–80.

16: MOTHERS' LITTLE HELPERS

257 **The earliest ads:** Heather Radke's brilliant essay "The Magic Bullet: How a Drug Called Miltown Ushered in an Age of Pill-Popping for Anxious Americans," in *Topic Magazine*, no. 16, "Fear Itself" (October 2018), includes adverts for Miltown from both the medical and women's press up to the 1960s: https:// www.topic.com/the-magic-bullet.

257 **". . . their husbands' advances":** D. Cooley, "The New Nerve Pills and Your Health," *Cosmopolitan*, January 1956, 68–75, quoted in Jeremy A. Greene and David Herzberg, "Hidden in Plain Sight: Marketing Prescription Drugs to Consumers in the Twentieth Century," *American Journal of Public Health* 100, no. 5 (2010): 798.

258 **sufferers risk being dismissed:** Faith Cotter, "When Tight Becomes Too Tight: A Helpful Primer on Vaginismus," *Jezebel*, January 23, 2015, https://jezebel.com /when-tight-becomes-too-tight-a-helpful-primer-on-vagin-1679485378; and Alexa Tsoulis-Reay, "What It's Like to Have Severe Vaginismus," *The Cut*, April 21, 2015, https://www.thecut.com/2015/04/what-its-like-to-have-severe-vaginismus .html.

259 **loosen up with a few drinks:** Kate Lloyd, "'It Destroys Lives': Why the Razor-Blade Pain of Vaginismus Is So Misunderstood," *The Guardian*, August 31, 2020, https://www.theguardian.com/lifeandstyle/2020/aug/31/pain-vag inismus-destroys-lives-misunderstood-common-conditions-surgery-treatment.

259 **"...I don't feel that way, Doctor":** Henry B. Safford, "Tell Me, Doctor," *Ladies' Home Journal*, September 1956, 50, 55, 125, quoted and discussed in Jonathan Metzl, "'Mother's Little Helper': The Crisis of Psychoanalysis and the Miltown Resolution," *Gender and History* 15, no. 2 (August 2003): 251–52.

260 **"...no organic etiology":** Wallace Laboratories, advertisement for Meprospan, *Journal of the American Medical Association*, 1960, New York Academy of Medicine Library. See Radke, "Magic Bullet," https://www.topic.com/the-magic -bullet.

260 **misdiagnosed with "hysteria":** See Colin T. Talley, "The Emergence of Multiple Sclerosis, 1850–1970: A Puzzle of Historical Epidemiology," *Perspectives in Biology and Medicine* 48, no. 3 (Summer 2005): 383–95.

261 **predominantly affected men:** Naomi Chainey, "How Sexism Is Hindering Medical Research," *Sydney Morning Herald*, February 6, 2018, https://www .smh.com.au/lifestyle/health-and-wellness/how-sexism-is-hindering-medical -research-20180206-h0uy60.html.

261 **misdiagnosed as somatization disorder:** L. A. Rolak, "Multiple Sclerosis: It's Not the Disease You Thought It Was," *Clinical Medicine and Research* 1, no. 1 (2003): 57–60; Jon Stone et al., "Systematic Review of Misdiagnosis of Conversion Symptoms and 'Hysteria,'" *British Medical Journal*, October 13, 2005, https://www.bmj.com/content/bmj/331/7523/989.full.pdf.

261 **"...to assuage doctors' anxieties":** M. M. Glatt, "The Abuse of Barbiturates in the United Kingdom," United Nations Office on Drugs and Crime, 1962, https://www.unodc.org/unodc/en/data-and-analysis/bulletin/bulletin_1962-01 -01_2_page004.html.

261 **"hypochondriacs and neurotics":** National Health Service (Prescription Charges), HC Deb, November 29, 1956, vol. 561, cc661-726, https://api.parlia ment.uk/historic-hansard/commons/1959/jan/26/prescription-charges.

262 **tranquilizer use skyrocketed:** Ali Haggett, *Desperate Housewives, Neuroses, and the Domestic Environment, 1945–1970* (London: Routledge, 2012), 151.

262 **"...chemically induced tranquility":** I. Atkin, "The Lotus-Eaters; or Stress, Neurosis, and Tranquilizers," *The British Medical Journal*, December 26, 1959, 1478.

263 **"...for the physician":** "The Battered Parent Syndrome," Miltown advertisement. c. 1960, New York Academy of Medicine Library. See Radke, "Magic Bullet," 2018, https://www.topic.com/the-magic-bullet.

263 **small-print side effects:** For an incredible selection of vintage pharmaceutical advertisements for Serax, Valium, Librium, and many other psychoactive drugs, see "Benzodiazepine Vintage Advertising," Benzodiazepine Information Coalition, https://w-bad.org/vintageads.

264 **roles as wives and mothers:** Betty Friedan, "Introduction to the Tenth Anniversary Edition," *The Feminine Mystique* (New York: W. W. Norton, 1974).

264 **"...accept them with good grace":** *Newsweek*, March 7, 1960, quoted in Friedan, "The Problem That Has No Name," *The Feminine Mystique*, 20.

264 **"...puzzling their doctors...for years":** Friedan, *The Feminine Mystique*, 2.

265 **labeled "housewife's fatigue":** Friedan, *The Feminine Mystique*, 18.

265   **It felt less painful this way:** Friedan, *The Feminine Mystique*, 23.

265   **". . . nation and a culture":** Friedan, *The Feminine Mystique*, 18.

265   **"NOW is dedicated to . . .":** Betty Friedan, "The National Organization of Women's Statement of Purpose," adopted at NOW's first national conference in Washington, DC, on October 29, 1966, https://now.org/about/history/state ment-of-purpose.

Today, NOW represents the "grassroots arm" of the women's movement, through members and chapters across all US states and the District of Columbia. NOW's purpose is to "take action through intersectional grassroots activism to promote feminist ideals, lead societal change, eliminate discrimination, and achieve and protect the equal rights of all women and girls in all aspects of social, political, and economic life." NOW's six core issues are reproductive rights and justice, ending violence against women, economic justice, LBGTQIA rights, racial justice, and a constitutional equality amendment. See https://now.org.

265   **"women without men":** bell hooks (1988), "Black Women: Shaping Feminist Theory," in *Feminist Theory: From Margin to Center*, 2nd ed. (London: Pluto Press, 2000), 2.

265   **". . . my children and my house":** hooks, quoting Friedan in *Feminist Theory*, 1.

265   **of thought, of action:** hooks, *Feminist Theory*, 1–2.

266   **". . . live on the margin":** hooks, "Preface to the First Edition," *Feminist Theory*, xvii.

266   **". . . anything exclusively female":** Robert A. Wilson, *Feminine Forever* (London: Mayflower-Dell, 1966), 17.

267   **". . . this living decay":** Wilson, *Feminine Forever*, 38.

267   **both female and male sex hormones:** For a fascinating account of the biochemical and scientific discoveries of "heterosexual hormones," and the way these discoveries transformed the dualistic nature of sex difference in endocrinology, see "The Birth of Sex Hormones," chapter 2, of Nelly Oudshoorn's groundbreaking book *Beyond the Natural Body: An Archeology of Sex Hormones* (London: Routledge, 1994). See also Nancy Langston, "The Retreat from Precaution: Regulating Diethylstilbestrol (DES), Endocrine Disruptors, and Environmental Health," *Environmental History* 13, no. 1 (January 2008): 43–44.

267   **". . . keeps her from changing":** Wilson, *Feminine Forever*, 47.

268   **". . . estrogen makes women adaptable . . .":** Wilson, *Feminine Forever*, 55.

269   **"expenses of writing 'Feminine Forever'":** Gina Kolata with Melody Petersen, "Hormone Replacement Study a Shock to the Medical System," *New York Times*, July 10, 2002, https://www.nytimes.com/2002/07/10/us/hormone -replacement-study-a-shock-to-the-medical-system.html; see also "Wilson Versus Living Decay," in Gary Null and Barbara Seaman, *For Women Only!: Your Guide to Health Empowerment* (New York: Seven Stories Press, 1999), 751–52.

269   **any prescription medications:** Daniel Carpenter, *Reputation and Power: Organizational Image and Pharmaceutical Regulations at the FDA* (Princeton, NJ: Princeton University Press, 2010), 600–1.

269   **feminists embraced estrogen therapy:** See Judith A. Houck, "'What Do These Women Want?': Feminist Responses to *Feminine Forever*, 1963–1980," *Bulletin of the History of Medicine* 77, no. 1 (Spring 2003): 103–32.

270   **"ever experience the menopause":** Wilson, *Feminine Forever*, 156.

270 **to use successfully:** Margaret Sanger, "Birth Control on the March," October 1952, Margaret Sanger Papers, Sophia Smith Collection, Margaret Sanger Microfilm S72:0713, https://www.nyu.edu/projects/sanger/webedition/app /documents/show.php?sangerDoc=236511.xml.

271 **criminal offense in Massachusetts:** For full accounts of the inception, development, and trialing of the combined oral contraceptive pill, see Elizabeth Seigel Watkins, "The Genesis of the Pill," in *On the Pill: A Social History of Oral Contraceptives, 1950–1970* (Baltimore: Johns Hopkins University Press, 1998); Lara V. Marks, *Sexual Chemistry: A History of the Contraceptive Pill* (New Haven, CT: Yale University Press, 2001); Nelly Oudshoorn, "The Transformation of Sex Hormones into the Pill," chap. 6, in *Beyond the Natural Body: An Archeology of Sex Hormones* (London: Routledge, 1994); and Pamela Verma Laio, "Half a Century of the Oral Contraceptive Pill: Historical Review and View to the Future," *Canadian Family Physician* 8 (December 2012). See also "The Birth Control Pill: A History," Planned Parenthood Federation of America, https://www.plannedparenthood.org/files/1514/3518/7100/Pill_History_Fact Sheet.pdf; Drew C. Prendergrass and Michelle V. Raji, "The Bitter Pill: Harvard and the Dark History of Birth Control," *Harvard Crimson*, September 28, 2017, https://www.thecrimson.com/article/2017/9/28/the-bitter-pill; and "The Puerto Rico Pill Trials," *American Experience*, PBS, https://www.pbs.org/wgbh /americanexperience/features/pill-puerto-rico-pill-trials.

271 **". . . cage of ovulating females":** McCormick quoted in Barbara Seaman, *The Greatest Experiment Ever Performed on Women: Exploding the Estrogen Myth* (New York: Seven Stories Press, 2003), 29.

271 **"We all jumped on it quickly . . .":** Delia Mestre quoted in Ray Quintanilla, "Puerto Ricans Recall Being Used as Guinea Pigs for 'Magic Pill,'" *Chicago Tribune*, April 11, 2004. https://www.chicagotribune.com/news/ct-xpm -2004-04-11-0404110509-story.html.

272 **"causes too many side-effects . . .":** Edris Rice-Wray, "Field Study with Enovid as a Contraceptive Agent," *Proceedings of a Symposium on 19–Nor Progestational Steroids* (Chicago: G. D. Searle, 1957), quoted in Watkins, *On the Pill*, 32.

272 **"emotional super-activity . . .":** Annette B. Ramírez de Arellano and Conrad Siepp, *Colonialism, Catholicism, and Contraception: A History of Birth Control in Puerto Rico* (Chapel Hill: University of North Carolina Press, 1983), 166, quoted in Nelly Oudshoorn, *Beyond the Natural Body: An Archeology of Sex Hormones*, 130.

272 **". . . every sense psychologically":** Dr. Pincus, "Discussion of Oral Methods of Fertility Control," *Report of the Proceedings of the Sixth International Conference on Planned Parenthood* (London: International Planned Parenthood Federation, 1959). Excerpt reprinted in Jay Katz with Alexander Capron and Eleanor Swift Glass, "A Case Study of Oral Contraception," in *Experimentation with Human Beings: The Authority of the Investigator, Subject, Professions and State in the Human Experimentation Process* (New York: Russell Sage Foundation, 1972), 747.

272 **". . . decisions for ourselves?":** Mestre quoted in Quintanilla, "Puerto Ricans Recall Being Used as Guinea Pigs for 'Magic Pill.'"

273 **No autopsies were ever conducted:** Milton Silverman and Philip R. Lee, *Pills, Profits, and Politics* (Berkeley: University of California Press, 1974), 99–100.

273 **La operación, as it was known:** Katherine Andrews, "The Dark History of Forced Sterilization of Latina Women," Panoramas Scholarly Platform,

University of Pittsburgh, October 30, 2017, https://www.panoramas.pitt.edu /health-and-society/dark-history-forced-sterilization-latina-women.

273 **without parental consent:** Claudia Goldin and Lawrence F. Katz, "The Power of the Pill: Oral Contraceptives and Women's Career and Marriage Decisions," *Journal of Political Economy* 110, no. 4 (2002): 731.

274 **contraceptives for "mature minors":** Goldin and Katz, "The Power of the Pill," 731.

274 **"... doctors are listening intently":** Richard D. Lyons, "New Data on the Safety of the Pill," *New York Times*, September 7, 1969, quoted in Watkins, *On the Pill*, 84.

274 **Premarin for menopause symptoms:** Seaman, *The Greatest Experiment Ever Performed on Women*, 14–16.

275 **"... millions of healthy women":** Statement of Dr. Hugh Davis, Hearings Before the Subcommittee on Monopoly of the Select Committee on Small Business, US Senate, 91st Cong., 2nd session on Present Status of Competition in the Pharmaceutical Industry, pt. 15 (January 14, 15, 21, 22, and 23, 1970), Oral Contraceptives (Volume 1), *Competitive Problems in the Drug Industry* (printed for the use of the Select Committee on Small Business, 1970), 5295.

275 **"... rather than redistribute resources?":** Regina Sigal, "Politics of the Pill," *Off Our Backs* 1, no. 1 (February 27, 1970), 3.

275 **male pill reported:** Andy Extance, "Why the Male Pill Still Doesn't Exist," *The Atlantic*, July 13, 2016, https://www.theatlantic.com/health/archive/2016/07 /why-the-male-pill-still-doesnt-exist/490985.

275 **"acceptability" of the male pill:** See Holly Grigg-Spall, "The Pill Is Linked to Depression—and Doctors Can No Longer Ignore It," *The Guardian*, October 3, 2016, https://www.theguardian.com/commentisfree/2016/oct/03/pill-linked -depression-doctors-hormonal-contraceptives. See also "Acceptability of Drugs for Male Fertility Regulation: A Prospectus and Some Preliminary Data," World Health Organization Task Force on Psychosocial Research in Family Planning, *Contraception* 21, no. 2 (February 1980): 121–34.

275 **thrust upon women:** See Lisa Campo-Engelstein, "Contraceptive Justice: Why We Need a Male Pill," Virtual Mentor, *American Medical Association Journal of Ethics* 14, no. 2 (February 2012): 146–51.

275 **"Let's see how you feel ...":** For footage of members of DC Women's Liberation interrupting the Nelson hearings, see the National Women's Health Network history video "The Pill Hearings," National Women's Health Network, https://www.nwhn.org/pill-hearings/.

276 **"... more important than our lives!":** "Senate Hearings on the Pill," *American Experience*, PBS, https://www.pbs.org/wgbh/americanexperience/features /pill-senate-holds-hearings-pill-1970.

276 **"... reasons behind that suppression":** Sigal, "Politics of the Pill."

276 **"... antiseptically directing our lives":** Opening statement of DC Liberation's women's hearings, March 1970, quoted in Null and Seaman, *For Women Only!*, 726.

276–77 **Links between pill hormones and depression:** An oft-cited study of over one hundred thousand Danish women, published in 2016, asked, "Is use of hormonal contraception associated with treatment of depression?" Findings showed that, within six months after first taking the pill, 34 percent of women taking the progesterone-only pill, and 23 percent of women on the combined pill, were more likely to have been prescribed antidepressants. See C. W. Skovlund, L. S. Mørch, L. V. Kessing, and Ø. Lidegaard, "Association of Hormonal Contraception with Depression," *JAMA Psychiatry* 73, no. 11 (2016): 1154–62.

277 **shrinking the hypothalamus:** Vicky Spratt, "Hysterical Women: Why Is Hormonal Contraception Still Failing Us?," *Refinery29*, September 9, 2020, https://www.refinery29.com/en-gb/2020/09/10005772/side-effects-of-the-contraceptive-pill.

277 **on our minds and lives:** Grigg-Spall, "The Pill Is Linked to Depression."

277 **Progestin levels were decreased:** Sharon Snider, "The Pill: 30 Years of Safety Concerns," *FDA Consumer* 24, no. 10 (December 1990): 10.

277 **manufacturers had to follow suit:** Null and Seaman, *For Women Only!*, 731.

17: OUR BODIES, OUR SELVES

279 **"... his control and supposed expertise":** Boston Women's Health Collective, *Women and Their Bodies: A Course* (Boston, 1970), 7, https://www.ourbodiesour selves.org/cms/assets/uploads/2014/04/Women-and-Their-Bodies-1970.pdf.

280 **"... learning with our sisters":** Boston Women's Health Collective, "Course Introduction," in *Women and Their Bodies*, 3, https://www.ourbodiesourselves .org/cms/assets/uploads/2014/04/Women-and-Their-Bodies-1970.pdf.

281 **carried out the abortions:** The Jane Collective helped an estimated eleven thousand women end their pregnancies between 1969 and 1973. To read the story of Jane, the women who were involved, and the women who were helped, see Laura Kaplan, *The Story of Jane: The Legendary Underground Feminist Abortion Service* (Chicago: University of Chicago Press, 1997). Kaplan became a member of Jane in 1971 and helped found a women's health center in Chicago. After moving to rural Wisconsin, Kaplan supported women during homebirths and established a shelter program for female victims of domestic violence. She is now on the board of the National Women's Health Network, and she gives lectures about Jane and works with community health projects.

281 **Downer felt "awestruck":** Carol Downer quoted in Hannah Dudley-Shotwell, *Revolutionizing Women's Healthcare: The Feminist Self-Help Movement in America* (New Brunswick, NJ: Rutgers University Press, 2020), 16.

282 **precancerous cervical cells:** "May Edward Chinn," in Wini Warren, *Black Women Scientists in the United States* (Bloomington: Indiana University Press, 1999), 26–28.

282 **enabled early detection:** See Ilana Löwy, *A Woman's Disease: The History of Cervical Cancer* (Oxford: Oxford University Press, 2011), 114–15.

282 **women's experiences as patients:** Carol Downer, "Sex Discrimination Against Women as Medical Patients," address to the American Psychological Association meeting, Hawaii, September 5, 1972, CWLU Herstory Project: A History of Chicago Women's Liberation, https://www.cwluherstory.org/classic -feminist-writings-articles/covert-sex-discrimination-against-women-as-medical -patients.

283 **"... forced us into subservience":** Barbara Ehrenreich and Deirdre English, *Witches, Midwives, and Nurses: A History of Women Healers*, 2nd ed. (1973; New York: Feminist Press, 2001), 100.

284 **Geraldine "Gerri" Santoro:** Amanda Arnold, "How a Harrowing Photo of One Woman's Death Became an Iconic Pro-Choice Symbol," *Vice*,

October 26, 2016, https://www.vice.com/en_us/article/evgdpw/how-a-har rowing-photo-of-one-womans-death-became-an-iconic-pro-choice-symbol.

285　"... making their own decisions": J. Temkin, "The Lane Committee Report on the Abortion Act," *Modern Law Review* 37, no. 6 (November 1974): 659–60.

285　diagnoses of pregnancy: Jesse Olszynko-Gryn, "The Feminist Appropriation of Pregnancy Testing in 1970s Britain," *Women's History Review* 28, no. 6 (2019): 872.

286　glare of professional opinion: See Olszynko-Gryn, "The Feminist Appropria- tion of Pregnancy Testing in 1970s Britain," 869–94.

286　"... government thinks we need": *Women and Abortion: The Women's Abortion and Contraceptive Campaign's Evidence to the Lane Commission* (London: WACC, 1972), quoted and discussed in Olszynko-Gryn, "The Feminist Appropriation of Pregnancy Testing in 1970s Britain," 873.

287　"Feminism gave me my body...": Interview with Dr. Jan McKenley, "The Feelings Behind the Slogans: Part 4," Sisterhood and After: The Women's Lib- eration Oral History Project, British Library, https://www.bl.uk/collection -items/the-feelings-behind-the-slogans-part-4.

　　　　Sisterhood and After is part of a wider Leverhulme Trust–funded project, which created "an original and extensive history of feminist change-makers of the 1970s and 1980s." The project website, hosted by the British Library, in- cludes an amazing selection of interviews, transcripts, biographies, and articles on a range of issues affecting women's lives, including consciousness-raising, body experience, health and reproduction, sex education, and the politics of therapy. McKenley's interview, "The Feelings Behind the Slogans," is in four parts. To access this rich and fascinating resource, go to https://www.bl.uk/ sisterhood.

　　　　Margaretta Jolly's book *Sisterhood and After: An Oral History of the UK's Women's Liberation Movement* (Oxford University Press, 2019) draws on the oral history project to cast "new light on feminist critiques of society and on the lives of prominent and grassroots activists."

287　National Black Women's Health Project: See Sandra Morgan's discussion of the work of Avery and the development of the NBWHP in "On Their Own: Women of Color and the Women's Health Movement," chap. 3, in *Into Our Own Hands: The Women's Health Movement in the United States, 1969–1990* (New Brunswick, NJ: Rutgers University Press, 2002), 41–51.

288　conference's rallying cry: Fannie Lou Hamer, "I'm Sick and Tired of Being Sick and Tired" (1964), as published in *Speeches of Fannie Lou Hamer: To Tell It Like It Is* (Jackson: University Press of Mississippi, 2013). The speech is avail- able to read online on Iowa State University's Archives of Women's Political Communication site: https://awpc.cattcenter.iastate.edu/2019/08/09 /im-sick-and-tired-of-being-sick-and-tired-dec-20-1964.

　　　　At a rally for the Mississippi Freedom Democrat Party at Williams Institu- tional Church in Harlem, New York, with Malcolm X, Hamer delivered a speech explaining how, after an intense struggle to claim her right to vote, she was jailed with several other Black women for sitting in a segregated bus station in Charleston, South Carolina. While in jail, she was violently beaten, which left her with irreversible damage to her eye, kidneys, and leg. See Debra Michals, ed., "Fannie Lou Hamer (1917–1977)," National Wom-

en's History Museum, https://www.womenshistory.org/education-reso
urces/biographies/fannie-lou-hamer.

288 **Sixty percent of Black women in Sunflower County:** Dorothy Roberts discusses Hamer's experiences and the prevalence of the covert, nonconsensual
sterilization of Black women in the 1970s in "The New Reign of Sterilization
Abuse," *Killing the Black Body* (1997; 2017), 89–98.

288 **"the uterus collector":** Project South: Institute for the Elimination of Poverty
and Genocide, OIG Report, September 14, 2020, https://www.scribd.com
/document/476013004/OIG-Complaint#from_embed; Izzie Ramirez, "An
ICE Nurse Revealed That a US Detention Center Is Performing Mass Hysterectomies," *Refinery29*, September 15, 2020, https://www.refinery29.com
/en-gb/2020/09/10025368/ice-hysterectomies-immigration-whistleblower-project
-south.

289 **proposed that Black women:** J. T. Witherspoon and V. W. Butler, "The Etiology of Uterine Fibroids, with Special Reference to the Frequency of Their Occurrence in the Negro: An Hypothesis," *Surgery, Gynecology and Obstetrics* 58
(1934): 57–61; see also Ranell L. Myles, "Unbearable Fruit: Black Women's Experiences with Uterine Fibroids" (dissertation, Georgia State University, 2013),
https://scholarworks.gsu.edu/sociology_diss/72.

289 **"acted like water to a thirsty seed . . .":** Byllye Avery, "Equal, But Still Not on
the Same Level," *Contact*, no. 98, "National Black Women's Health Project:
Empowerment Through Wellness" (August 1987): 4.

289 **". . . waking up inside":** Felicia Ward, "I Met Lillie . . . and I Discovered Myself, or How Self-Help Programmes Are Born," *Contact* no. 98, 6.

290 **". . . carry around all that junk":** Ward, "I Met Lillie . . . and I Discovered
Myself," 7.

290 **"exercise control over their own lives":** Byllye Avery, "Equal, But Still Not on
the Same Level," 4.

291 **BWHI is leading change:** See the website of the Black Women's Health Imperative to find out more about the organization's signature programs, special
initiatives, policy development, and publications dedicated to "improving the
health and wellness" of the 21 million Black girls and women living in the US
today: https://bwhi.org/who-we-are.

291 **longer than men to be referred:** Dorothea Z. Lack, "Women and Pain:
Another Feminist Issue," *Women and Therapy* 1, no. 1 (1982): 55–64.

293 **criteria were spectacularly biased:** Sean H. Yutzy and Brooke S. Parish,
"Somatoform Disorders," in *The American Psychiatric Publishing Textbook of
Psychiatry*, 5th ed., ed. Robert E. Hales et al. (Washington, DC: American
Psychiatric Publishing, 2008), 609–22.

293 **vomiting, and painful extremities:** Ekkehard Othmer and Cherilyn DeSouza,
"A Screening Test for Somatization Disorder (Hysteria)," *American Journal of
Psychiatry* 142, no. 10 (1985): 1146–49.

294 **not been rigorously tested:** Leila McNeil, "The Woman Who Stood Between
America and a Generation of 'Thalidomide Babies,'" *Smithsonian Magazine*, May 8, 2017, https://www.smithsonianmag.com/science-nature
/woman-who-stood-between-america-and-epidemic-birth-defects-180963165.

294 **Distaval was so "outstandingly safe":** "Thalidomide in the Market Place,"
Objects and Stories, Science Museum, December 11, 2019, https://www
.sciencemuseum.org.uk/objects-and-stories/medicine/thalidomide.

295   **life-threatening condition:** Katherine A. Liu and Natalie A. DiPietro Mager, "Women's Involvement in Clinical Trials: Historical Perspective and Future Implications," *Pharmacy Practice* 14, no. 1 (January–March 2016): 708.

295   **". . . in ALL pregnancies":** Advert for desPLEX (DES) by Grant Chemical Company (1957), in Amanda Arnold, "The Devastating Effects of a 1940s 'Wonder Pill' Haunt Women Generations Later," *Vice*, June 5, 2017, https://www.vice.com/en_us/article/zmbvp9/des-daughters-the-devastating-effects-of-a-1940s-wonder-pill-haunt-women-generations-later.

295   **". . . pregnancy more normal":** Nancy Langston, "The Retreat from Precaution: Regulating Diethylstilbestrol (DES), Endocrine Disruptors, and Environmental Health," *Environmental History* 13, no. 1 (January 2008): 50.

295   **impotence and breast growth:** Langston, "The Retreat from Precaution," 50–51.

296   **"the indiscriminate use of DES . . .":** Belita Cowan, interview with Tania Ketenjian (September 1999) in Gary Null and Barbara Seaman, *For Women Only!: Your Guide to Health Empowerment* (New York: Seven Stories Press, 1999), 967.

296   **". . . can make a difference":** Belita Cowan, interview with Tania Ketenjian (September 1999) in Null and Seaman, *For Women Only!* (1999), 967.

296   **"no cases have been reported . . .":** Lawrence K. Altman, "Rare Cancer Seen in 41 Homosexuals," *New York Times*, July 3, 1981, https://www.nytimes.com/1981/07/03/us/rare-cancer-seen-in-41-homosexuals.html.

297   **"omission of women as a focus . . .":** Susan Blumenthal, "A World Without AIDS for American Women," amfAR, June 20, 2014, https://www.amfar.org/world-without-aids-for-american-women (originally published in the *Huffington Post*).

297   **". . . women of all ages":** "Women's Health, Report on the Public Health Service Task Force on Women's Health Issues," *Public Health Reports* 100, no. 1 (January–February 1985): 76.

297   **". . . therapies have not been determined":** "Women's Health, Report on the Public Health Service Task Force on Women's Health Issues," *Public Health Reports*, 80.

298   **". . . affect women's health differently . . .":** "Women's Health, Report on the Public Health Service Task Force on Women's Health Issues," *Public Health Reports*, 81.

299   **men as the normative standard:** Bernadine Healy, "The Yentl Syndrome," *New England Journal of Medicine* 325, no. 4 (July 25, 1991): 275.

299   **"nonspecific chest pain":** See Caroline Criado-Perez's discussion of Yentl syndrome in *Invisible Women: Exposing Data Bias in a World Designed for Men* (London: Vintage, 2019), 217–20.

299   **"Yentl syndrome pervades medicine . . .":** Healy, "The Yentl Syndrome," 274.

300   **"require, rather than recommend":** Blumenthal, "A World Without AIDS for American Women"; and Blumenthal, "Writing a New National Prescription to Improve Women's Health: History, Progress and Challenges Ahead," *HuffPost* blog, April 1, 2017, https://www.huffpost.com/entry/writing-a-national-prescr_b_8251238.

        See also "History of Women's Participation in Clinical Research," National Institutes of Health Office of Research on Women's Health, https://orwh.od.nih.gov/toolkit/recruitment/history.

300 **different-but-equal needs:** As Healy writes, "We must awaken fully to these facts and address the diseases of women as different from the diseases of men but of equal importance, even when they also affect men": Healy, "The Yentl Syndrome," 275.

300 **". . . disease to the interventionist":** Lucy Candib, "Women, Medicine, and Capitalism," in Boston Women's Health Collective, *Women and Their Bodies: A Course*, 7.

301 **". . . without the stuffing":** William Boly, "Raggedy Ann Syndrome," *Hippocrates Magazine* (July–August 1987); Philip M. Boffey, "Fatigue 'Virus' Has Experts More Baffled and Skeptical Than Ever," *New York Times*, July 28, 1987, https://www.nytimes.com/1987/07/28/science/fatigue-virus-has-experts-more-baffled-and-skeptical-than-ever.html; and Mike Mariani, "A Town for People with Chronic-Fatigue Syndrome," *New Yorker*, September 3, 2019, https://www.newyorker.com/culture/personal-history/a-town-for-people-with-chronic-fatigue.

301 **"run out of town . . .":** Boly quoting Incline resident Chris Guthrie in "Raggedy Ann Syndrome," *Hippocrates Magazine*.

302 **benign myalgic encephalomyelitis:** Colin McEvedy and A. W. Beard, "Concept of Benign Myalgic Encephalomyelitis," *British Medical Journal* 1 (January 3, 1970): 11–15.

302 **hysteria, hypochondria, and psychological delusions:** Liliana Dell'Osso et al., "Historical Evolution of the Concept of Anorexia Nervosa and Relationships with Orthorexia Nervosa, Autism, and Obsessive-Compulsive Spectrum," *Neuropsychiatric Disease and Treatment* 12 (July 7, 2016): 1651–60.

303 **official name: fibromyalgia:** For a history of the clinical definitions of fibromyalgia, see Gerald N. Grob, "The Rise of Fibromyalgia in 20th Century America," *Perspectives in Biology and Medicine* 54, no. 4 (Autumn 2011): 417–37; and Don L. Goldenberg, "Fibromyalgia: Why Such Controversy?," *Annals of the Rheumatic Diseases* 54 (1995): 3–5.

303 **fibromyalgia was quickly characterized:** Kirsti Malterud, "Women's Undefined Disorders—A Challenge for Clinical Communication," *Family Practice* 9, no. 3 (September 1992): 299–303; and Nortin M. Hadler, "If You Have to Prove You Are Ill, You Can't Get Well: The Object Lesson of Fibromyalgia," *Spine* 21, no. 20 (1996): 2397–400.

303 **"affective spectrum disorder":** James I. Hudson et al., "Comorbidity of Fibromyalgia with Medical and Psychiatric Disorders," *American Journal of Medicine* 92 (April 1992): 363–67; J. I. Hudson and H. G. Pope, "The Concept of Affective Spectrum Disorder: Relationship to Fibromyalgia and Other Syndromes of Chronic Fatigue and Chronic Muscle Pain," *Baillière's Clinical Rheumatology* 8, no. 4 (November 1994): 839–56; and Don L. Goldenberg et al., "Understanding fibromyalgia and its related disorders" (teleconference report prepared by the CME Institute of Physicians Postgraduate Press), *Primary Care Companion to the Journal of Clinical Psychiatry* 10, no. 2 (2008): 133–44.

304 **". . . Maybe it's all in your head":** Norma C. Ware, "Suffering and the Social Construction of Illness: The Delegitimation of Illness Experience in Chronic Fatigue Syndrome," *Medical Anthropology Quarterly* 6, no. 4 (1992): 352.

304 **"Medicine's focus on objective factors . . .":** Diane E. Hoffmann and Anita J. Tarzian, "The Girl Who Cried Pain: A Bias Against Women in the Treatment of Pain," *Journal of Law, Medicine, and Ethics* 29 (2001): 23.

306   **by patient communities:** Dr. Anne Peled, "Being Your Own Advocate for Better Breast Cancer Treatment Options," *Resensation* 22 (October 2020), https://www.resensation.com / breast-reconstruction-and-neurotization-after-mastectomy-blog/becoming-your-own-best-advocate.

CONCLUSION: BELIEVE US

318   **neglect—in medical research and funding—is directly responsible:** Ruth Bonita and Robert Beaglehole, "Women and NCDs: Overcoming the Neglect," *Global Health Action* 7, no. 1 (2014), doi:10.3402/gha.v7.23742.

INDEX

ABOUT THE AUTHOR

Elinor Cleghorn has a background in feminist culture and history, and her critical writing has been published in several academic journals, including *Screen*. After receiving her PhD in humanities and cultural studies in 2012, Elinor worked for three years as a postdoctoral researcher at the Ruskin School of Art at the University of Oxford on an interdisciplinary arts and medical humanities project. She has given talks and lectures at the Tate Modern, ICA London, and the British Film Institute, where she has been a regular contributor to the education program, and she has appeared on the BBC Radio 4 discussion show *The Forum*. In 2017, she was shortlisted for the Fitzcarraldo Editions Essay Prize, and she has since written creatively about her experience of chronic illness for publications including *Ache* (UK) and *Westerly* (AUS). She is a freelance writer and lives in Sussex.